HOMEOPATHY FOR PREGNANCY, BIRTH, AND YOUR BABY'S FIRST YEAR

Also by Miranda Castro
THE COMPLETE HOMEOPATHY HANDBOOK

HOMEOPATHY FOR PREGNANCY, BIRTH, AND YOUR BABY'S FIRST YEAR

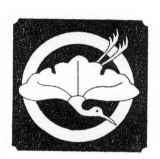

Miranda Castro *F. S. Hom.*

St. Martin's Press
NEW YORK

HOMEOPATHY FOR PREGNANCY, BIRTH,
AND YOUR BABY'S FIRST YEAR.

Library of Congress Cataloging-in-Publication Data

Castro, Miranda
Homeopathy for pregnancy, birth, and your baby's first year/
Miranda Castro.
p.   cm.
ISBN 0-312-08809-4
1. Obstetrics, Homeopathic–Popular works.   2. Pregnancy–
Popular works.   3. Infants–Diseases–Homeopathic treatment.
I. Title.
RX476.038   1993
618.2'4–dc20   92-28880
                                                                     CIP

First published in Great Britain by Macmillan London Limited under
the title *Homeopathy for Mother and Baby*.

20 19 18 17 16 15 14 13 12 11

Note to the reader:

It is advisable to seek the guidance of a physician before
implementing the approach to health suggested in this book. It is
essential that any reader who has any reason to suspect that she or
her baby suffers from illness check with her doctor before attempting
to treat it with this method. Neither this nor any other book should
be used as a substitute for professional prenatal care, or medical care
or treatment.

For Robert

CONTENTS

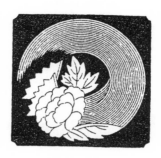

ACKNOWLEDGEMENTS

I am very grateful for the teaching I have received from all the babies in my life – both my own baby and those of my friends as well as the hundreds of baby patients I have been fortunate enough to treat over these past ten years in my capacity as a homeopath. This, and the feedback I have had from their mothers, has enabled me to explore and consolidate my beliefs around pregnancy, birth and parenthood. In the initial stages of writing this book I talked to many parents with a view to quoting their anecdotes. Sadly, I haven't been able to do this as the book became unwieldily long but I wove in their spirit as I wrote, using their comments and suggestions. I'd like to thank each one who shared their pregnancy, birth and parenting stories with me: they were funny in parts, sad in others, always interesting, informative and touching. Many thanks to Carol Boyce, Clare Palmer, Collette Barnard, David Orme, Frances Monte, Hazel Orme, Jane Howard, Jenner Roth, Maggie McKenzie, Maggi Sikking Jackson, Rachel Packer, Terry Cooper and Tony Dowmunt.

Thanks also to those who did spadework for me – typing and research – including Frances Monte, Claudia Benson, Helen Tye, Sue Clarke and Sue Mellis; to Jane Harter and Sue Morrison for reading through the manuscript and giving me their invaluable feedback; to Barbara Levy and Felicity Rubinstein for believing in me; to Hazel Orme for her patience and her unlimited, unconditional support; to all at Macmillan for helping to make this book what it is. I wish this baby a long and useful life.

INTRODUCTION

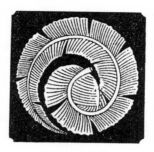

Having a baby has been the most rewarding challenge of my life – so far! My child has taught me much about myself – about the mother *and* the child in me, about my strengths and my weaknesses, and as he grows and changes so I learn more.

I became happily pregnant in 1978, and I loved it. I loved the feeling of a life taking shape inside me, of his swimmings and turnings. I loved the shape my body took, my big, soft roundness. I felt cocooned.

And . . . I was convinced that Daniel would just fit into my life, that it would carry on much as it had done, with a baby in it, sleeping in a corner in his basket. I wish I had known that almost every aspect of my life would change to some degree.

I apparently had a urinary-tract infection when I was three months' pregnant – I felt perfectly well and had not one symptom but I was scared into taking antibiotics by my doctor. Having grown up with naturopathic and homeopathic medicine I had rarely been to a doctor in my life, and found it perplexing to be treated as if I were ill. I felt lousy after the antibiotics for quite some time. I wish I had been better prepared when I went for my first pre-natal visit.

I was irrationally scared that my baby would be stillborn. My doctor said that I shouldn't worry – the figures of stillbirths were very low. I wish that I had known I needed to take my fears seriously, that they related to feelings, still unresolved, from an abortion I had had the year before.

Daniel was born two days before Christmas. I had a hospital birth because I wanted to know that pain relief was on hand in case I needed it. When I expressed my fears about my ability to cope with the pain I was told not to worry, that women the world over dropped their babies behind bushes and carried on working. I wish I had known that the birth would hurt. Not that the horror stories were true but that it might be incredibly hard work and not a little painful.

My labour *was* long, hindered by my fear and anxiety and because I wasn't allowed to eat. I finally accepted an epidural and relaxed into a deep sleep. My body then did its job well, freed from tension. I pushed Daniel out in a haze of exhaustion – by this point I had forgotten that I was going to have a baby. I don't know who was more surprised, him, me or his father. I felt an unexpected, primitive welling up of love of a new kind for me, a powerful response to this new life, newly in *my* life: motherlove. Birth was a miracle for me.

Motherhood was a huge shock, an explosion of mixed emotions. I had so much to adapt to, seemingly so quickly, that I found myself frequently chasing my own tail as I struggled to understand what to do next! I wish I had known it would be such hard work.

I remember a nurse handing me my baby a few hours after the birth and telling me that he was ready for his first feed and then walking away. I remember just feeding him, but awkwardly and with some difficulty, and the bad habits we developed then stayed with us long enough to cause my nipples to crack and bleed. I wish I had known that breastfeeding and mothering are both learnt skills! I got help from a La Leche League counsellor and then settled down to enjoy breastfeeding. I loved the closeness and the convenience.

I remember changing him for the first time and marvelling at his little body. I remember his baby smell and exquisitely soft skin. I also remember picking him up and holding his delicious, tiny, naked body when he was two days old. His eyes opened wide in surprise as this cute little fountain of wee spurted all over us! I remember laughing! My baby brought much unexpected fun and laughter into my life.

Daniel thrived until he contracted whooping cough at a year old. Homeopathic treatment helped him through it and over it and I used it also for his accidents and injuries, for everyday coughs and colds – and for those of his friends. Motherhood led me further into homeopathy because I needed help for my baby. The effectiveness of that treatment led me to take professional training and to specialise in working with mothers and babies. I wanted to work with a system of medicine that I could teach others to use, albeit in a limited way.

Homeopathy is a wonderful system of medicine for women in their childbearing years when anxiety about the side effects of orthodox medicines often leads them to suffer rather than seek medical help for minor aches and pains. Worse still, in an attempt to give their children the best care possible mothers find themselves giving one course of antibiotics after another for relatively minor complaints. Many parents are questioning this and are looking for more natural ways to look after themselves and their children when they fall ill.

This book is a natural extension of my wish to empower patients to help themselves. It is not intended to replace your doctor but rather to encourage you to think twice before giving, say, antibiotics for a 'teething cough' or Calpol for a fever. I hope that you will take a little time to become familiar with the process of working out a good remedy – the results will be rewarding. My aim is that you use orthodox medicines only when absolutely necessary so that your children grow up strong, vital, healthy and able to withstand ordinary, everyday stress. Finally, I wish you well in your exploration of this effective route to creating health.

Miranda Castro,
January 1992

HOW TO USE THIS BOOK

The goal of this book is to enable you to use homeo-pathic medicines safely and effectively at home during pregnancy, childbirth and in the post-natal year, both for yourself and your baby.

Many homeopathic first-aid books currently available have attempted to simplify the process of finding a remedy (as homeopathic medicines are called) to make homeopathy more accessible. This has resulted in some disappointment, as many people have found their attempts to use this form of natural medicine to be a hit-or-miss affair. This book aims to right this error by mimicking the method that a professional homeo-path uses. To this end chapters 1 and 6 focus on taking a case history, working out a remedy and prescribing. Chapter 2 looks at many of the practical aspects of preparing for pregnancy, birth and the post-natal year, and chapters 3, 4 and 5 deal with the complaints common to each of those times.

Chapter 1: Understanding and Using Homeopathy

This chapter looks at the history and theory of homeo-pathy, including its guiding principles and the myths that surround it; clear guidelines on taking a 'case history', on working out a remedy, on how and when to prescribe – including complaints you can't treat as well as those you can treat yourself – and a list of symptoms to watch out for that would necessitate your seeking professional help (Cause for Concern, p. 23). This part ends with 12 sample cases which bring all of the above theory to life.

Chapter 2: Preparing for Life after Birth

This part discusses many of the issues that come up during pregnancy, birth and the post-natal period, many of which can be addressed in pregnancy to gain a sense of perspective and to be better prepared, especially for life after birth. Issues that need to be looked at for you to be able to enjoy this all important time include your choices regarding medical treat-ment, medical tests and interventions (before, during and after birth) and how to cope with them, the pros and cons of breastfeeding and bottle-feeding, general advice to help you look at how you are going to maintain (or even improve if necessary) your strength and health during this time in your life; and a job description of parenthood!

Chapters 3, 4 and 5: Pregnancy, Birth and the Post-natal Period

Each of these sections starts with a look at what happens to your body because many changes take place – during pregnancy, birth and post-natally – all of which can affect your health. Then the complaints common to each of these periods are listed. Each complaint includes clear guidelines on how you can deal with it yourself and suggestions of practical measures that may be helpful or downright important for healing to take place, and pointers to help you decide when to seek professional help.

Chapter 6: The Materia Medicas and Repertories

This part of the book is divided into two sections: the external remedies (drops, lotions, creams and oint-ments) and internal remedies (tablets taken by mouth). Each has a Materia Medica – an alphabetically arranged list of descriptions of the remedies, and a Repertory – an index of the symptoms and complaints listed in the Materia Medica. As a homeopath, my tools for prescribing are the Materia Medica and Repertory. What I present here is a simplified form of these books where they apply to home prescribing, translated where possible into lay-person's terms.

You will need to read chapter 1 to be able to use this section, and, although it may take some time and effort to get the hang of it, it is worth persevering. I hope that the results will encourage you to pursue this most rewarding system of healing.

· 1 ·
UNDERSTANDING AND USING HOMEOPATHY

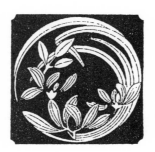

THE HISTORY OF HOMEOPATHY

SAMUEL HAHNEMANN (1755–1843)

Samuel Hahnemann, the founder of homeopathy, was born in Meissen in Saxony on 10 April 1755 into an era of change and political upheaval. The Seven Years' War, the French Revolution and the Napoleonic Wars threw Europe into turmoil; the Industrial Revolution brought social change and technological and scientific advances; there was also a revolution in thought – the political, spiritual and intellectual movement now known as the Enlightenment. The freedom of thought and opinion it encouraged was important for the birth and development of homeopathy.

Hahnemann was born into a poor and devout family who encouraged their son in his education. He qualified as a doctor in 1791 and practised medicine in Leipzig for about nine years, but he became increasingly disillusioned by the cruel and ineffective treatments of his time (blood-letting, purging, poisonous drugs with horrendous side effects) and gave up his practice, concentrating instead on study, research, writing and translation.

One of the major works he translated was Dr William Cullen's *A Treatise on Materia Medica*. Cullen (1710–90) was an Edinburgh teacher, physician and chemist, and his book included an essay on Peruvian bark or *Cinchona* (which homeopaths call *China*), from which quinine, the treatment for malaria, is derived. Cullen attributed *Cinchona*'s ability to cure malaria, with its symptoms of periodic fever, sweating and palpitations, to its bitterness. Hahnemann, sceptical of this explanation, tested small doses on himself:

I took by way of an experiment, twice a day, four drachms of good *China*. My feet, finger ends, etc., at first became quite cold; I grew languid and drowsy; then my heart began to palpitate, and my pulse grew hard and small; intolerable anxiety, trembling, prostration throughout all my limbs; then pulsation, in the head, redness of my cheeks, thirst, and, in short, all these symptoms which are ordinarily characteristic of intermittent fever, made their appearance, one after the other, yet without the peculiar chilly, shivering rigor. Briefly, even those symptoms which are of regular occurrence and especially characteristic – as the stupidity of mind, the kind of rigidity in all the limbs, but above all the numb, disagreeable sensation, which seems to have its seat in the periosteum, over every bone in the whole body – all these made their appearance. This paroxysm lasted two or three hours each time, and recurred, if I repeated this dose, not otherwise; I discontinued it and was in good health.

In other words, Hahnemann observed that *Cinchona* produced in a healthy person the symptoms of malaria, the very disease that it was known to cure, a discovery which was a cornerstone in the development of homeopathy.

In the fifth century BC, Hippocrates, the 'father of medicine', wrote that there were two methods of healing: by 'contraries' and by 'similars'. Although country people throughout the world have always used the principle of cure by 'similars' successfully in their own folk-medicines, the standard medical assumption has always been that if the body produced a symptom the appropriate treatment would be an antidote, an opposite or 'contrary' medicine to that symptom. For example, constipation would be treated with laxatives, which produce diarrhoea.

During the sixteenth century, Paracelsus, a German doctor known as the 'father of chemistry', made new departures in medicine and pharmacology based on chemical experiments and direct observation of nature. He set the stage for the germ theory by stating that the causes of disease were external, seed-like factors introduced into the body through air, food and drink. He believed in the natural recuperative power of the human body and saw nature in every person as a vital spirit. He investigated the law of similars and by using only one medicine at a time and giving careful attention to dosage, noted that a very small dose could overcome a great disease.

Hahnemann embarked on further experiments which confirmed this principle. By observing the symptoms any substance produced when given to a healthy person, Hahnemann found the healing properties of that substance. This testing procedure was called 'proving'.

He referred to it as *similia similibus curentur*, or 'let like be cured with like'; this principle became the first law of a system of healing he called 'homeopathy', from the Greek *homoios* (similar) and *pathos* (suffering or disease), in order to differentiate it from orthodox medicine, which he called 'allopathy', meaning 'opposite suffering'.

Over several years he conducted many provings on his family and friends, and also studied accounts of the symptoms shown by victims of accidental poisonings. Finally he set up in medical practice again, but with a different basis for his prescriptions. He used the material he had gathered from the provings and for each of his patients looked for the *similimum* – the remedy whose 'symptom picture',

based on the provings, most matched that of the patient. His methods were met with disbelief and ridicule from his colleagues, but the patients flowed in and his astonishing results verified his theory.

He also differed from conventional practitioners in giving only one remedy at a time. In an age when apothecaries made fortunes by mixing numerous substances, many of which were highly noxious, this earned him many enemies.

Hahnemann did not stop there: dissatisfied with the side effects of his medicines, he experimented with smaller and smaller doses. He found, however, that when he diluted a medicine sufficiently to eradicate the side effects, it no longer effected a cure. He developed a new method of dilution: instead of simply stirring the substance after each dilution he shook it vigorously. This shaking he called 'succussion' and the resultant liquid a 'potentised remedy'. He found now that not only did the remedy lack side effects but the more he diluted it using succussion, the more effectively his remedy cured. He believed that the shaking released the strength or energy of the substance and dissipated its toxic effects.

Hahnemann numbered the potentised remedies according to the amount of times they had been diluted: a remedy diluted six times (taking out one hundredth of the liquid each time and adding 99/100 alcohol) was called a 6C (see p. 6). Initially he prescribed remedies that had been diluted up to the sixth potency; then he experimented with the higher dilutions, finding them more effective still. Eventually he prescribed up to the 30th potency, and his followers took dilution even further.

This process of dilution incurred further derision from the medical establishment, who could not explain, and therefore could not accept, how anything so dilute could have any effect. Yet despite opposition, homeopathy survived and spread remarkably quickly – because it was remarkably effective.

Samuel Hahnemann lived before the germ theory of disease had been proposed, before thermometers, the X-ray and antibiotics made medicine appear increasingly 'scientific'. Yet he himself was an innovative scientist of sufficient intellect and culture to combine science and metaphysics. Consciously and unconsciously, he drew on the traditions of German folk-medicine, alchemy and magic, as well as the developments in chemistry, pathology, pharmaceutics and medicine which were beginning to make diagnosis and treatment both more accurate and more humane. In later life he became a religious free-thinker, believing that God permeated every living thing, and that he was divinely chosen and guided in his work. His development of a safe and effective system of medicine has given the world a priceless gift.

Hahnemann's literary output was prodigious. He proved about a hundred remedies, wrote over seventy original works, translated many texts on a wide range of subjects and also corresponded widely. In 1810 he published the first edition of *The Organon of Rational Medicine* (later *The Organon of the Healing Art*), which ran to six editions, each one modified and expanded. In it he set out clearly the homeopathic philosophy. In the same year, when Leipzig was besieged in the Napoleonic campaigns, his treatments of the survivors of the siege and the victims of the great typhus epidemic that followed were highly successful and further increased his reputation.

Between 1811 and 1821 Hahnemann published his *Materia Medica Pura* in six volumes; this represented the results of his provings – thousands of symptoms for sixty-six remedies. In 1828 came *Chronic Diseases and Their Homeopathic Cure*, in which he elaborated on the philosophy of *The Organon*, added more remedies, discussed the use of higher potencies and introduced the concept of 'miasms' to account for the failure of some patients to respond to treatment with remedies which clearly matched their symptoms. Among such people he found a family history of certain diseases and was able to link a tendency to a particular condition to the patient's 'inherited' health. He developed a way of treating these blocks to health homeopathically (see Miasms, p. 7).

In 1831 cholera swept through central Europe. Hahnemann advocated the remedy *Camphor* in the early stages and *Cuprum metallicum, Veratrum album, Bryonia alba* or *Rhus toxicodendron* in the later stages. He also stressed that clothing and bedding should be heated to destroy 'all known infectious matters' and advised cleanliness, ventilation and disinfection of the rooms, and quarantine. (These ideas were far ahead of his time: the work of Pasteur on the germ theory of disease and that of Lister on disinfection was still to come.) Cholera was more successfully treated with homeopathy than with orthodox medicine; mortality rates varied between 2.4 and 21.1 per cent compared with 50 per cent or more with conventional treatment.

He gave lectures about his theory at the university, which often deteriorated into violent tirades against current medical practices earning him the nickname 'Raging Hurricane'. A few medical practitioners were prepared to go against mainstream opinion, trained under him and took his teachings out into the world.

In the 1820s, when homeopathy arrived in the USA, the state of orthodox medicine was, if anything, worse than it was in Europe. The practice of almost completely draining the body of blood (four-fifths was let) was advocated, even for children. A drug know as 'Calomel' (*Mercurius chloride*), which had been introduced originally to cure syphilis, was used as a standard purgative; its side effects were loss of teeth, seizure of the jaws and death from mercury poisoning.

Homeopathy was easily accepted, and flourished. Homeopaths were seen to be well-educated, hard-working people, and the metaphysical background appealed to many church people. It was adopted in particular by followers of Swedenborg (1689–1772), a visionary who believed himself a vehicle for a new religious revelation. His writings appealed to people who were studying the new sciences, such as Darwinism, and who were concerned about the conflict between science and orthodox religion. For many homeopaths this blend of reason and mysticism was ideal.

In 1846 the American Medical Association was founded, which adopted a code of ethics forbidding its members to consult homeopaths. Local and state medical societies were told to purge themselves of homeopaths and their sympathisers, but homeopathy had already made a positive mark on orthodox medicine: blood-letting abated, medical training improved and several homeopathic remedies found their way into allopathic prescribing. Public demand for homeopathic treatment continued.

The 1860s through to the 1880s saw the flowering of American homeopathy. Practitioners proved every conceivable remedy, often at great cost to their own health. There were some fifty-six homeopathic hospitals, thirteen lunatic asylums, nine children's hospitals and fifteen sanatoriums. The homeopathic training colleges, unlike their allopathic counterparts, excluded neither women nor black people.

In 1826 a young well-connected English doctor called Frederick Quin studied with Hahnemann and on his return to London set up a homeopathic practice, treating many famous people, including Dickens and Thackeray. He established the British Homoeopathic Society (later the Faculty of Homoeopathy), and in 1849 founded the London Homoeopathic Hospital, where, during the cholera outbreak of 1854, deaths were a mere 16.4 per cent, compared with the 50 per cent average for other hospitals. The Board of Health suppressed this fact, explaining, 'The figures would give sanction to a practice opposed to the maintenance of truth and the progress of science.'*

After the Crimean War a medical bill was introduced in Parliament to outlaw homeopathy, but Quin's friends in the House of Lords secured a saving amendment.

*Pinchuck and Clark, *Medicine for Beginners*, Writers and Readers, London, 1984.

If Quin was the practical and fashionable force behind homeopathy in Britain, the two most influential writers and teachers were Robert Dudgeon, who translated Hahnemann's texts into English, and Richard Hughes, a mild man with a conciliatory attitude towards the medical establishment as well as a rigorous and scientific attitude towards homeopathy. Queen Adelaide, wife of King William IV, brought homeopathy from her native Saxony to the British royal family. The royal family maintains an active involvement in homeopathy to this day. The Queen has her own consultant homeopath and carries her 'black box' of remedies with her on all her travels.

THE TWENTIETH CENTURY

By the time of Hahnemann's death in 1843, homeopathy was established throughout the world, although the mutual antagonism and distrust between homeopaths and allopaths continued to hinder its progress.

Developments in medicine around the close of the nineteenth century strengthened the orthodox camp: science had proved the existence of microbes, the old practices Hahnemann had condemned were diminishing, and powerful drugs were being developed. The pharmaceutical industry, helped by the power of advertising, became an effective and wealthy lobbying force behind allopathic medicine. Meanwhile the homeopathic establishment was weakened by internal division, and the public – and many homeopaths – were drawn to the side that could put its case most clearly.

The American Medical Association moved to close many homeopathic teaching institutions and mounted a huge anti-homeopathy propaganda campaign. Consequently, by 1918 the number of homeopathic hospitals in the USA had dwindled to seven. Great optimism accompanied the introduction of penicillin: doctors thought that a medical nirvana had been reached. They regarded the taking of a homeopathic case as too time-consuming – the five-minute prescription and a cure for every ill had arrived. Little did they realise that it was the dawn of a medical nemesis.

Homeopathy has spread rapidly throughout the world. It is popular over Asia, particularly in India where it is now officially recognised as a separate branch of medicine and is fully supported by the government. Although it is poorly represented in some European countries, other parts of Europe show a fast-growing interest. In France and Germany homeopathic medicines are readily available in most pharmacies and there are homeopathic consultants at some hospitals. Homeopathy is highly respected in many South American countries, with Mexico, Argentina and Brazil at the forefront. It is spreading in Australia, New Zealand, Greece and Israel although it is non-existent in the Arab states.

In 1946, when the National Health Service was established, homeopathy was included as an officially approved method of treatment and in Britain today its popularity is increasing rapidly. It is still practised under the auspices of the National Health in five hospitals in Bristol, Liverpool, Glasgow, Tunbridge Wells and London, and by some GPs, although the limit of time on consultations often means that antibiotics are handed out with the homeopathic medicines just in case the latter do not work.

Professional homeopaths run private practices and many participate in almost-free clinics for the needy. The Society of Homoeopaths, the organisation which represents the professional homeopath in this country, promotes the highest standards. From small beginnings in 1974, the number of registered members – who use the initials R.S.Hom. (Registered member) or F.S.Hom. (Fellow) after their names – increases annually and a dozen colleges train several hundred professional homeopaths each year.

PRINCIPLES AND CONCEPTS

The highest ideal of therapy is to restore health rapidly, gently, permanently; to remove and destroy the whole disease in the shortest, surest, least harmful way, according to clearly comprehensible principles.

So it was that Samuel Hahnemann, in *The Organon*, defined his goals for a new system of medicine. It is hard to imagine a description that could express more concisely the needs of both practitioner and patient.

The principles of homeopathy represent a complete view of the processes of health and disease. Since 1810, when *The Organon* was first published, they have proved resistant to major reinterpretation and are crucial to successful prescribing.

The Similimum or Law of Similars

This basic principle of homeopathy – *similia similibus curentur* or 'let like be cured with like' – states that any substance that makes you ill can also cure you: anything that can produce symptoms of disease in a healthy person can cure a sick person with similar symptoms.

By 'symptom' the homeopath means those changes that are felt by the patient (subjective) or observed by someone else (objective), which may be associated with a particular disease, or state of disease, and which are the outward expression of that state.

Provings

'Proving' is the name given to the homeopathic method of testing substances to establish their 'symptom pictures'. Since Hahnemann's first proving in 1790, hundreds of others have been carried out and their results collated in the great Materia Medicas (see below). In the 1940s, the Americans organised a programme of re-proving remedies, but it was abandoned when identical symptoms were elicited all over again.

Today, healthy volunteer provers of new, potentially medicinal substances are divided into two groups, with one group being given the unnamed substance and the other a placebo. It is always a double-blind trial: neither the provers nor the conductor of the proving knows at the time who is taking what. The remedies are sometimes tested in their diluted – potentised – form or, if they are not poisonous, in crude doses (in the 'mother tincture', see Potencies, p. 6). All symptoms – physical, emotional and mental – are noted in detail, then gathered schematically and common themes noted.

Apart from such provings two other sources are used:

Accidental provings provide a rich source of valuable information that might not otherwise be available. Homeopaths have been able to add symptom pictures of substances such as deadly nightshade, the remedy *Belladonna*, or snake venom, such as *Lachesis*, to the Materia Medica by drawing on detailed accounts of accidental poisonings. Because these substances can cause serious conditions, they also have the ability to cure them, and so are of great value.

Cured symptoms After a remedy has been successfully prescribed, symptoms cured by it which did not emerge either in the provings or in the accidental provings are noted. If the remedy consistently cures these symptoms in many people, then they are added to its symptom picture.

The Materia Medica

The Materia Medica (Latin, meaning medical matter or material) lists the symptom pictures of each remedy as discovered in the provings. The many hundreds of remedies are arranged alphabetically and the symptoms of those remedies are arranged according to body area. New remedies are constantly being discovered and added.

The professional homeopath works with a number of Materia Medicas compiled by different homeopaths, each reflecting their own personal experience. They all have the same basic information, but the individual homeopath may interpret the material slightly differently. Within this vast amount of information certain patterns emerge and it is these patterns with which the homeopath becomes familiar. He or she will memorise the strong symptoms or keynotes of every remedy.

The Repertory

This is an index of symptoms from the Materia Medica listed in alphabetical order and thereby providing a valuable cross-referencing system. A good Repertory is essential as it is impossible to memorise the vast number of symptoms in the Materia Medica.

The Single Remedy

The classical homeopath gives one remedy at a time to gauge its effect more precisely than would be possible if two or more remedies were given together. Indeed, the remedies were all originally proved separately and it is consequently not known how they interact if mixed; combined remedies should only be considered once they have been proved in combination.

However, this most difficult aspect of homeopathic prescribing deters many people. Finding a single remedy to match the patient's symptoms is a constant challenge and can involve an enormous amount of hard work. The lazy, busy or misguided homeopath may mix several remedies together in the hope that one may work, a hit-or-miss approach which is not true classical homeopathy, as Hahnemann defined it, and shows a lack of understanding of the fundamental principles.

The Infinitesimal Dose

The more a remedy is diluted and succussed (vigorously shaken), the stronger it becomes as a cure (see p. 6). The concept of the infinitesimal dose is one of the great stumbling blocks for a conventionally trained scientific mind. Sceptics scoff at the idea that a very dilute solution of sea salt – beyond the point where there is any salt measurable in the solution – is capable of curing a wide range of complaints, from cold sores, hayfever and headaches to depression (see *Natrum muriaticum*, p. 226). Logically, it does seem unlikely that a substance that can cause high blood pressure in its crude form could become a strong and effective agent for healing when it is so dilute. However, a pharmacological law states that although a large dose of poison can destroy life, a moderate dose will only paralyse and a very small dose will actually stimulate those same life processes.

New discoveries in physics are beginning to explain this phenomenon. One theory is that the succussion creates an electrochemical pattern which is stored in the dilutant and which then spreads like liquid crystal through the body's own water. Another hypothesis suggests that the dilution process triggers an electromagnetic imprinting which directly affects the electromagnetic field of the body.

Potencies

There are two scales for diluting substances: the decimal and the centesimal. In all cases the starting remedy – a 'tincture' or 'mother tincture' – is made by steeping the substance itself in alcohol and then straining it.

For the decimal scale, one-tenth of the tincture is added to nine-tenths alcohol and shaken vigorously; this first dilution is called a 1X. The number of a homeopathic remedy reflects the number of times it has been diluted and succussed: for example, *Sulphur 6X* has been diluted and succussed six times.

The centesimal scale is diluted using one part in a hundred of the tincture (as opposed to 10) and the letter C is added after the number (although in practice homeopaths have omitted the C and just use the numbers for the centesimal scale).

Paradoxically, a 6X is called a low potency and 200(C) a high potency – the greater the dilution, the greater the potency.

The most commonly used potency in the decimal scale is the 6X, although the 9X, 12X, 24X and 30X are used by some. In the centesimal scale those low potencies most commonly used are the 6, 12 and 30. The higher potencies – 200, 1M (diluted one thousand times), 10M (ten thousand times) and CM (one hundred thousand times) – are highly respected by homeopaths and should not be used by the home prescriber.

'Inert' substances (such as Lycopodium, the tiny spore of the club moss) are ground for several hours with a pestle and mortar until they become soluble. This process, called 'trituration', is used for metals as well as other substances that do not dissolve easily to prepare them for succussion.

The Whole Person

The concept of treating the 'whole person' is an essential element of classical homeopathy. The basis of this belief is that symptoms, diseases or pains do not exist in isolation, but are a reflection of how the whole person is coping with stress. It is the *whole* person that counts, not just the physical body but also the mental and/or emotional 'bodies'. The homeopath looks beyond the 'presenting complaint', beyond the label of the disease (for example, 'tonsillitis', 'migraines' or 'food poisoning') to the 'totality of symptoms' experienced. The prescription is individualised to fit the whole person.

As far as first-aid prescribing is concerned, it *is* possible to prescribe on a single symptom such as, for example, chilblains or mouth ulcers, but it is always preferable to find a remedy that matches more of a person's symptom picture, taking into account as many pieces of the jigsaw as possible.

Constitution and Susceptibility

I often hear people say enviously about a friend, 'He smokes like a chimney, drinks like a fish, works like a maniac and has never had a day's illness in his life. It's not fair. I struggle constantly to stay healthy and need nine hours' sleep a night, otherwise I get sick. Why?'

The answer lies in the constitution. The person who works all hours and smokes and drinks as if there were no tomorrow has a strong constitution – and may well be wasting his 'inheritance', because there *will* come a time when it will run out, when even *he* will get sick.

In *The Science of Homeopathy* George Vithoulkas defines the constitution as 'the genetic inheritance tempered or modified by our environment', that is, a person's fundamental structure – their state of health *and* their temperament. A strong constitution can withstand considerable pressure without falling ill; a weak constitution has a greater susceptibility to illness.

Susceptibility is simply the degree to which a person is vulnerable to an outside influence. In an epidemic not everyone will be affected, but those who are we call 'susceptible'. Their predisposition is due to an underlying constitutional weakness, which is either inherited or due to past and/or current stress (mental, emotional or physical).

If your grandparents all died of old age and your parents have been healthy all their lives; if your birth was planned and your mother was healthy throughout her pregnancy (didn't smoke, drink, etc.); if your parents' marriage is happy and your birth was uneventful, then your constitution should be of the strongest.

If, on the other hand, all your grandparents died at early ages of cancer or heart disease, one of your parents had tuberculosis as a child and the other suffered from asthma and eczema, then your chances of inheriting a weak constitution are greater. You can still escape the worst of a poor inheritance if your parents' marriage is happy, if they have taken care of their own health, and brought you up with plenty of love and a good diet.

And that is where alternative medicine comes in. Many people come to a homeopath for 'constitutional treatment', to improve their general health rather than wait until they fall ill. The value of constitutional treatment is that it boosts the weak constitution and decreases its susceptibility to disease. Homeopathy strengthens the body's vitality and its ability to respond to stress without recourse to other medicines.

The Vital Force

Homeopaths believe that a balancing mechanism keeps us in health, provided that the stresses on our constitution are neither too prolonged nor too great. Hahnemann called it the 'vital force' and he believed it to be that energetic substance, independent of physical and chemical forces, that gives us life and is absent at our death.

The human organism, indeed any living thing, has a unique relationship with its environment, which biologists refer to as 'homeostasis'. This means that a healthy living being is self-regulating, with an innate (protective) tendency to maintain its equilibrium and compensate for disruptive changes. Homeopaths believe that the vital force produces symptoms to counteract stresses and makes adjustments, moment by moment throughout our lives, to keep us healthy and balanced. These symptoms, then, are simply the body's way of telling us how it is coping with stress. Obvious examples are shivering when cold, perspiring when overheated and eating or drinking when hungry or thirsty, reactions which help to ensure the regulation of a constant, life-preserving environment within the body. Disease 'attacks' only when this vital force is weakened.

Homeopathic medicines act as a catalyst, the remedy stimulating the body's own vital force to heal itself. They do not weaken the defence mechanism by suppressing it as do many orthodox medicines. The correct homeopathic treatment not only alleviates the symptoms but enables the patient to feel that life is once again flowing harmoniously.

Acute and Chronic Disease

Acute disease is self-limiting; it is not deep-seated and, given time, will usually clear of its own accord. Some acute illnesses, such as pneumonia, meningitis or nephritis, for example, are very serious and can, although rarely, be fatal. These are not within the scope of the home prescriber and always need expert advice.

An acute disease has three definite stages: *the incubation period*, when there may be no symptoms of disease; *the acute phase*, when the recognisable symptoms surface; *the convalescent stage*, when a person usually improves. Coughs, colds, flu, food poisoning and children's illnesses such as chickenpox are all examples of acute illnesses. Well-chosen homeopathic remedies will speed up recovery, alleviate pain and ensure that there are no complications. (See pp. 22 and 23 as well as the complaints sections of chapters 3, 4 and 5 for the acute illnesses or complaints you can and cannot treat using this book.)

Chronic disease is more deep-seated than acute disease. It develops slowly, continues for a long time and is often accompanied by a general deterioration in health. The development of the disease does not take a predictable course; neither is it possible to say for how long it will last. An acute disease that is followed by complications can develop into a chronic, long-term illness.

Arthritis, heart disease, cancer and mental illness are all examples of chronic disease. Homeopaths believe that the current increase in incidence of these conditions is in part due to chemical stresses, including the overuse of orthodox medicines and environmental pollution.

Miasms

In his early years in practice, Hahnemann was puzzled to find that some patients failed to respond to their constitutional remedies and others who improved relapsed after only a short time. He collected these 'difficult' cases together and after much careful study found a common factor in the presence of certain diseases in their personal or family history, which he realised must constitute blocks to health preventing the indicated constitutional remedy from working. He called the blocks 'miasms' and developed a comprehensive and complex theory around them. His insights have enabled the professional homeopath to assess through the history of a patient (both personal and inherited) their likely constitutional strength and often to predict the sort of blocks that they might encounter during the course of constitutional treatment.

Hahnemann defined three basic miasms which he believed to be the underlying causes of chronic disease, each of which predisposes a person to a particular range of health problems which he also defined at length. The three miasms were: *Psora*, which he associated with suppressed skin diseases and with leprosy; *Sycosis*, associated with suppressed gonorrhoea; and *Syphilis*, associated with suppressed syphilis. Homeopaths have since added many more including tuberculosis, radiation and heavy metals. The treatment of miasms is always a matter for the professional homeopath, not for self-treatment.

The Laws of Cure

The Laws of Cure were formulated by Constantine Hering (a doctor, homeopath and a follower of Hahnemann), who based them on a lifetime's observation of the processes involved when sick patients became well. Throughout his years of practice he was able to draw the following conclusions:

- As someone becomes well, symptoms move from the innermost organs of the body (those most vital to life) to the outer organs. Therefore, cure moves from within to without. For example, someone with heart disease (serious, life-threatening) may experience stomach or bowel problems during the process of cure.
- Cure also takes place from above to below, so that symptoms usually 'drip off' the body, starting from the head and clearing downwards, with the hands and the feet (sometimes simultaneously) being the last to be affected (with, say, a skin eruption).
- Symptoms that have been suppressed in the past often resurface during the process of cure and usually do so in the reverse order from their original sequence. For example, if a patient with heart disease had been successfully treated with orthodox medicines for a stomach ulcer before the heart condition, then the appearance of stomach symptoms (less severe than in the original complaint) would be welcomed as a sign that the old suppressed symptoms were being cleared out.

The suppression of a disease usually leads to a more deep-seated illness surfacing. For example, many children whose eczema has been 'successfully' treated with steroids may suffer from asthma later in life. These two events are seen by the orthodox medical profession as having only a casual connection, whereas the homeopath believes that the suppression of the eczema has caused the asthma. Successful homeopathic treatment involves the eczema reappearing at some point.

It is also possible to suppress with homeopathic medicines by treating a single symptom and not therefore taking into account the whole person.

Homeopaths use the Laws of Cure to monitor treatment, to check whether the cure is going in the 'right' direction. These laws apply to the treatment of chronic complaints but occasionally also to acute prescribing. As far as acute treatment or home prescribing is concerned, a very well-selected constitutional remedy will occasionally push to the surface old symptoms that may have been forgotten. These will clear of their own accord. It is important not to prescribe another remedy and by so doing encourage the chronic condition to go back 'in' again.

Health and Disease

Health is more than simply the absence of disease. *I* believe it is a sense of well-being, of feeling good, of being in balance, that is hard to dislodge. It is, above all, the ability to withstand stress.

When we are physically healthy we have strength and flexibility, and a reservoir of energy to draw on should we need it. When we are emotionally healthy we can acknowledge and express our feelings and by so doing maintain rewarding relationships. When we are mentally healthy we can think clearly, formulate ideas, solve problems and make decisions easily.

Disease limits our personal freedom; a broken leg, for example, limits physical freedom by making it difficult to walk. Depression can limit emotional freedom because it is difficult to interact with other people. Mental exhaustion after, say, a taxing exam makes it difficult to concentrate and make decisions and therefore limits our mental freedom. If you fall ill it is often useful to ask yourself how and why that illness is limiting you.

The orthodox medical view, or germ theory, of disease is that illness is a 'bad' thing. An alternative medical view is that disease is a 'good' thing, alerting the body to the necessity of taking some time to recuperate or to have a good clear-out.

I believe that disease is neither good nor bad. The disease we succumb to provides us with information about our personal weaknesses, about how we are living our lives and how we are coping with stress. It alerts us to the existence of something that needs attention.

Building Health – Preventive Medicine

The desire to rid the body of disease is a healthy attitude, although any approach that involves building health and therefore preventing disease or ill-health will, of course, be of greater benefit in the long term than any temporary suppression of the symptoms alone. How we approach illness, as well as the treatment we choose, deserves some thought.

The presence of disease or pain often creates anxiety, which in turn can lead to fear and panic. Most of us have consulted an authoritative figure (a doctor) to allay our anxiety by putting a name to what is happening to our bodies, and to determine how it must be treated. The danger here is that, in looking outside ourselves for the answers and in asking too few questions, we experience a loss of personal control with consequent feelings of helplessness. We give up responsibility for our own health to the people 'in charge' and we become real patients, or, as I see it, victims. We find that we feel unable to confide misgivings, to express our instincts about our own health, or to explore other options. We become passive consumers of medical care.

As patients, how can we redress the balance? The first step is to become informed, by reading and talking to people who are sympathetic to our views (and doubts), and who may have had similar experiences. We must also learn to ask for what we need, to make realistic demands of health-care professionals, and to seek the help of doctors and specialists, both orthodox and alternative, who are willing to communicate with us, who are able to acknowledge that we, the patients, have a part to play in our own healing processes, and who are therefore able to give us the information we need, and deserve, about what they think is happening.

By taking responsibility for what happens to our bodies we can begin to create for ourselves the balance we want in our lives, and tune into our own feelings, or inner sense, of what is wrong. By developing a positive approach towards creating a healthy life we can move away from automatically taking a defensive position towards illness.

Stress

We all vary in our ability to adapt to and cope with stress. Understanding our own stress limits is tremendously important.

I divide stress into two main categories: healthy stress and unhealthy stress. Healthy stress pushes you to perform better and achieve more than usual in certain circumstances: for example, to work all hours in your job during a crisis or to gain that little extra from your body during a race (or during labour!). Unhealthy stress brings you too near to that 'last straw' state where your own coping mechanisms are overstretched, when your performance level starts to drop. You make mistakes. You fall ill.

Under stress our bodies let us know when the pressure is too great by producing the symptom(s) of illness. And when symptoms surface on one level, other levels are often affected. For example, a head injury (physical) can initially cause shock (emotional) and amnesia (mental) as well as pain (physical). A difficult, aggressive boss can create an emotionally stressful environment for his staff, who may produce physical ailments such as headaches, indigestion or neck pain as a response to suppressed emotions. (The suppression of any emotion can be harmful: it takes a lot of energy to suppress joy and will be as stressful as holding in rage.)

We respond to different stresses in different ways, according to our age and resources. Giving birth at forty is a bigger physical stress than doing so at twenty when a woman's body is more supple and she has greater energy resources – but an older, more mature woman may find herself less emotionally stressed by motherhood.

The body operates as a unit, with the physical, emotional, mental and spiritual working together to maintain a balance. Each aspect needs nourishment, but mental and emotional nourishment is often lacking in our society. Because of the widespread rejection of religion many people do not have a time of peace or quiet in their lives to reflect or just *be*. To still the mind and let the cares of life drift away is a deeply healing process. You can do this by meditating, daydreaming, painting and writing, walking and enjoying nature or through prayer.

You can also nourish yourself with food, sleep, massage, spending time with friends or family members who accept you as you are, who will listen when needed, and provide you with loving support and advice. Laughter is one of nature's great healers. Letting go of the serious business of living and having fun is essential to maintaining health.

Recognising and Dealing with Stress

Learn to recognise the first symptoms of being overstressed, when the body shows early-warning signs but before illness develops. Being ill can be a fruitful way of coping with stress although, of course, disease itself can be stressful, especially if you take antibiotics or homeopathic remedies *and* carry on. You need to stop, rest and allow time for self-healing.

As a home prescriber, it is important to understand that disease is a response to stress. Identifying the stress is the first step: you can use the stress symptom and the response to prescribe on. Some people are sensitive to physical stresses, for example, to changes in the weather, always falling ill with a cold when the warm summer weather first changes to cold. Others are more vulnerable to emotional stress, and find it hard to cope with upsets at home or at work.

The more we understand about how we react to stress the better able we are to deal with it and choose how to respond to it.

Get to know your own stress response. What can you cope with? What are your limits? How do you recognise them? How can you stretch your limits when you have to? What nourishes you? How do *you* balance the stress in *your* life? Assess your reserves and strengths for dealing with it; look at ways in which you can balance it. Avoid unnecessary stress. Learn to offload, delegate, say no – and ask for support and help.

Remember that you are an important person in your own life. You need to look after yourself so that you can do your job(s) well – so that you can be a healthy mother/father/friend/employee/homeopath or whatever!

MYTHS AND MISAPPREHENSIONS

Many homeopaths, believing that the explanation of how homeopathy works is secondary to its success, have traditionally refused to reveal the names of the medicines they give. This and the lack of information they have provided about their practice has led to an aura of secrecy in which myths abound. Let's look at a few of them.

MYTH: 'HOMEOPATHY IS SAFE'

In the same way that homeopathy can cure – often dramatically and permanently – it can also cause harm. Potential dangers are:

Unintentional Provings

If you take a homeopathic remedy for too long it is possible to 'prove' the remedy – that is, to suffer again from the symptoms that the remedy was supposed to cure. If the remedy was correct, your symptoms may improve initially but worsen again if you continue to take it. Worse still, if the remedy did not fit your picture – was not right for you – you may experience symptoms you haven't had before.

This is a danger with self-prescribing or over-the-counter prescribing, where there is no professional homeopath to monitor the symptoms. In my first year in practice a woman rang me one day in a frantic state, desperate for help. She told me the following story:

I asked for help at a homeopathic chemist for thrush, from which I had suffered for several months, and was prescribed *Nux Vomica 30* over the counter and told to take it three times daily. After a few days I experienced a marked improvement in my condition, so I carried on taking it.

After a week of no further changes my symptoms started to get worse, so I carried on taking it. I finished the bottle of pills and went back to the pharmacy and told them my thrush was now as bad as when I had started to take the remedy. They gave me another bottle of *Nux Vomica 30* and told me to continue with the treatment. It is now two months since I started on this remedy and my thrush is unbearable. It is so bad I can't sleep at night and I am irritable all the time. Please help me.

I advised her to stop taking the pills and to antidote the remedy with strong coffee and camphorated ointment (to counteract the effect of the proving) and within twenty-four hours she was back to her old self, having slept well for the first time in a month. The thrush was back to where it had been before she took the *Nux Vomica* – annoying but manageable – and she took a course of acupuncture treatment to deal with the remaining thrush.

It is important not to overuse homeopathic medicines.

Confusion of the Symptom Picture

If a remedy has not been prescribed on the whole person it will work in a limited way, curing a restricted number of symptoms. Some symptoms remain and you may end up giving one remedy after another to try to 'get rid' of them. The whole picture becomes so changed that it is difficult to find the *similimum* (that single remedy that was needed in the beginning).

The professional homeopath has different ways of dealing with this phenomenon to get back to the original symptom picture: if you find that you are prescribing one remedy after another with only limited effect, then get professional homeopathic help.

Suppression

A homeopathic remedy can cure a specific symptom such as a skin eruption in the same way as, for example, the application of a hydrocortisone cream. This will only occur if the remedy has been prescribed on the skin complaint (single symptom) without taking into account the whole person and/or the cause. The effect is to push the disease further into the body (see Laws of Cure, p. 8). Constitutional treatment will often begin with the original symptom resurfacing. Suppression is not common with homeopathic treatment but *is* possible. In self-prescribing, if your complaint disappears but *you* feel much worse in yourself (your moods and your energy) then it is likely that you have made a poor choice of remedy. Antidote it (see p. 21) and take professional homeopathic advice.

MYTH: 'HOMEOPATHY IS A FORM OF HERBALISM'

This is the commonest myth of all. While it is certainly true that some homeopathic remedies are based on plants, and that, as in homeopathy, the herbalist prescribes on the individual, the principles that govern the two therapies are quite different.

Many plants have known healing properties; herbalism, used for thousands of years, is concerned with the known sphere of action of a plant based on its chemical constituents as well as its known healing qualities. Homeopathy is based on different principles (see pp. 4–10). The remedies are not used in the material dose; nor are they based solely on plants, using also poisons, metals and disease products. Homeopaths generally prescribe one remedy at a time rather than the mixtures of plant tinctures that herbalists employ.

MYTH: 'HOMEOPATHY IS A FORM OF VACCINATION'

People often say that they understand homeopathy to be like a vaccination in that the patient is given a small quantity of the disease they already have to make him immune to it. Homeopathy and vaccination have only *similar*, not the *same*, concepts, and have very different practices. Vaccines stimulate the immune system directly to produce specific antibodies *as if* that person had contracted a particular disease; in so doing they stress the immune system. They are tested on animals and then humans to verify their safety, and even then children and adults can suffer serious side effects.

A homeopathic remedy works differently by affecting an individual's energy patterns – the vital force – and stimulating the body to heal itself. It is administered orally in a diluted (and safe) dose whereas most vaccinations are introduced directly into the bloodstream, thereby bypassing the body's natural defence system and stressing it in a way that is not fully understood. Homeopathic medicines are not tested on animals and when correctly used do not have side effects.

MYTH: 'HOMEOPATHIC REMEDIES ARE PLACEBOS'

This myth can be rephrased to read 'You need to believe in it for it to work', which is nonsense to anyone who has experienced or prescribed a successful homeopathic cure for a head injury or a middle-ear infection in a baby.

A placebo is an unmedicated pill which the patient believes contains something that will cure him or her. Homeopathic medicines work on babies and animals, neither of whom are susceptible to the placebo effect. Research has ruled out the placebo effect and shown over and over again that homeopathy is effective and *does* work.

Many people recognise the experience of consulting a practitioner who inspires belief and hope, leaving them feeling buoyant and encouraged. But if this initial rapport is not backed up with good solid prescribing, then no amount of positive 'transference' will effect a cure.

MYTH: 'HOMEOPATHY IS MYSTERIOUS AND UNSCIENTIFIC'

Homeopathic medicines are prepared in a pharmacy or a laboratory, involving a technique subject to precise and clearly stated controls. Preparation does not involve mysterious and secret processes which put it into the realm of white magic or alchemy.

The homeopathic principles constitute a unified hypothesis whose validity is tested empirically: cured patients confirm the hypothesis. Harris Coulter discusses this issue at great length in his book *Homoeopathic Science and Modern Medicine: The Physics of Healing with Microdoses*, and also describes many of the trials that have been conducted over the past fifty years or so using plants, animals and humans as controls to prove the effectiveness of homeopathic medicines.

TAKING THE CASE HISTORY

It is well worth the effort to approach first-aid prescribing seriously by teaching yourself how to take a case history and how to work out a remedy. That is the major concern of this book: to help you to prescribe, where possible, in the same way as a professional homeopath. Many homeopathic first-aid books take a 'symptomatic approach', directing you to a remedy on the strength of one symptom or complaint. This is not thorough enough and the results cannot be guaranteed. In this book, therefore, I have taken the more classical approach of looking at the whole person in a detailed way.

If you fall ill and wish to prescribe for yourself it is important to remember that it may be difficult to be objective about your own symptoms: you may be fooled into prescribing the wrong remedy. For example, you may feel quite calm in yourself while those around you have experienced an increase in your levels of irritability and touchiness; and/or you may already have forgotten the drenching you had the day before you fell ill. It can be useful to talk through your symptoms with your partner or a friend before you self-prescribe. Some people are competent at knowing exactly what their 'symptom picture' is and are clear about the stresses that led up to their illness; others need more help. If you need it, get help from your local homeopath.

Before you begin to take the case, check that the complaint is within the scope of this book (see pp. 22 and 23 as well as Complaints, pp. 79–104, 107–15, 117–60).

Don't attempt to prescribe for a chronic disease; these always need professional attention.

THE SYMPTOM PICTURE

This is a detailed account of what is wrong with you as a whole person when you fall ill. Your symptoms – the signs or indications of your being ill – are an expression of need and a call for help from your body. A homeopathic prescriber is a symptom sleuth! For a remedy to work well you need to match, as accurately as possible, your symptom picture with a *remedy picture* – the collection of symptoms produced by the remedy in its proving, as set out in the Materia Medica. It doesn't have to be identical, merely similar. You won't need to experience *all* the symptoms of the remedy for it to work! Symptoms are divided into three main categories: general, mental/emotional and physical complaints. You will need one or more from each main category of symptom. See pp. 14–15 for the case-taking chart.

I have used the word *complaint* throughout the book to mean the disease itself, or rather its label – for example, 'sore throat' or 'cough'. The symptoms are the visible signs of the complaint, or, the complaint expresses itself through the symptoms. Say your child is complaining of a barking cough that is worse at night and better for sitting up: the complaint is the cough and the symptoms are barking, worse at night and better for sitting up.

Understanding and treating the cause is fundamental to homeopathic practice. It is helpful to identify the stresses that affect us, so that we can avoid them or take action before we actually fall ill.

All disease is caused by stress, which can be physical, emotional or mental. Different people are sensitive to different stresses at different times in their lives: cold, heat, changes in weather, mental strain, etc. The diseases people develop will also vary according to their individual weaknesses.

Stress symptoms may be general, in which case you will find them in the Repertory under Complaints from (and in the Materia Medica under General Symptoms, Complaints from). Perhaps your child always becomes ill with, say a cold or a cough or an earache, if the weather changes from warm to cold: begin by looking in the Repertory under Complaints from/after: Change of weather to cold.

Stress symptoms may be specific, in which case you will find them listed as a Cause under the complaint itself. For example, some children (and adults) are sensitive to falls. If they bang their heads they suffer from headaches. In the Repertory (p. 264) under Headache, Causes, head injury you will find *Natrum sulphuricum* (*Nat-s.*) listed. If you turn to *Natrum sulphuricum* in the Materia Medica (pp. 229–30) you will find that under the physical complaint 'Headache', head injury is listed as the 'cause'.

It is vital to build a strongly indicated stress symptom into your picture. Once you are familiar with particular patterns you need not wait for the complaints to prescribe. For example, if you have a child who is sensitive to bangs on the head and *Natrum sulphuricum* has cured in the past, you can give it automatically (after *Arnica* has dealt with the bruising) to prevent a headache from developing.

Similarly, you can give *Calcarea carbonica* to a baby who has a cough and cold *and* you suspect that she is teething once again *and Calcarea carbonica* has helped her before under similar circumstances. You can even give it before the cough develops. If she is restless, has a runny nose and you know she is teething, the remedy will help her teethe without becoming sick.

Your observations are very important: you are not simply looking for aches and pains, you need to gain a picture of the *differences* from the normal state of health. Gathering information is not always easy. Look for clear, strongly marked symptoms: vague, 'well . . . sometimes' symptoms are not useful unless they present a 'changeable' symptom picture in themselves.

Certain symptoms are always present in any given disease and are indicated in its name. For example, pain during urination is usually called cystitis; conjunctivitis refers to inflamed, bloodshot eyes. As homeopathy does not treat the labelled disease alone but the individual who is sick, and since no two cases of cystitis are exactly the same, every labelled disease (or complaint) is accompanied by symptoms peculiar to the individual who has it, which differ from those of another individual with the same 'disease'. It is the individual symptoms which guide us to the remedy that will help.

Simply to write 'headache' or 'cough' is not enough. If you look up either of these symptoms in the Repertory you will find many remedies listed. It is the particular symptoms of the patient's headache or cough that enable you to begin to narrow down the choice of remedies, to individualise the prescription. One person with a headache may have a throbbing forehead that feels better for fresh air, while another will have sharp pains in the temples that are better for warmth and lying down. Different remedies are called for.

NOTE-TAKING

It is essential that you write down the symptoms, and that you record the remedy that you give as well as its result. Even if you write only a few words plus the date, the name and potency of the remedy, that will suffice to remind you should the same problem recur. I suggest you open a loose-leaf file marked 'Health' and use it for keeping interesting articles as well as notes on your home prescribing. You can file photocopies of the case-taking chart (pp. 14–15) and the repertorising chart (p. 17) so that you always have 'blanks' to hand should you need them.

First Impressions

Give some attention to your first impressions about what is happening as they are an important and reliable source of information. Say your child wakes up in the night screaming. You go into her room. What do you immediately smell and see? What note do you hear in her scream? Is it one of pain or fright? Or perhaps your best friend has flu, she's pregnant and has asked you to come and help. You walk into the room and what do you see before she has organised herself to be sociable with you? Is the room tidy or messy? Is it hot or cold? Does she look sad and tired before she makes an effort to be 'fine'?

If remedies do come to mind as you are talking, do not ignore them but write them in the margin: those instincts can be inspired. Generally speaking, it is better to forget about working out a remedy while you take notes; the analytical part comes later. Con-centrate on using your senses to pick up clues and on being receptive to what you are hearing.

What do you smell?

The smell is often the first thing you notice on walking into a sick person's room. Smell the head/neck/hands of a feverish or sick child and you will find that sweat can smell sour or just plain offensive. Smell the breath, too. Other discharges can also smell 'interesting': the stools or urine of a teething baby can smell sour; vomit can also be very smelly. If the smell is strong and you can describe it clearly, write it down and use it as a symptom.

What do you see?

In the case of an illness, note the colour and expression on your patient's face. Has the colour drained from it or is it flushed? Is the expression anxious or obviously in pain (suffering)?

Look for clues: drinks not drunk; covers piled high or, alternatively, kicked off; restlessness; log-like patients who groan if you sit on the edge of the bed and disturb them and so on. You may learn more by looking than your patient is aware of.

What do you feel?

Touch the skin to find out whether there is sweat. If so, is it hot or cold, clammy or profuse? A dry skin with a fever (sweat, absent), for example, is an important symptom. Check to see if some parts of the body are sweaty and others aren't. Perhaps your patient is complaining of an inner, burning heat while the skin feels cold to the touch.

What do you hear?

Some sick children moan or grind their teeth in their sleep; others might whine for attention if they think you are not listening and stop when you enter the room (and vice versa!). Listen to the tone of the voice. Is it anxious or sad or angry?

Let your patient talk, if they are old enough, without any interruption from you if possible. This in itself can be healing, and can also provide you with information. For example, the *Lachesis* patient talks incessantly, jumping from one subject to another, while the *Bryonia* patient will not want to talk at all.

Questions

Ask yourself (or your 'patient') general rather than specific questions.

General	Specific
How am I/are you feeling?	Am I/are you feeling sad?
How painful is it?	Does it hurt a lot?
Describe the pain?	Is it throbbing?
Does heat or cold help or make it worse?	Is it better for heat?

Some people will reply negatively when asked about themselves or their symptoms: 'I'm not well'; 'He's not bad'; 'It isn't much better'; 'It doesn't hurt that much'. These replies do not tell you what is actually happening. Questions like 'How are you, then?', 'What *are* you feeling?' can sometimes help, but people who speak in negatives often need careful questioning to tell you what is wrong. In answer to 'It doesn't hurt that much', you could ask 'Is the pain stopping you from doing anything?' (that is, 'How serious is it?'). Then you can go on to give a list of different types of pain and if your patient alights on one, saying 'That's it!', then write it down. If they are not sure, go on to another question.

Finally, remember . . .

Do not discount anything. What other information do you have about that person? What has been going on in her life lately that might be part of why she is feeling sick now? What have you been told by her mother/father/child/neighbour? Have you given this person a first-aid remedy before, say, for a flu? Did the remedy work well? If that remedy worked marvellously, consider whether it might be indicated again. The case-taking chart and questionnaire below will help you take a good case history.

Name: **Date:**

Complaint (headache, cough, etc.) ....
When did it start?...
Did it start suddenly/slowly? ....
Caused by ....
....
....
Symptoms ....
....
....
Better...
....
....
Worse...
....
....

General symptoms...
....
....
Better...
....
....
Worse...
....
....

Mental/emotional state/symptoms...
....
....

Other physical symptoms...
....

Have you had this before? *If this is a recurring chronic complaint then* **don't** *treat yourself* (see p. 7). Check that this complaint is within the scope of this book (see the complaints section of the appropriate chapter). Seek professional advice if necessary.

Think carefully about what happened in the days/weeks prior to falling ill and list the stresses, especially those that preceded the complaint. Check the stress list in the Repertory under 'Complaints from' (p. 269).

List everything you can think of that relates to the complaint – especially its strongest symptoms, the type of pain and accompanying discharges, etc.

Is there anything that affects the complaint, anything that makes it better or makes it worse: heat, cold, fresh air, pressure, drinking (hot or cold drinks), draughts, time of day or night, lying down, noise, movement, sleep, etc.?

These symptoms are related to a person, whether well or ill: they may or may not change during an illness. They relate to how you feel generally as opposed to how your complaint is reacting. For example, you may feel worse for cold and better for heat (general symptoms) – you want to be wrapped up with the heating on – *but* your headache is worse for heat and better for cold and fresh air so you have to sit beside an open window.

Do you feel better or worse for heat or cold or fresh air? Are you generally better in the morning or at night? And so on.

Read through some of the 'General Symptoms' sections in the Materia Medica to get an idea of what you're looking for.

Describe the emotions/moods if you can, using the checklist opposite to help you.

Use the checklist opposite to help you.

Physical symptoms List any other physical symptoms that you've noticed. Use this checklist to jog your memory. Underline and/or add additional symptoms.

Head	headache, dizziness, hair loss, faintness
Eyes	inflamed, watering, sensitive to light, styes, pupils dilated/contracted
Ears	earache, hearing
Nose	common cold, catarrh, nosebleeds, sense of smell, cracks
Face	expression, colour, lips dry/cracked, cold sores
Mouth	ulcers, dryness, excess saliva, taste
Teeth	toothache, teething, abscess
Tongue	colour, cracks, indented on edges
Throat	sore throat, voice lost, hoarseness
Stomach	appetite (likes/dislikes), thirst, nausea, vomiting, colic, indigestion
Chest	cough, croup, palpitations, breastfeeding problems
Bowels	constipation, diarrhoea, stools (colour/consistency), piles, worms, flatulence
Urination	pain (cystitis), retention, bedwetting
Periods	painful, heavy, late
Neck/back	stiff neck, glands swollen, backache, sciatica
Arms/legs	joint pain, cramps, clumsy, weak ankles, chilblains, corns
Sleep	unrefreshing, restless, insomnia, nightmares
Energy	exhaustion, sluggish, apathetic, anaemia
Skin	prickly heat, boils, hives, thrush, blisters
Fever	with or without sweating, flu
Sweat	smelly, profuse, scanty, localised, generalised
Discharges	colour, consistency
Stressed by	(complaints from) change of weather, getting wet, getting chilled, injury, emotions, etc.
Injuries	see under each heading – bruises, burns, etc.
Symptoms	side, onset (slow/sudden)
Pains	general, labour pains

Emotional state List any emotional symptoms that you have noticed. Use this as a checklist to jog your memory. Underline and/or add additional symptoms.

absent-minded
affectionate
angry
anxious
apathetic
aversion (being alone/touched/
    hugged/consolation/children
    or partner etc.)
biting (children)
broody
capricious
cheerful

childish
clingy
concentration, poor
confused
conscientious
critical
dazed
delirious
denial
depressed
desire (for company/to be alone/
    to be carried)

despair
despondent
dictatorial
disappointment
discontented
disobedient
dreamy
dwells on the past
euphoric
excitable
exhilarated
expressions (anxious/suffering
    etc.)
fearful
forgetful
gentle
gloomy
guilt
hitting (children)
homesick
humiliation
hurried
idealistic
impatient
impulsive
indecisive
indifferent
introspective
introverted
irritable
jealous
joking
jumpy
lack of self confidence
lazy
lively
lonely

loss of libido
melancholic
memory weak
mild
mischievous
moaning/complaining
moody
morose
panic
quarrelsome
rage
resentful
restless
screaming
self-confidence, lack of
sensitive (to light/music/noise/
    pain)
sentimental
shock
shy
sighing
slowness
sluggish
spiteful
stubborn
stupor
sulky
sympathetic
talkative
tantrums
tearful
tidy
uncommunicative
unforgiving
weary
whiny

Babies and children

Babies and small children cannot describe what they are feeling so you need to be especially observant to find the symptoms that will lead you to a successful prescription. Remember, you are looking for any changes from their normal (healthy) patterns of behaviour. Be aware of your child's patterns of health so that changes, when they are ill, are clear to you.

You may need to do lots of looking and feeling and smelling with babies as well as using your intuition to get a sense of how ill your baby really is. See p. 23 for when to seek expert help. If you are at all unsure, do not delay in getting help and reassurance.

With very young babies you need to check out the following: bowels, skin (including temperature and sweating), sleep, discharges, stresses, energy, eyes, tongue, digestion (colic) and emotions.

WORKING OUT THE REMEDY

Having taken your case history, follow these steps to select your remedy: choose your symptoms; repertorise; differentiate. Once you become familiar with this process you will be able to take short cuts but it is worth getting to grips with even if it does feel tedious initially. These steps are brought to life in the sample cases on pp. 23–8.

1   Choose Your Symptoms

Go through your case and underline the symptoms that stand out clearly and strongly. It is best to leave vague and unclear symptoms alone for the moment: you may use them later if you can't make up your mind between two or more remedies.

Wherever possible, choose at least three strong symptoms, one from each symptom group: one general symptom, one mental/emotional symptom and one physical symptom. You *can* prescribe on a single symptom but this is rarely successful. If you work out a remedy based on a symptom from each of these groups you can be confident that it has a good chance of working. If you add in a stress symptom you can be even surer of your prescription. The more symptoms that fit the remedy picture the better.

2   Repertorise

'Repertorising' sounds much more complicated than it is. List the symptoms you've chosen on a separate piece of paper or on a copy of the Repertorising chart. Then look up each one in the Repertory and list the remedies that occur under each symptom, or alternatively tick them off on the repertorising chart. When you have completed the list you will be able to see which remedy, or remedies, occurs most often – which contains all or most of the symptoms on your list. As you become more familiar with the remedy pictures you will learn to recognise the remedy your patient needs without repertorising.

3   Differentiate

In some cases only one remedy will contain all your symptoms. Go to the Materia Medica and read through the remedy picture to check that it fits. If it does, prescribe that remedy, following the potency and dosage guidelines set out on pp. 19–20.

Often, however, more than one remedy will contain all your symptoms, or several remedies will have most of your symptoms and none will have all of them. If more than one remedy is indicated according to the repertorising chart, choosing between them can be difficult; it is one of the skills that makes a competent homeopath. Read through each of the remedies that has all or most of the symptoms and pick the one that fits best.

If you can't find a remedy that fits your picture, then go back to your chart and see if you have missed any remedies. Check your case for missed symptoms. Add these to your list and repertorise them. Then read through any new remedies that emerge through this process. Repeat these steps until you find a remedy that fits. If you are really stuck, you may have to go back to square one and take the case history again from scratch.

NB Your general and emotional/mental symptoms may point to a remedy that does not list the physical complaint you are suffering from in its picture. For example, you have flu and are feeling restless, irritable, hot and bothered and extremely thirsty. You find that *Sulphur* comes up strongly for your mental/ emotional and general symptoms but isn't listed under Flu in the Repertory. The closest remedy is *Bryonia* but when you read the *Bryonia* picture you don't recognise yourself. When you read *Sulphur* you immediately think 'that's it' and are able to identify a number of other symptoms which are characteristic of you whether you are well or not, for example, you hate to stand and have always suffered from hot feet. You check your tongue and find that it also fits the *Sulphur* description.

Even though the remedy doesn't have flu as one of the physical symptoms, because it is 'constitutional', and because it is strongly indicated for *you*, that is, for your emotional and general picture, it will work.

PRESCRIBING

Never rush into prescribing for someone else. Don't think that you have to give a remedy just because you have the book and someone wants you to. If you don't feel right about working out a remedy for someone you don't know very well, or are unsure about what remedy to give, then don't do it. Suggest they go to a professional homeopath or to their GP. If you are thinking of prescribing for yourself then proceed cautiously because it is notoriously difficult to prescribe accurately if you are feeling unwell.

If you are already under the care of a professional homeopath, it is preferable that they are consulted before you prescribe. It is better to give nothing than to interfere with what may be an aggravation (see p. 21) and therefore not fully understood by you. However, in an accident or an emergency you can take the indicated remedy (*Arnica*, *Aconite* or *Hypericum*, for

REPERTORISING CHART

Symptoms:

No.	ACO.	AESC.	AGAR.	ALL-C.	ALU.	ANT-C.	ANT-T.	AP.	ARG-N.	ARN.	ARS.	ASAR.	BAR-C.	BELL.	BELL-P.	BOR.	BRY.	CALC-C.	CALC-F.	CALC-P.	CALC-S.	CALEN.	CANTH.	CARB-A.	CARB-V.	CAST.	CAUL.
1.																											
2.																											
3.																											
4.																											
5.																											
6.																											
7.																											
8.																											
9.																											

No.	CAUST.	CHAM.	CHEL.	CHIN.	CIMI.	CINA.	COCC.	COCC-C.	COFF.	COLCH.	COLOC.	CON.	CUPR.	CYPR.	DIOS.	DROS.	DULC.	EUP-P.	EUPHR.	FERR-M.	GELS.	GLON.	HAM.	HEP-S.	HYP.	IGN.	IP.
1.																											
2.																											
3.																											
4.																											
5.																											
6.																											
7.																											
8.																											
9.																											

No.	JAB.	KALI-B.	KALI-C.	KALI-M.	KALI-P.	KALI-S.	KREOS.	LAC-C.	LAC-D.	LACH.	LED.	LIL-T.	LYC.	MAG-C.	MAG-M.	MAG-P.	MERC-C.	MERC-S.	NAT-C.	NAT-M.	NAT-P.	NAT-S.	NIT-AC.	NUX-M.	NUX-V.	OP.	PETR.
1.																											
2.																											
3.																											
4.																											
5.																											
6.																											
7.																											
8.																											
9.																											

No.	PHO-AC.	PHOS.	PHYT.	PODO.	PULS.	PYR.	RHE.	RHOD.	RHUS-T.	RUMEX.	RUTA.	SAB.	SARS.	SEC.	SEP.	SIL.	SPO.	STAP.	STRAM.	SUL.	SUL-AC.	SYMPH.	TAB.	THU.	URT-U.	VER-A.	ZINC.
1.																											
2.																											
3.																											
4.																											
5.																											
6.																											
7.																											
8.																											
9.																											

NB PHOTOCOPY THIS CHART SO THAT YOU HAVE A STOCK FOR WHENEVER YOU NEED ONE example) immediately, but make sure that you seek additional professional help if needed and write down the remedy you took as well as its response for reference.

Whom to Prescribe For

When prescribing for adults, however close they may be to you, remember this rule: prescribe only if you are asked for help. Over-zealousness can be very off-putting and if you force a remedy on to someone the chances of its being sabotaged by antidoting (see p. 21) are very high. If there is an improvement, it will be attributed to coincidence. It is always possible to offer help and leave it at that. Don't get into the way of thinking that you can cure anybody and everybody of their complaints or impinge on other people's right to look after their own health in their own way.

If you are self-prescribing, it is advisable to discuss your remedy with a friend to make sure that you are not deluding yourself about your true state of body and mind.

Babies and children respond very well to homeopathic treatment. If they do not respond quickly to your first-aid prescribing, seek the advice of a professional homeopath.

REMEDY FORMS AVAILABLE

Homeopathic remedies are most commonly available as tablets made of sugar of cow's milk, or *Saccharum lactose*, commonly known as *sac lac*; this has been found to be the ideal medium for the potentised remedy. *Sac lac* comes in several forms: hard or soft tablets, globules or powders. Most homeopathic pharmacies will automatically make up remedies in the form of hard *sac lac* tablets unless they are specifically asked otherwise.

Listed below are the different forms a homeopathic remedy can take. In each case a few drops of the potentised remedy in alcohol are used to medicate (or moisten) the base substance.

Soft tablets (*sac lac*) dissolve quickly and easily under the tongue and are also easily crushed for administering to babies. (See p. 19.)

Hard tablets (*sac lac*) do not dissolve as easily as the soft tablets. They should be chewed and held in the mouth for a few seconds before being swallowed. They can also be crushed.

Globules (*sac lac*) are tiny round pills, like poppy seeds. A few grains should be dissolved on the tongue and not a lidful as is sometimes suggested (in theory one grain should suffice – a single dose is a single dose, it is not the size that counts).

Sucrose (*plain sugar*) is sometimes used, especially for pocket travel kits. A few grains should be dissolved on the tongue. They can (like the globules) be tipped on to the palm of the person taking the remedy, or straight on the tongue.

Liquid potencies Homeopathic remedies can be made up in liquid form for children or adults known to be allergic to cow's milk. The remedy is added to an alcohol base, supplied in dropper bottles; the dose is either administered neat on the tongue or diluted in water for babies and children, in which case 5 drops should be added to a little water and held in the mouth for a second or two before being swallowed.

Powders (*sac lac*) Most homeopathic pharmacies can make up remedies in powder form. These are wrapped individually in small squares of paper and are convenient if you need only a few doses of an unusual remedy that you are unlikely to want again, or if you need to send small quantities by mail, especially abroad. They should be dissolved on or under the tongue like soft tablets or added to a small amount of water and held in the mouth for a few seconds before swallowing.

Wafers Selected pharmacies can provide remedies in wafers, which, like powders, are wrapped individually. The wafers are made of rice paper, which is useful for people sensitive to milk *and* sugar.

Storing Remedies

Homeopathic remedies will keep their strength for years without deteriorating: remedies made over a hundred years ago still work well. They should be stored in a cool, dark, dry place with their tops screwed on tightly, well away from strong-smelling substances: strong smells cause the remedies to lose their potency. It is not a good idea to keep them in a bathroom cabinet alongside perfumes and cough mixtures, or in a spare-room cupboard with the mothballs. A sealed plastic container like an ice-cream tub is good for storing loose bottles or you may choose to purchase one of the ready-made kits available from many pharmacies, to your own specifications if you wish (see p. 301).

It is wise to keep all tablets out of the reach of children as a matter of course. If your child eats the entire first-aid kit in one glorious secret feast, do not panic. Your bank balance is the only thing that will suffer! A single dose at a time is a single dose, whether it is one pill or one bottle of pills. If your child eats a full bottle of, say, *Chamomilla* 6 or even 30 tablets it will have roughly the same effect as taking one tablet.

How to Take Remedies

Carefully tip a tablet into the lid of the bottle. If more than one falls out, tip the others back so that only one remains. Tip it on to the palm of the person taking the remedy and then replace the lid on the bottle. You can touch your own tablets, but if you are giving the remedy to someone else try to avoid touching it.

Never put back tablets that have fallen out on to the floor or anywhere else, or that you have given out and are unused. In so doing you may contaminate your stock. Always throw them away.

Soft tablets, powders, sucrose, globules and wafers should be dissolved under the tongue where they are absorbed into the bloodstream; if they are swallowed whole they become mixed with the stomach acids and work less effectively. Hard tablets should be chewed, held in the mouth for a few seconds and then swallowed. Liquid potencies can be dropped on to the tongue or diluted with a little water and held in the mouth for a few seconds before swallowing.

It is preferable not to eat, drink (except water), smoke or brush your teeth for 10–20 minutes before and after taking a remedy as this gives it the best possible chance of working, although in practice remedies given to toddlers who eat before and after still work well. The 10-minute gap makes sure that residues of food do not affect the action of the remedy.

Many homeopathic remedies available in the chemist or wholefood shop give dosage instructions on the bottle, suggesting different doses for adults (two tablets) and children (one tablet). This is questionable given that there isn't a measurable quantity of the medicine in the tablet. The size of the dose is immaterial; it is how often it is taken that counts. I instruct my patients to take one tablet, whatever their age.

Tablets for babies can be crushed between two spoons and the powder tipped dry on to the tongue. This is hard to spit out, unlike a tablet. A little water can be added to the crushed powder on the spoon, or the tablet can be dissolved in a clean glass with a little water. Stir it vigorously and then give as needed, a teaspoonful at a time. Scour the glass and the spoon (with boiled water) after use so that the next person to use them doesn't get an inadvertent dose of the remedy.

How Many Doses and How Often

Do
- prescribe according to the urgency of the case.
- stop on improvement.

- start again if the same symptoms return: repeat as needed.
- if you have given six doses and have had no response, stop and reassess the case or seek advice.
- change the remedy if the symptom picture changes.
- if the 'patient' is already receiving homeopathic treatment, consult the homeopath, if possible, before prescribing (unless it is an emergency).

Always seek professional help from your homeopath or GP if your symptoms recur or do not improve.

Having selected the remedy, you will need to decide on the dose. This depends on the urgency of the case: frequent doses for an acute illness that has come on suddenly and strongly, and less frequent doses for a slowly developing illness. Some earaches with severely distressed patients need the remedy to be repeated every five minutes; a head injury may need the remedy repeated every half-hour; and a slowly developing flu may need a remedy every four hours or three times a day. The dosage chart (p. 20) will help you to establish the frequency.

Once you see that a remedy has started to work – when you notice a definite reaction or change resulting from the remedy – continue with the same remedy but give it less often, increasing the gaps between the doses.

Once there is a *marked* improvement – a strong positive reaction having occurred – it is essential to stop the remedy. This is the absolute opposite of the instructions you receive when taking orthodox medicines (for example, antibiotics), where it is necessary to finish the whole course of tablets. A homeopathic remedy acts as a trigger, a catalyst: it stimulates the body to begin to heal itself, and once that has happened the body's own healing process will take over. In some cases, taking another tablet after this reaction has occurred can stop the remedy working and if too many are taken it is possible to start proving the remedy (see p. 5).

Prescribe up to six pills according to the urgency of the case. If you have given six pills and there has been no change whatsoever, then it is probably the wrong remedy, unless you are prescribing a 'tonic' or remedy that needs to be taken over the course of a week or so (like remedies for anaemia or exhaustion).

Which Potency?

Homeopathic remedies come in different potencies. The 6X, 6C, 12C and the 30C are all safe for the home prescriber. The 6X and the 6C are the most widely available; they are the best potencies to use for minor

DOSAGE CHART

Degree of seriousness	Potency	Dosage
Very serious		
Symptoms need immediate attention accompanied by great pain, e.g. earache; head or back injury; second- or third-degree burn; cystitis, labour pains, etc.	6C, 12C or 30C	one dose every 5–30 minutes
Serious		
Symptoms need help within about 24 hours and are not necessarily accompanied by pain, e.g. bad cough; abscess; food poisoning; vomiting, etc.	6C or 12C	one dose every 1–2 hours
Less serious		
Symptoms can wait a day or two to be treated, e.g. sore throat; flu; teething; chickenpox, etc.	6C or 12C	one dose every 4–8 hours
Not serious (i.e. tonic)		
Symptoms are usually mild and need longer-term treatment, e.g. anaemia; exhaustion, etc.	6X or 6C	one dose 3 times daily for up to 10 days

Stop on improvement. Repeat as needed.

NB *Alternating remedies*. I have occasionally suggested that you alternate remedies where, for example, two are indicated. This can happen after childbirth when you might want to take, say, *Arnica* for bruising and *Calendula* to speed the healing of an episiotomy. Instead of taking them both together it is better to alternate them as frequently as needed, every one to two hours if the soreness is severe, less often if it is tolerable, for several days if you're taking them as a tonic.

---

complaints. 12C is slightly stronger than 6C, and 30C is stronger still so fewer doses are needed. It tends to work faster and is useful for more serious complaints, such as bad burns or head injuries with concussion. If you are ordering a kit from a pharmacy I suggest you order the remedies in the 6C or 12C potency to start with. As you gain experience in prescribing, you'll begin to know when one of the other potencies is more appropriate.

Assessing the Response

A homeopathic remedy is like a pebble which creates healing ripples when thrown into your pond. The prescriber must get the 'pebble' as close to the middle of the 'pond' as possible, so that the 'ripples' reach out to every part of the patient. If you have given six doses and have had no significant response then the remedy you have chosen is likely to be wrong. Did you have more than one remedy to choose from? How did you make your choice? Check your symptoms. Read through the remedy pictures in the Materia Medica again. If you are convinced that your choice of remedy was correct, persevere for another three to six doses. If your prescription does not work, you may have missed the *real* cause or stress. Homeopaths will delve relentlessly until they uncover what it was that weakened an individual, causing them to become ill, so seek professional homeopathic advice if your complaint is particularly debilitating, and self-prescribing is not helping. If you are prescribing for someone else you should refer back to your notes to see whether you need any specific or extra information. For example, your friend has heartburn which is worse for eating: you realise that you don't know whether she is having difficulty swallowing liquids and whether hot or cold drinks help. Ask some more specific questions and gauge how strongly marked the symptoms are by the response you get. An unequivocal 'yes' or 'no' counts; a 'maybe' or a 'sometimes' doesn't.

Having reassessed the symptom picture, you may decide to select another remedy. The same guidelines apply again: give up to six doses, according to the urgency of the case. If you become unsure, however, it is better to stop prescribing and either get professional help or let nature take its course.

Write down exactly what you have done at each step, with notes to explain your reasons, plus the results of your own prescribing. (If you decide to do nothing and your patient gets better, make sure you write that down too.) Although it is hard to imagine, it is the easiest thing in the world to forget the one brilliant remedy you gave your baby for a cough, and here they are with another one six months later . . .

In an acute illness like an earache or a bruised head, one, two or three doses may be enough to begin the healing process. If you feel better *in yourself* you will get better even if your physical symptoms remain the same or get slightly and temporarily worse. If your symptoms improve for a while and then relapse, a repeat dose of the same remedy may be necessary – but *only* on return of the same symptoms. If the symptom picture changes, it is likely that you will need a different remedy.

The Homeopathic Aggravation

This is the term given to the worsening of symptoms that may occur after a constitutional remedy has been taken. This *can* happen during an acute illness and either the symptoms may worsen or an old symptom may surface temporarily (see Laws of Cure, p. 8). If an old symptom surfaces after a good prescription, wait to see if it will clear of its own accord. If it does, the remedy is still working . . . carry on waiting.

There may be a more general clearing out, or 'healing crisis' as it is often called, in the form of a streaming cold or diarrhoea. The aggravation can occur on a mental/emotional level with some patients feeling very weepy if, for example, it is suppressed grief that has caused a general lowering of their health and the physical complaint.

The higher potencies (200C and above) are especially renowned for their ability to cause aggravations and

that is one of the main reasons why a first-aid prescriber should stick to the lower ones.

Antidotes

The subject of antidotes always arouses heated discussion among homeopaths. There are those who believe that coffee strongly counteracts the action of a homeopathic remedy, while others believe that it has no effect whatsoever. I believe that it depends on the individual, often someone who is generally sensitive and finds coffee gives them insomnia and palpitations will experience coffee as an antidote. In this case it is wise to stop drinking it while the remedies are being taken and for a short time afterwards. If you are sensitive to coffee and stop drinking it while you are taking your remedy, note whether your symptoms return when you start drinking it again. If they do, you may have to stop drinking it and take another short course of the remedy to clear your symptoms once more.

The following all counteract the effects of a homeopathic remedy to some extent. They are not necessarily 'bad', but as the action of a remedy can last for as little as a few days or as long as a few months, they are strong enough to stop it working and should be avoided while it is being taken and for several weeks afterwards.

Camphor In 'tiger balm', deep-heat ointments and many lip salves

Coffee See above

Menthol/eucalyptus In cough mixtures, Karvol capsules, 'tiger balm', Fisherman's Friend, Vick, Olbas Oil, etc.

Peppermint In regular toothpaste and strong peppermint sweets. Natural, fresh mint in cooking and the odd cup of peppermint tea is fine. Alternatives to ordinary, minty toothpaste are fennel toothpaste (available at most health-food shops), salt water or bicarbonate of soda. A solution of *Calendula* is an efficient mouthwash, both at home and at the dentist (see External Materia Medica)

Any strong-smelling or strong-acting substance will affect a homeopathic remedy. Some people have found that a spicy curry will have an adverse effect, as might a night of heavy drinking.

An emotional or physical shock can also stop a remedy working; for some people this can mean a piece of bad news; for others a visit to the dentist with the stress and strain of treatment.

If your remedy has 'stopped working' (you took it and your symptoms cleared for a time and have now returned), ask yourself if you have antidoted the remedy. If you think you have, then repeat your last remedy: sometimes a single repeat is enough.

And Finally . . .

I would encourage anyone who is taking homeopathic prescribing seriously to enroll for a short homeopathic first-aid course. Many adult education colleges run courses and most homeopathic practitioners also run their own on a private basis. Being signed on with a local homeopath is also important as you will have someone who knows your case (or those of your children) with whom you can check before you self-prescribe. I encourage my patients to ring in with a list of symptoms if, for example, their child has flu, and make sure that it is all right to give, say, *Gelsemium*, or whether it will interfere with the child's long-term constitutional treatment. This also enables them to confirm their choice of remedy in the early stages of getting to know the remedy pictures.

I also strongly advise you to take a first-aid course with the St John Ambulance or the Red Cross to learn the mechanics of first-aid.

COMPLAINTS YOU CAN TREAT USING THIS BOOK

It is important to understand fully the difference between acute and chronic disease so that you know which illnesses you may safely and appropriately treat and which you must take to a professional homeopath (or your GP). For an explanation of the differences between the two see p. 7.

The complaints sections in each chapter will tell you whether the particular complaint you wish to treat is within your scope as a home prescriber, *before* you attempt to work out a remedy. A good general first-aid book or family medical encyclopaedia will give you more detailed information about the complaints themselves. If the complaint has an obvious cause it is important to remove or avoid specific stresses (for example, don't let your child get chilled if you know that it leads to earache). Once you become ill use common-sense measures and take sensible care of yourself to avoid more serious symptoms developing.

Having established that your complaint *is* within the scope of this book, you can start to work out the remedy you need.

Your complaint may be treatable either by internal or external remedies, or both. You can establish this in each case by looking up your symptoms in the Repertories (pp. 168 and 264).

A criticism levelled at many homeopathic first-aid books is that they encourage people to take their lives in their own hands by treating serious illnesses at home. I believe that the treatment of chronic complaints is inadvisable. *Never* treat serious injuries or complaints yourself. If in any doubt seek expert advice. Cause for Concern, p. 23, lists general alarm symptoms, and specific alarm symptoms to watch out for are indicated in the individual complaints sections throughout the book.

DISEASES AND CONDITIONS NOT COVERED BY THIS BOOK

This book does not cover *chronic diseases*; these are complex conditions and need careful diagnosis and treatment at all stages. The homeopathic treatment of chronic disease often requires a long-term commitment so that the homeopath can treat underlying weaknesses in the constitution.

The following symptoms are not dealt with in this book:

Asthma is a life-threatening, deep-seated chronic disease which needs careful management to cure it. Acute attacks of asthma can be alleviated by homeopathic remedies, but these should always be prescribed by a professional homeopath who is in charge of the whole case and prescribing constitutional remedies between attacks so that their severity and frequency is lessened

Frequently recurring symptoms, such as flu, diarrhoea and coughs, which have no obvious cause and occur as often as every week

Hayfever see Asthma, above

Lumps and bumps: cysts, growths or warts anywhere on or in the body must always be taken to a professional homeopath

Persistent abdominal pain

Persistent constipation can mask a more serious, underlying complaint that needs professional treatment. If it is simply the result of poor diet (lots of low-fibre junk food) then the first step is to make the necessary dietary changes

Serious degenerative diseases such as cancer, hepatitis, heart disease and AIDS

Skin symptoms, including eczema, psoriasis, dermatitis, should never be tackled by the first-aid prescriber. Read the Laws of Cure (p. 8) to understand the dangers of suppressing a skin disease

Ulcers, anywhere except occasional mouth ulcers which you can treat yourself

CAUSE FOR CONCERN

The following symptoms may indicate serious illness and signal that you should seek immediate professional help. Some also appear in the remedy pictures, for example the laboured breathing of an *Antimonium tartaricum* cough and the delirium of a *Belladonna* fever. If you are worried about the general state of either yourself or your baby, call for help and then give the indicated homeopathic remedy. Further treatment may not be needed if the remedy works. In some instances, where the picture is very clear and/or you know from past experience that your patient is not seriously ill, you will be able to give the remedy and wait for improvement. If your baby does not show rapid signs of improvement you should call for help.

SEEK HELP IF THERE IS
Bleeding: unexplained, from any part of the body, including the skin
Breathing: rapid – over 50 breaths per minute at rest in children under two;
shallow or laboured (difficult)
Chest pain: severe
Convulsions
Delirium
Fever: above 104°F/40°C;
high, with a slow pulse (normal adult pulse is about 90 beats a minute and 120 in a child);
persistent, lasting for longer than 24 hours in a baby
Mental confusion, uncharacteristic
Neck stiff, especially if accompanied by severe headache
Pain that is severe, especially if accompanied by one or more of the other symptoms in this section
Stools, pale – grey or almost white
Urination profuse, accompanied by a great thirst
Urine dark and scanty/bloody (certain foods when eaten in quantity can change the colour of urine; beetroot for example, can turn urine red. This is nothing to worry about)
Vomiting, unexpected, repeated which comes on some time after the onset of a viral infection (i.e. a childhood illness)
Weakness, extreme
Wheezing, severe
Yellowing of the skin or whites of the eyes

If you are concerned about a baby of up to a year old, even if you can't put your finger on why, you should telephone your doctor or homeopath. If neither is available you can always take your child to the nearest hospital casualty department for reassurance.

In addition to the above causes for concern seek help for your baby if there is:
Blueness around the lips or face – whether temporary or not
Breathing difficulty with or without wheezing
Convulsion
Pain – your baby is obviously in pain and you don't know where the pain is
Sudden rash – small red or purple spots *or* bruises
Unconsciousness or unusual drowsiness or listlessness without drowsiness
Unusual pallor which doesn't change – especially if it is all over the body
A combination of two or more of the following:
high fever
irritability or drowsiness
an altered cry (especially if it is high-pitched or a weak moaning)
diarrhoea and/or vomiting
dry mouth and tongue
sunken eyes
sunken or bulging fontanelle
refuses feeds/drinks
dislikes bright lights (unusual)
passes much less urine than usual
passes blood in stools
vomits green fluid
stops focusing – eyes glaze over
'grunts' with each breath
has visible 'dips' in the chest when breathing

If your baby seems ill, even if he or she does not have any easily identifiable symptoms, always trust your instincts and get help.

Always seek professional help if the symptoms recur or do not improve.

SAMPLE CASES

The following cases will bring the process of first-aid prescribing to life for you. Keep in mind the steps with which you need to be familiar to prescribe successfully:

1 **Check that your complaint is within the scope of this book** by looking up the appropriate section, for example, Complaints in pregnancy (pp. 79–104) if you are pregnant and want to prescribe on, say, anaemia. Take note of the practical advice, the Dos and Don'ts before you move on to work out a remedy.
2 **'Take the case'.** Choose your symptoms (using the case-taking chart on pp. 14–15).

3 Repertorise them (using the repertorising chart on p. 17).
4 **Differentiate** between remedies if more than one is indicated, by reading through the remedy pictures in the Materia Medica until you find the one that 'fits' best.
5 **Prescribe** (see p. 16).

PREGNANCY

Case 1

Food poisoning

You are four months' pregnant, over the nausea and exhaustion of the first three months and really enjoying this time. You are taken out for your birthday and wake up some time after midnight with a nasty attack of food poisoning – it must have been the meat casserole that only you ate. You don't know whether to sit on the toilet or lean over it because you feel like vomiting and passing diarrhoea at the same time. The diarrhoea is very painful and utterly exhausting. You feel faint after vomiting, and, in spite of being thirsty, can only keep down small sips of water. You are terribly anxious that it might be affecting the baby and feel like death at the same time. You don't want to be on your own even for a minute. Your partner scribbles down the following symptoms: (see Chart 1)

Complaint Food Poisoning
  When did it start? Suddenly. Midnight
  Caused by Meat
Symptoms Diarrhoea – painful. Vomiting – feels faint after
General symptoms Thirsty for sips
Emotional state Anxious, worse when alone
Other physical symptoms Exhaustion from diarrhoea

Arsenicum fits most symptoms; even though it is missing from 'Onset of complaint, sudden' it doesn't matter as you would expect acute food poisoning to come on suddenly. You will need to repeat the remedy frequently, every 15–30 minutes and you can expect it to work quickly if it is the right one, within an hour or less.

If it doesn't help, reassess the whole picture. It may be that you are vomiting a few minutes after drinking and not immediately, which would lead you to think of taking *Phosphorus*.

Case 2

Exhaustion

After the third month of pregnancy, when the morning sickness passes, you still feel tired more or less all the time with dips in the day when you just can't move a limb. Sleep doesn't help much. Eating temporarily perks you up but it doesn't last. You feel apathetic, indifferent to everything and snappy. You bite the head off anyone who tells you what to do – especially if it contradicts what you want to do.

You rouse yourself to jot a few symptoms down in a desultory way as follows: (see Chart 2)

Complaint Exhaustion
  Caused by Pregnancy
  Worse Slightest exertion
General symptoms Appetite lost in pregnancy. Better after eating.
Emotional state Apathetic. Angry from contradiction. Repertorising the above symptoms comes up with *Sepia* followed by *Natrum carbonicum* and *Phosphorus*. You are able to cross *Natrum carbonicum* off your shortlist because you are a person who feels the cold acutely. When you read the *Sepia* emotional state and the general symptoms you immediately identify yourself with the saggy individual who's gone off sex and remember how when you had to run for the bus a few days previously you felt quite invigorated for a few hours after.

If this stage of repertorising hadn't helped you to come up with a remedy, you would have had to list some more symptoms, possibly getting some help with this and repertorising again, until a picture emerged.

Case 3

Anaemia

You are seven months' pregnant and, after a glowing first six months, are starting to feel as though you've had enough. A routine check by the doctor identified anaemia, so your doctor prescribed iron tablets anyway. You became constipated from taking the tablets, which has continued even though you stopped taking them a week ago. You look very pale.

You've been getting on badly with your partner who is working all hours to be able to take time off after the birth. You feel neglected and resentful but think you should keep your negative feelings to yourself, that it wouldn't be right to 'dump' them. You have noticed that you've been snapping at the people you work with more than usual and finding the noise levels in the office almost unbearable – you just want peace and quiet.

You have had a lot of abdominal pain in the past month; you have an active baby who is prone to delivering kicks that belong on the sports field! You are getting very fed up with it. You repertorise the following (knowing that it is a limited collection of symptoms): (see Chart 3)

Complaint Anaemia
Symptoms Face pale
Emotional state Resentful. Sensitive to noise
Other physical symptoms Constipation. Abdominal pain

Just as you thought, many remedies are indicated including *Calcarea carbonica, Kali carbonicum, Lycopodium, Natrum muriaticum, Nux vomica, Staphysagria* and *Zincum*. On reflection you realise that you are feeling very resentful towards your partner and the baby. You feel primarily battered by the baby and abandoned by your partner. And because you haven't talked about these feelings you have become touchy, erupting angrily over trivial things.

You prioritise the symptoms 'resentful' and 'abdominal pain', which leaves you with *Staphysagria*. On reading through the picture it is clear to you that you need an urgent dose of *Staphysagria* and some time to come clean with your nearest and dearest. You guess that if you let go of your grudges your bowels will clear out too.

BIRTH

Case 1

Labour

In labour you find yourself coping really well although your baby is posterior. You are finding the backache manageable and are coping well with the contractions. You take *Arnica* from time to time and the odd *Kali phosphoricum* when you get tired. Then you hit a rough patch: your midwife tells you that you are (only) 3cm dilated when you thought you were much further along. Your back begins to hurt more with contractions, you feel tired and suddenly discouraged – almost despairing. As you take a dive your contractions weaken in sympathy. In between contractions, with the help of your partner, you jot down the following symptoms and scribble the remedies listed next to them:

Labour pains in the back: *Cham., Cimi., Coff., Gels., Kali-c., Nux-v., Puls., Sep.*
Labour pains, weak: *Bell., Cimi., Gels., Kali-c., Nat-m., Op., Puls., Sec.*
With exhaustion: *Bell., Caul., Cham., Kali-c., Kali-p., Nat-m., Nux-v., Op., Puls., Sec., Sep., Ver-a.*

The remedies that are present in each symptom are *Kali carbonicum* and *Pulsatilla*. You check the main entry for Exhaustion in the Repertory and see that *Chamomilla, Gelsemium, Nux vomica, Pulsatilla* and *Sepia* are also listed. You need some more symptoms. You know that you've been sweating profusely since the pains increased in intensity and that you have been more sensitive than usual to cold; you add the

following symptoms to your jottings, writing only those remedies which agree with your shortlist:

Sweat – profuse; *Kali-c., Sep.*
Worse for cold: *Kali-c., Nux-v., Puls., Sep.*
Despair in labour: *Coff., Gels., Sep.*

So, it's a showdown between *Kali carbonicum* and *Sepia* even though *Kali carbonicum* isn't 'despairing'. Your partner reads each picture quickly and there's no contest, you are being manipulative and anxious and not at all saggy. A few doses of *Kali carbonicum* restore your emotional equilibrium and help to ease the back pain – enough to establish effective labour once again.

NB I have included this case to demonstrate that it is possible to repertorise and prescribe 'on the back of an envelope', without filling in a chart, especially in a situation where you don't have a lot of time.

POST-NATAL – MOTHER

Case 1

Post-natal depression and afterpains

You were warned about this but you didn't believe it. You've had the baby you always wanted, had a perfect first few days and then vooom! On the fifth day after the birth a black cloud descends. You feel tearful, all the time, the least little thing sets you off. You'd really rather others weren't so sympathetic. Your milk came in yesterday and your breasts are like footballs, huge, hard and painful. Your baby fed every 1½ hours last night, your nipples are beginning to crack and you are absolutely exhausted. As if this weren't enough you are still getting some afterpains, especially when you feed. You are a generally chilly, sweaty type and are finding that you are sweating more than ever since the birth. You repertorise the following symptoms: (see Chart 4).

Complaint Depressed. Tearful
  Worse Consolation
General symptoms Sweat profuse
  Worse Cold
Other physical symptoms After pains. Breasts painful.
  Nipples cracked

Silica and *Sepia* come out as having the most symptoms in the repertorising. This surprises you: you expected *Sepia* to be the remedy, based on an occasion in your pregnancy when you needed it. You read the *Silica* picture in the Materia Medica and are able to add some other symptoms to confirm this remedy as your choice. Your episiotomy scar is taking a long time to heal – you had thought that as long as you took lots of *Arnica* and bathed it with *Calendula* it would heal quickly and it hasn't. You wonder about *Silica* being a good constitutional remedy for you since you are generally stubborn and tenacious, you feel the cold, have sweaty feet that smell and had constant chest colds as a child. If it is a good remedy you can be assured that it will work quickly and effectively on your physical symptoms and your emotional state.

Case 2

Flu not needing treatment

Your baby is ten months old when you go down with an attack of flu. You've been back at work for six months now, leaving the baby with a full-time nanny from 8.30 a.m. until 6.30 p.m. You have been working extremely hard with very little time off these past six months: your time 'off' has been taken up with being a mother, and your precious bundle still wakes once or twice at night. You feel achy, weak and exhausted and although your symptoms are unpleasant they are not severe. You agree (reluctantly!) to rest in bed for a few days and then to take a week off to recuperate fully. Your nanny will continue to look after the baby in the day and your partner agrees to the evenings *and* the night shifts until you are recovered.

You do not need homeopathic treatment. It might be necessary to review the situation if you didn't recover easily at any stage of this illness. It isn't wise to take a homeopathic remedy and carry on working when all your body needs is a very good rest.

Case 3

Flu needing treatment

You are a single parent with two children – a toddler of two and a half and a baby. You go down suddenly with a severe bout of flu: every bone in your body aches, you have a fever, feel depressed and angry and extremely chilly. You have no one to help with the children, although a friend offers to shop for you. Homeopathic treatment in this case is appropriate because of the severity of the symptoms, and also because of your situation – it just isn't possible to take two weeks off. You choose the following symptoms: (see Chart 5)

Complaint Flu
    Symptoms Pains in bones
General symptoms Exhaustion. Fever
    Worse Exertion. Cold
Emotional state Angry. Depressed

On repertorising, you find that *Arsenicum, Nux vomica* and *Rhus toxicodendron* are all strongly indicated but when you read through the picture in the Materia Medica it doesn't quite fit. You are not restless.

You search for other symptoms. You are *very* thirsty for cold drinks, in spite of feeling generally worse for getting cold. You are very shaky in your whole body with the pains. You add the following symptoms:

Thirsty. Likes cold drinks. Flu with shivering

You then read through *Bryonia, Eupatorium perfoliatum, Phosphorus* and *Pyrogen* and decide to take *Eupatorium* because of the terrible pains, because you also have a headache and aren't sweating much with the fever. You ask a friend to buy some from the local whole-food shop on her way home.

Don't forget to look to the practical advice (DOs and DON'Ts) in each instance as well as taking the appropriate homeopathic remedy.

BABIES

Case 1

An accident/head injury

Your nine-month-old baby climbs onto the sofa while you answer the telephone. It's her first serious climbing expedition, hugely aided by a pile of cushions. You just miss saving her from falling backwards off the sofa head first and unfortunately, she catches the back of her head on a pile of wooden bricks. She's in great distress but the skin hasn't been broken and you know it wasn't a serious enough fall to warrant a visit to casualty. An egg is fast developing – a swelling where the fall was broken by the edge of a brick.

Your first prescription must be for Shock, Head injury and Bruising. In the Repertory you will find that *Arnica* is the only remedy that is listed for all three of these symptoms. You give her a single dose of *Arnica 12* and she falls asleep. The swelling goes right down and you don't worry about it any more.

Over the next week you suspect that she is teething because she is more bad-tempered than usual and wakes frequently at night screaming. She asks to be carried but soon starts screaming again after you pick her up. Nothing comforts her for long. You begin to feel exasperated – your happy, contented baby has turned into a 'ratbag' and you find the nights especially trying. You repertorise her symptoms (teething, angry, capricious) and give her *Chamomilla*. It has no effect whatsoever. You are convinced that she is teething and so you persevere with it for a few days. She continues to be difficult, both day and night, and you are running out of sympathy and energy.

Since *Chamomilla* was so strongly indicated and didn't work you know that it is the wrong remedy and you begin to wonder if she *is* teething. It is unlikely that she has a sore throat or earache as she has no fever but you wonder if you should get your GP to check her just in case. You decide to go over your notes again. And then you have a brainwave: you notice that her irritability started on the day that she had her fall. So much was happening that day with your other children that you didn't connect the two events. You know that she is in pain and you know that she fell, so you wonder whether she has a headache from the head injury (a surprisingly common but difficult-to-diagnose symptom in pre-verbal infants). You give a single dose of *Natrum sulphuricum 30* and as it dissolves in her mouth she smiles angelically again. That night she sleeps and regains her former good nature.

Case 2

Chickenpox not needing treatment

Your nine-month-old baby develops mild cold symptoms about 10 days after having been in contact with your nephew who has chickenpox. You feel sure your baby is incubating chickenpox and watch carefully. You decide not to prescribe for the cold as it isn't preventing him from feeding or sleeping. After a couple of days he throws a fever of 102°F/39°C and although a bit miserable continues to drink well and sleep a lot. When awake he wants attention and lots of cuddles and as long as these are forthcoming is reasonably happy. About a dozen spots appear well scattered all over his body which quickly scab over and don't seem to itch much. You remember reading that young babies can have chickenpox very mildly and decide not to treat yours as he is coping with it well on his own.

Case 3

Chickenpox needing treatment

Your one-year-old develops chickenpox, starting with the typical cold symptoms. A high fever develops and you start to worry when delirium quickly sets in. The baby feels burning hot to the touch and doesn't want to eat but is unusually thirsty. The spots come out all over the body – there are hundreds of them and they are very red and itchy. Nothing seems to help the itching but they are much worse for heat. They seem to be painful because he cries after scratching. A right-sided earache develops and a dry cough, which prevents him from sleeping. You decide to work out a remedy. He is now very distressed, restless and irritable. Homeopathic treatment is appropriate in this case to ease the pain, control the fever and help the baby deal with this very unpleasant 'attack'. You write up

the case using the case-taking and repertorising charts and choose the following symptoms: (see Chart 6)

> *Complaint* Chickenpox
>> *Symptoms* Rash – itchy
> *General symptoms* Thirsty
>> *Worse* Heat
> *Emotional state* Delirious. Irritable.
> *Other physical symptoms*
>> Earache – right side
>> Dry cough
>> Fever – burning heat

Belladonna and *Sulphur* are both well indicated but when you read them up in the Materia Medica you eliminate *Sulphur*, because it has left-sided earaches and it doesn't have the delirium of *Belladonna*. You note that your baby's pupils are dilated and a little wild-looking and that the measles rash in a *Belladonna* infant itches and burns and rightly assume that it is possible for the chickenpox rash to do likewise, which confirms your choice. You hold *Sulphur* in reserve in case *Belladonna* doesn't help.

Case 4

Cough/cold

Your six-month-old baby has a cough and cold. It started four days ago. The day previously, you had both been out shopping when it had rained unexpectedly and she was drenched even though you ran home as fast as you could. Then her nose started running that evening and she coughed in the night. In the morning your baby was pale and pathetic and didn't want any solids, only to breastfeed, and to be carried and cuddled. She has been more or less like this for the past three days, not letting you do anything and regressing emotionally, crying every time you put her down. Where she would formerly take the odd bottle of water she won't drink and is pretty listless, her nose is running with lots of thick, yellow-green catarrh and she has a loose cough in the mornings which is dry at night. It is worse when lying down at night and if the room is overheated. She also seems more whiny and clingy if too hot. Oddly enough, when you had to go out yesterday to do some shopping together she was a bit better: her nose stopped running, she coughed less and was more lively. There is no fever and no sweating. Using the case-taking chart you choose the following symptoms and repertorise the ones not in brackets. (See Chart 7)

> *Complaint* Cough (and cold)
>> *When did it start?* (4 days ago)
>> *Cause* (Getting wet)
>> *Symptoms* Dry at night, loose at mornings

Better Fresh air

Worse Lying down

General symptoms Thirstless. Pale. Complaints from getting wet. (Listless/appetite lost.)

Better Fresh air

Worse Heat

Emotional state Whiny. Tearful. Desires to be carried.

Other physical symptoms Common cold with thick, yellow-green nasal catarrh.

On repertorising (see p. 16) you find that *Pulsatilla* is indicated under each symptom, and no other remedies are strongly indicated. You give *Pulsatilla* knowing that it will help quite quickly. In the unlikely event that it doesn't you will need to go through the case again and repertorise choosing different symptoms, or seek the advice of a professional homeopath.

Case 5

Teething

Your baby is eight months old and teething . . . again. A friend has recommended the homeopathic 'teething granules', but you know better than to give a routine hit-or-miss prescription and when you tried them once in the middle of the night in desperation they had no effect.

Usually a contented, easy-going baby, he has been more fractious of late and waking at night when previously he slept straight through. Unlike many of his friends of the same age, your baby only has two teeth – and these were produced with great difficulty. His father had difficulty teething as a baby also. You feel desperate at the thought of endless broken nights ahead. When you go to him at night all that is wanted is a drink and a cuddle and he goes quickly back to sleep. However, you notice that his head is unusually sweaty and that his sweat smells sour.

His bowels have been upset for the past three weeks, with diarrhoea that smells sour and contains undigested food. He has also been more prone to catching colds over the past few months and they seem to be running into each other so that the poor child has a constantly runny nose.

Recently he has been more stubborn about what he wants although generally very placid. You choose the following symptoms: (see Chart 8)

Complaint Teething painful and slow.

Symptoms With diarrhoea – stools sour, undigested

General symptoms Sweat on head, sour. Catches colds easily

Emotional state Stubborn

Calcarea carbonica has each of these symptoms. On reading through the picture in the Materia Medica you recognise your easy-going baby in many of the general and emotional symptoms. This remedy will not only help him through the pains of the teething and clear up the diarrhoea and runny nose but will also help the teeth to come through faster. Don't worry if you have to repeat it fairly frequently during the teething year: your baby may need it.

Symptoms:

#	Symptom	ACO.	ABSC.	AGAR.	ALL-C.	ALU.	ANT-C.	ANT-T.	AP.	ARG-N.	ARN.	ARS.	ASAR.	BAR-C.	BELL.	BELL-P.	BOR.	BRY.	CALC-C.	CALC-F.	CALC-P.	CALC-S.	CALEN.	CANTH.	CARB-A.	CARB-V.	CAST.	CAUL.
1.	FOOD POISONING											✓														✓		
2.	" " - CAUSE MEAT											✓														✓		
3.	ONSET - SUDDEN	✓													✓													
4.	DIARRHOEA - PAINFUL											✓																
5.	VOMITING - FAINT AFTER											✓																
6.	THIRSTY FOR SIPS											✓																
7.	ANXIOUS	✓							✓			✓		✓	✓✓				✓✓		✓✓					✓		
8.	" - WORSE WHEN ALONE											✓																
9.	EXHAUSTION - CAUSE DIARRHOEA											✓														✓		

#	Symptom	CAUST.	CHAM.	CHEL.	CHIN.	CIMI.	CINA.	COCC.	COCC-C.	COFF.	COLCH.	COLOC.	CON.	CUPR.	CYPR.	DIOS.	DROS.	DULC.	EUP-P.	EUPHR.	FERR-M.	GELS.	GLON.	HAM.	HEP-S.	HYP.	IGN.	IP.
1.	FOOD POISONING																											
2.	" " - CAUSE MEAT																											
3.	ONSET - SUDDEN																											
4.	DIARRHOEA - PAINFUL		✓								✓							✓										
5.	VOMITING - FAINT AFTER																											
6.	THIRSTY FOR SIPS																											
7.	ANXIOUS	✓			✓			✓			✓																	
8.	" - WORSE WHEN ALONE																											
9.	EXHAUSTION - CAUSE DIARRHOEA		✓																									

#	Symptom	JAB.	KALI-B.	KALI-C.	KALI-M.	KALI-P.	KALI-S.	KREOS.	LAC-C.	LAC-D.	LACH.	LED.	LIL-T.	LYC.	MAG-C.	MAG-M.	MAG-P.	MERC-C.	MERC-S.	NAT-C.	NAT-M.	NAT-P.	NAT-S.	NIT-AC.	NUX-M.	NUX-V.	OP.	PETR.
1.	FOOD POISONING																											
2.	" " - CAUSE MEAT																											
3.	ONSET - SUDDEN																											
4.	DIARRHOEA - PAINFUL													✓			✓✓											
5.	VOMITING - FAINT AFTER																											
6.	THIRSTY FOR SIPS																											
7.	ANXIOUS			✓	✓✓						✓			✓✓✓					✓					✓	✓			
8.	" - WORSE WHEN ALONE																											
9.	EXHAUSTION - CAUSE DIARRHOEA																						✓✓					

#	Symptom	PHO-AC.	PHOS.	PHYT.	PODO.	PULS.	PYR.	RHE.	RHOD.	RHUS-T.	RUMEX.	RUTA.	SAB.	SARS.	SEC.	SEP.	SIL.	SPO.	STAP.	STRAM.	SUL.	SUL-AC.	SYMPH.	TAB.	THU.	URT-U.	VER-A.	ZINC.
1.	FOOD POISONING				✓																							
2.	" " - CAUSE MEAT				✓																							
3.	ONSET - SUDDEN																											
4.	DIARRHOEA - PAINFUL																											
5.	VOMITING - FAINT AFTER																											
6.	THIRSTY FOR SIPS																											
7.	ANXIOUS	✓				✓				✓					✓	✓	✓		✓		✓	✓						
8.	" - WORSE WHEN ALONE	✓																										
9.	EXHAUSTION - CAUSE DIARRHOEA	✓													✓						✓						✓	

Symptoms:

#	Symptom	ACO.	AESC.	AGAR.	ALL-C.	ALU.	ANT-C.	ANT-T.	AP.	ARG-N.	ARN.	ARS.	ASAR.	BAR-C.	BELL.	BELL-P.	BOR.	BRY.	CALC-C.	CALC-F.	CALC-P.	CALC-S.	CALEN.	CANTH.	CARB-A.	CARB-V.	CAST.	CAUL.
1.	EXHAUSTION					✓	✓	✓	✓	✓	✓						✓	✓	✓		✓				✓	✓		
2.	" – IN PREGNANCY					✓															✓							
3.	" – WORSE SLIGHTEST EXERTION													✓			✓	✓										
4.	APPETITE LOST – IN PREGNANCY																											
5.	BETTER AFTER EATING																											
6.	APATHETIC					✓	✓	✓																		✓		
7.	ANGRY FROM CONTRADICTION																											
8.																												
9.																												

#	Symptom	CAUST.	CHAM.	CHEL.	CHIN.	CIMI.	CINA.	COCC.	COCC-C.	COFF.	COLCH.	COLOC.	CON.	CUPR.	CYPR.	DIOS.	DROS.	DULC.	EUP-P.	EUPHR.	FERR-M.	GELS.	GLON.	HAM.	HEP-S.	HYP.	IGN.	IP.
1.	EXHAUSTION	✓		✓		✓		✓			✓	✓	✓								✓	✓						
2.	" – IN PREGNANCY																											
3.	" – WORSE SLIGHTEST EXERTION												✓															
4.	APPETITE LOST – IN PREGNANCY	✓																										
5.	BETTER AFTER EATING																											✓
6.	APATHETIC								✓														✓					
7.	ANGRY FROM CONTRADICTION																										✓	
8.																												
9.																												

#	Symptom	IAB.	KALI-B.	KALI-C.	KALI-M.	KALI-P.	KALI-S.	KREOS.	LAC-C.	LAC-D.	LACH.	LED.	LIL-T.	LYC.	MAG-C.	MAG-M.	MAG-P.	MERC-C.	MERC-S.	NAT-C.	NAT-M.	NAT-P.	NAT-S.	NIT-AC.	NUX-M.	NUX-V.	OP.	PETR.
1.	EXHAUSTION		✓		✓									✓				✓	✓	✓	✓				✓			
2.	" – IN PREGNANCY																											
3.	" – WORSE SLIGHTEST EXERTION									✓											✓							
4.	APPETITE LOST – IN PREGNANCY																				✓							
5.	BETTER AFTER EATING																				✓							
6.	APATHETIC											✓						✓	✓						✓		✓	
7.	ANGRY FROM CONTRADICTION												✓															
8.																												
9.																												

#	Symptom	PHO-AC.	PHOS.	PHYT.	PODO.	PULS.	PYR.	RHE.	RHOD.	RHUS-T.	RUMEX.	RUTA.	SAB.	SARS.	SEC.	SEP.	SIL.	SPO.	STAP.	STRAM.	SUL.	SUL-AC.	SYMPH.	TAB.	THU.	URT-U.	VER-A.	ZINC.
1.	EXHAUSTION	✓	✓			✓				✓						✓	✓				✓						✓	✓
2.	" – IN PREGNANCY															✓					✓						✓	
3.	" – WORSE SLIGHTEST EXERTION	✓	✓							✓							✓											
4.	APPETITE LOST – IN PREGNANCY															✓												
5.	BETTER AFTER EATING		✓																									
6.	APATHETIC	✓	✓		✓											✓			✓									
7.	ANGRY FROM CONTRADICTION															✓												
8.																												
9.																												

Symptoms:

	ACO.	AESC.	AGAR.	ALL-C.	ALU.	ANT-C.	ANT-T.	AP.	ARG-N.	ARN.	ARS.	ASAR.	BAR-C.	BELL.	BELL-P.	BOR.	BRY.	CALC-C.	CALC-F.	CALC-P.	CALC-S.	CALEN.	CANTH.	CARB-A.	CARB-V.	CAST.	CAUL.
1. ANAEMIA												✓						✓		✓					✓		
2. FACE PALE					✓	✓						✓						✓							✓		
3. RESENTFUL																											
4. SENSITIVE TO NOISE	✓											✓	✓														
5. CONSTIPATION		✓			✓													✓									
6. ABDOMINAL PAIN									✓					✓		✓											
7.																											
8.																											
9.																											

	CAUST.	CHAM.	CHEL.	CHIN.	CIMI.	CINA.	COCC.	COCC-C.	COFF.	COLCH.	COLOC.	CON.	CUPR.	CYPR.	DIOS.	DROS.	DULC.	EUP-P.	EUPHR.	FERR-M.	GELS.	GLON.	HAM.	HEP-S.	IGN.	IP.
1. ANAEMIA				✓																✓						
2. FACE PALE						✓							✓	✓						✓						
3. RESENTFUL																									✓	
4. SENSITIVE TO NOISE				✓						✓		✓														
5. CONSTIPATION	✓																							✓		
6. ABDOMINAL PAIN				✓																						
7.																										
8.																										
9.																										

	IAB.	KALI-B.	KALI-C.	KALI-M.	KALI-P.	KALI-S.	KREOS.	LAC-C.	LAC-D.	LACH.	LED.	LIL-T.	LYC.	MAG-C.	MAG-M.	MAG-P.	MERC-C.	MERC-S.	NAT-C.	NAT-M.	NAT-P.	NAT-S.	NIT-AC.	NUX-M.	NUX-V.	OP.	PETR.
1. ANAEMIA			✓		✓													✓	✓				✓				
2. FACE PALE													✓						✓	✓							✓
3. RESENTFUL													✓						✓								
4. SENSITIVE TO NOISE			✓																					✓	✓	✓	
5. CONSTIPATION			✓										✓		✓					✓					✓	✓	
6. ABDOMINAL PAIN																			✓								
7.																											
8.																											
9.																											

	PHO-AC.	PHOS.	PHYT.	PODO.	PULS.	PYR.	RHE.	RHOD.	RHUS-T.	RUMEX.	RUTA.	SAB.	SARS.	SEC.	SEP.	SIL.	SPO.	STAP.	STRAM.	SUL.	SUL-AC.	SYMPH.	TAB.	THU.	URT-U.	VER-A.	ZINC.
1. ANAEMIA	✓	✓			✓													✓		✓	✓						
2. FACE PALE	✓																							✓		✓	✓
3. RESENTFUL															✓✓												
4. SENSITIVE TO NOISE													✓	✓				✓									✓
5. CONSTIPATION					✓									✓	✓			✓		✓							✓
6. ABDOMINAL PAIN									✓						✓✓												
7.																											
8.																											
9.																											

Symptoms:

#	Symptom	ACO.	AESC.	AGAR.	ALL-C.	ALU.	ANT-C.	ANT-T.	AP.	ARG-N.	ARN.	ARS.	ASAR.	BAR-C.	BELL.	BELL-P.	BOR.	BRY.	CALC-C.	CALC-F.	CALC-P.	CALC-S.	CALEN.	CANTH.	CARB-A.	CARB-V.	CAST.	CAUL.
1.	DEPRESSED					✓					✓								✓		✓				✓			
2.	TEARFUL								✓						✓		✓		✓		✓							
3.	AVERSE CONSOLATION																											
4.	SWEAT PROFUSE								✓						✓				✓						✓	✓		
5.	WORSE FOR COLD				✓							✓		✓	✓		✓				✓							
6.	AFTER PAINS										✓																	
7.	BREASTS PAINFUL															✓	✓	✓										
8.	NIPPLES CRACKED																									✓		
9.																												

#	Symptom	CAUST.	CHAM.	CHEL.	CHIN.	CIMI.	CINA.	COCC.	COCC-C.	COFF.	COLCH.	COLOC.	CON.	CUPR.	CYPR.	DIOS.	DROS.	DULC.	EUP-P.	EUPHR.	FERR-M.	GELS.	GLON.	HAM.	HEP-S.	HYP.	IGN.	IP.
1.	DEPRESSED	✓	✓	✓	✓								✓						✓		✓	✓						
2.	TEARFUL	✓	✓																								✓	✓
3.	AVERSE CONSOLATION																									✓		
4.	SWEAT PROFUSE				✓																✓				✓			
5.	WORSE FOR COLD	✓		✓	✓						✓						✓								✓	✓		
6.	AFTER PAINS		✓		✓							✓													✓			
7.	BREASTS PAINFUL																											
8.	NIPPLES CRACKED	✓																										
9.																												

#	Symptom	JAB.	KALI-B.	KALI-C.	KALI-M.	KALI-P.	KALI-S.	KREOS.	LAC-C.	LAC-D.	LACH.	LED.	LIL-T.	LYC.	MAG-C.	MAG-M.	MAG-P.	MERC-C.	MERC-S.	NAT-C.	NAT-M.	NAT-P.	NAT-S.	NIT-AC.	NUX-M.	NUX-V.	OP.	PETR.
1.	DEPRESSED					✓				✓			✓	✓					✓	✓	✓				✓		✓	
2.	TEARFUL													✓						✓	✓							
3.	AVERSE CONSOLATION												✓							✓						✓		
4.	SWEAT PROFUSE			✓	✓									✓					✓									✓
5.	WORSE FOR COLD		✓	✓	✓												✓								✓	✓		
6.	AFTER PAINS			✓																								
7.	BREASTS PAINFUL																		✓									
8.	NIPPLES CRACKED																											
9.																												

#	Symptom	PHO-AC.	PHOS.	PHYT.	PODO.	PULS.	PYR.	RHE.	RHOD.	RHUS-T.	RUMEX.	RUTA.	SAB.	SARS.	SEC.	SEP.	SIL.	SPO.	STAP.	STRAM.	SUL.	SUL-AC.	SYMPH.	TAB.	THU.	URT-U.	VER-A.	ZINC.
1.	DEPRESSED	✓				✓				✓						✓				✓							✓	✓
2.	TEARFUL					✓		✓		✓						✓	✓			✓							✓	
3.	AVERSE CONSOLATION															✓	✓											
4.	SWEAT PROFUSE	✓														✓	✓				✓						✓	
5.	WORSE FOR COLD	✓	✓		✓	✓	✓	✓								✓	✓											
6.	AFTER PAINS					✓				✓			✓		✓													
7.	BREASTS PAINFUL																											
8.	NIPPLES CRACKED			✓												✓	✓		✓									
9.																												

Symptoms:

#	Symptom	ACO.	AESC.	AGAR.	ALL-C.	ALU.	ANT-C.	ANT-T.	AP.	ARG-N.	ARN.	ARS.	ASAR.	BAR-C.	BELL.	BELL-P.	BOR.	BRY.	CALC-C.	CALC-F.	CALC-P.	CALC-S.	CALEN.	CANTH.	CARB-A.	CARB-V.	CAST.	CAUL.
1.	FLU											✓						✓										
2.	" – WITH PAINS IN BONES																											
3.	EXHAUSTION					✓	✓	✓	✓			✓		✓				✓	✓		✓				✓	✓		
4.	FEVER	✓						✓	✓			✓						✓										
5.	WORSE FOR COLD			✓								✓			✓		✓	✓			✓							
6.	" " EXERTION											✓														✓		
7.	DEPRESSED									✓		✓							✓			✓			✓			
8.	ANGRY											✓			✓			✓										
9.																												

#	Symptom	CAUST.	CHAM.	CHEL.	CHIN.	CIMI.	CINA.	COCC.	COCC-C.	COFF.	COLCH.	COLOC.	CON.	CUPR.	CYPR.	DIOS.	DROS.	DULC.	EUP-P.	EUPHR.	FERR-M.	GELS.	GLON.	HAM.	HEP-S.	HYP.	IGN.	IP.
1.	FLU																	✓	✓			✓						✓
2.	" – WITH PAINS IN BONES																											✓
3.	EXHAUSTION	✓		✓		✓					✓		✓	✓								✓	✓					
4.	FEVER		✓		✓														✓			✓	✓		✓		✓	✓
5.	WORSE FOR COLD	✓			✓	✓					✓							✓							✓	✓		
6.	" " EXERTION							✓																				
7.	DEPRESSED	✓	✓		✓	✓															✓	✓			✓			✓
8.	ANGRY	✓																							✓	✓		
9.																												

#	Symptom	JAB.	KALI-B.	KALI-C.	KALI-M.	KALI-P.	KALI-S.	KREOS.	LAC-C.	LAC-D.	LACH.	LED.	LIL-T.	LYC.	MAG-C.	MAG-M.	MAG-P.	MERC-C.	MERC-S.	NAT-C.	NAT-M.	NAT-P.	NAT-S.	NIT-AC.	NUX-M.	NUX-V.	OP.	PETR.
1.	FLU																											
2.	" – WITH PAINS IN BONES																									✓		
3.	EXHAUSTION			✓	✓						✓							✓	✓	✓	✓							
4.	FEVER			✓																					✓	✓	✓	
5.	WORSE FOR COLD			✓	✓	✓											✓								✓	✓		
6.	" " EXERTION				✓																							
7.	DEPRESSED								✓				✓	✓				✓	✓	✓	✓		✓					✓
8.	ANGRY			✓		✓								✓							✓					✓		
9.																												

#	Symptom	PHO-AC.	PHOS.	PHYT.	PODO.	PULS.	PYR.	RHE.	RHOD.	RHUS-T.	RUMEX.	RUTA.	SAB.	SARS.	SEC.	SEP.	SIL.	SPO.	STAP.	STRAM.	SUL.	SUL-AC.	SYMPH.	TAB.	THU.	URT-U.	VER-A.	ZINC.
1.	FLU					✓				✓																		
2.	" – WITH PAINS IN BONES					✓				✓																		
3.	EXHAUSTION	✓	✓		✓	✓										✓	✓	✓	✓		✓						✓	✓
4.	FEVER		✓		✓	✓	✓									✓	✓				✓						✓	
5.	WORSE FOR COLD	✓	✓		✓	✓				✓	✓						✓	✓										
6.	" " EXERTION																		✓									
7.	DEPRESSED	✓								✓						✓					✓						✓	✓
8.	ANGRY															✓			✓		✓							
9.																												

REPERTORISING CHART — CHART 6. CHICKEN POX

Symptoms:

#	Symptom	ACO.	AESC.	AGAR.	ALL-C.	ALU.	ANT-C.	ANT-T.	AP.	ARG-N.	ARN.	ARS.	ASAR.	BAR-C.	BELL.	BELL-P.	BOR.	BRY.	CALC-C.	CALC-F.	CALC-P.	CALC-S.	CALEN.	CANTH.	CARB-A.	CARB-V.	CAST.	CAUL.
1.	CHICKEN POX	✓					✓	✓							✓													
2.	" " - RASH ITCHES																											
3.	THIRSTY	✓										✓			✓			✓										
4.	WORSE FOR HEAT						✓	✓				✓																
5.	IRRITABLE						✓	✓	✓							✓	✓				✓	✓			✓	✓	✓	
6.	DELIRIOUS																											
7.	EARACHE - RIGHT SIDE																											
8.	COUGH - DRY	✓										✓			✓		✓	✓	✓		✓							
9.	FEVER - BURNING	✓							✓			✓			✓													

#	Symptom	CAUST.	CHAM.	CHEL.	CHIN.	CIMI.	CINA.	COCC.	COCC-C.	COFF.	COLCH.	COLOC.	CON.	CUPR.	CYPR.	DIOS.	DROS.	DULC.	EUP-P.	EUPHR.	FERR-M.	GELS.	GLON.	HAM.	HEP-S.	HYP.	IGN.	IP.
1.	CHICKEN POX																											
2.	" " - RASH ITCHES																											
3.	THIRSTY		✓														✓											
4.	WORSE FOR HEAT																								✓			
5.	IRRITABLE	✓	✓				✓															✓			✓			
6.	DELIRIOUS																											
7.	EARACHE - RIGHT SIDE																											
8.	COUGH - DRY												✓		✓											✓	✓	✓
9.	FEVER - BURNING		✓																		✓							

#	Symptom	JAB.	KALI-B.	KALI-C.	KALI-M.	KALI-P.	KALI-S.	KREOS.	LAC-C.	LAC-D.	LACH.	LED.	LIL-T.	LYC.	MAG-C.	MAG-M.	MAG-P.	MERC-C.	MERC-S.	NAT-C.	NAT-M.	NAT-P.	NAT-S.	NIT-AC.	NUX-M.	NUX-V.	OP.	PETR.
1.	CHICKEN POX																		✓									
2.	" " - RASH ITCHES																											
3.	THIRSTY																			✓	✓	✓						
4.	WORSE FOR HEAT					✓							✓	✓	✓													
5.	IRRITABLE			✓			✓						✓	✓	✓					✓				✓		✓		✓
6.	DELIRIOUS																											
7.	EARACHE - RIGHT SIDE																								✓			
8.	COUGH - DRY			✓							✓		✓							✓						✓		
9.	FEVER - BURNING																		✓									✓

#	Symptom	PHO-AC.	PHOS.	PHYT.	PODO.	PULS.	PYR.	RHE.	RHOD.	RHUS-T.	RUMEX.	RUTA.	SAB.	SARS.	SEC.	SEP.	SIL.	SPO.	STAP.	STRAM.	SUL.	SUL-AC.	SYMPH.	TAB.	THU.	URT-U.	VER-A.	ZINC.
1.	CHICKEN POX					✓				✓											✓							
2.	" " - RASH ITCHES					✓				✓											✓							
3.	THIRSTY		✓			✓										✓					✓						✓	
4.	WORSE FOR HEAT			✓												✓					✓	✓						
5.	IRRITABLE	✓	✓	✓						✓						✓	✓				✓	✓						✓
6.	DELIRIOUS																											
7.	EARACHE - RIGHT SIDE																											
8.	COUGH - DRY	✓	✓																									
9.	FEVER - BURNING		✓			✓				✓																		

REPERTORISING CHART

CHART 7. COUGH/COLD

Symptoms — Block 1

Symptoms	ACO.	AESC.	AGAR.	ALL-C.	ALU.	ANT-C.	ANT-T.	AP.	ARG-N.	ARN.	ARS.	ASAR.	BAR-C.	BELL.	BELL-P.	BOR.	BRY.	CALC-C.	CALC-F.	CALC-P.	CALC-S.	CALEN.	CANTH.	CARB-A.	CARB-V.	CAST.	CAUL.
1. COUGH - DRY/NIGHT: LOOSE/MORNING																											
2. " - WORSE LYING DOWN								✓		✓																	
3. THIRSTLESS						✓	✓	✓						✓													
4. COMPLAINTS - GETTING WET																		✓									
5. BETTER FOR FRESH AIR	✓							✓			✓					✓									✓		
6. WORSE FOR HEAT								✓	✓		✓										✓						
7. WHINY								✓																			
8. TEARFUL								✓						✓	✓	✓					✓						
9. DESIRES TO BE CARRIED																								✓			

Symptoms — Block 2

Symptoms	CAUST.	CHAM.	CHEL.	CHIN.	CIMI.	CINA.	COCC.	COCC-C.	COFF.	COLCH.	COLOC.	CON.	CUPR.	CYPR.	DIOS.	DROS.	DULC.	EUP-P.	EUPHR.	FERR-M.	GELS.	GLON.	HAM.	HEP-S.	HYP.	IGN.	IP.
1. COUGH - DRY/NIGHT: LOOSE/MORNING																											
2. " - WORSE LYING DOWN	✓							✓				✓															
3. THIRSTLESS						✓				✓											✓						
4. COMPLAINTS - GETTING WET	✓																										
5. BETTER FOR FRESH AIR																											
6. WORSE FOR HEAT																						✓					
7. WHINY																											
8. TEARFUL	✓	✓																						✓			
9. DESIRES TO BE CARRIED		✓				✓																					

Symptoms — Block 3

Symptoms	IAB.	KALI-B.	KALI-C.	KALI-M.	KALI-P.	KALI-S.	KREOS.	LAC-C.	LAC-D.	LACH.	LED.	LIL-T.	LYC.	MAG-C.	MAG-M.	MAG-P.	MERC-C.	MERC-S.	NAT-C.	NAT-M.	NAT-P.	NAT-S.	NIT-AC.	NUX-M.	NUX-V.	OP.	PETR.
1. COUGH - DRY/NIGHT: LOOSE/MORNING																											
2. " - WORSE LYING DOWN			✓										✓														
3. THIRSTLESS																								✓			
4. COMPLAINTS - GETTING WET																											
5. BETTER FOR FRESH AIR						✓				✓			✓	✓						✓							
6. WORSE FOR HEAT						✓				✓	✓	✓									✓						
7. WHINY																											
8. TEARFUL													✓							✓							
9. DESIRES TO BE CARRIED			✓							✓																	

Symptoms — Block 4

Symptoms	PHO-AC.	PHOS.	PHYT.	PODO.	PULS.	PYR.	RHE.	RHOD.	RHUS-T.	RUMEX.	RUTA.	SAB.	SARS.	SEC.	SEP.	SIL.	SPO.	STAP.	STRAM.	SUL.	SUL-AC.	SYMPH.	TAB.	THU.	URT-U.	VER-A.	ZINC.
1. COUGH - DRY/NIGHT: LOOSE/MORNING					✓																						
2. " - WORSE LYING DOWN					✓				✓						✓					✓							
3. THIRSTLESS	✓				✓																						
4. COMPLAINTS - GETTING WET					✓			✓					✓														
5. BETTER FOR FRESH AIR					✓																✓						
6. WORSE FOR HEAT					✓										✓					✓	✓						
7. WHINY					✓																						
8. TEARFUL					✓									✓	✓	✓										✓	
9. DESIRES TO BE CARRIED					✓																						

REPERTORISING CHART
CHART 8. TEETHING

Symptoms:

#	Symptom	ACO.	AESC.	AGAR.	ALL-C.	ALU.	ANT-C.	ANT-T.	AP.	ARG-N.	ARN.	ARS.	ASAR.	BAR-C.	BELL.	BELL-P.	BOR.	BRY.	CALC-C.	CALC-F.	CALC-P.	CALC-S.	CALEN.	CANTH.	CARB-A.	CARB-V.	CAST.	CAUL.
1.	TEETHING – PAINFUL	✓													✓	✓	✓		✓		✓							
2.	" – SLOW																		✓		✓							
3.	" – WITH DIARRHOEA																		✓									
4.	DIARRHOEA – STOOLS SOUR																		✓									
5.	" – WITH UNDIGESTED FOOD																		✓									
6.	SWEAT – ON HEAD																		✓									
7.	" – SOUR											✓							✓									
8.	CATCHES COLDS EASILY											✓		✓					✓		✓							
9.	STUBBORN							✓																				

#	Symptom	CAUST.	CHAM.	CHEL.	CHIN.	CIMI.	CINA.	COCC.	COCC-C.	COFF.	COLCH.	COLOC.	CON.	CUPR.	CYPR.	DIOS.	DROS.	DULC.	EUP-P.	EUPHR.	FERR-M.	GELS.	GLON.	HAM.	HEP-S.	HYP.	IGN.	IP.
1.	TEETHING – PAINFUL		✓																									
2.	" – SLOW																											
3.	" – WITH DIARRHOEA		✓																									
4.	DIARRHOEA – STOOLS SOUR																											
5.	" – WITH UNDIGESTED FOOD				✓																✓							
6.	SWEAT – ON HEAD																											
7.	" – SOUR										✓														✓			
8.	CATCHES COLDS EASILY																	✓							✓			
9.	STUBBORN		✓	✓	✓																							

#	Symptom	JAB.	KALI-B.	KALI-C.	KALI-M.	KALI-P.	KALI-S.	KREOS.	LAC-C.	LAC-D.	LACH.	LED.	LIL-T.	LYC.	MAG-C.	MAG-M.	MAG-P.	MERC-C.	MERC-S.	NAT-C.	NAT-M.	NAT-P.	NAT-S.	NIT-AC.	NUX-M.	NUX-V.	OP.	PETR.
1.	TEETHING – PAINFUL							✓							✓													
2.	" – SLOW																											
3.	" – WITH DIARRHOEA																											
4.	DIARRHOEA – STOOLS SOUR														✓													
5.	" – WITH UNDIGESTED FOOD																											
6.	SWEAT – ON HEAD																											
7.	" – SOUR														✓	✓		✓			✓							
8.	CATCHES COLDS EASILY			✓																	✓					✓		
9.	STUBBORN																											

#	Symptom	PHO-AC.	PHOS.	PHYT.	PODO.	PULS.	PYR.	RHE.	RHOD.	RHUS-T.	RUMEX.	RUTA.	SAB.	SARS.	SEC.	SEP.	SIL.	SPO.	STAP.	STRAM.	SUL.	SUL-AC.	SYMPH.	TAB.	THU.	URT-U.	VER-A.	ZINC.
1.	TEETHING – PAINFUL			✓		✓		✓									✓											
2.	" – SLOW																✓											
3.	" – WITH DIARRHOEA			✓													✓											
4.	DIARRHOEA – STOOLS SOUR			✓																	✓							
5.	" – WITH UNDIGESTED FOOD																											
6.	SWEAT – ON HEAD																✓											
7.	" – SOUR															✓	✓					✓						✓
8.	CATCHES COLDS EASILY															✓	✓											
9.	STUBBORN																											

· 2 ·
PREPARING FOR LIFE
AFTER BIRTH

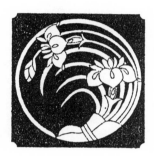

PREGNANCY

Pregnancy is a time when you can predict nothing. There are no rules. The outcome is unknown and largely unseen. The first-time mother has special delights and difficulties in store for her because this is a completely new experience.

Although subsequent babies are often easier – women know, roughly speaking, what they are letting themselves in for and feel more self-confident – here again, every pregnancy and every birth is different, there are no rules.

Pregnancy can be a time of pleasure if a woman is healthy and happy or a time of misery if she is ill or if there is too much stress in her life. You can do a great deal to help yourself with the physical changes, if they cause discomfort or pain, and the stresses, both practically and homeopathically. I have included both practical and homeopathic advice in this book. Homeopathic treatment is ideal in pregnancy because, provided you follow the guidelines set out in this book, it is safe. It can't harm you or your baby as there are no dangers of toxic side effects.

Much of the advice in this book applies to your partner as well as to you, for just as pregnancy can be a glorious time for many partners, it can be difficult for others. Partners can feel trapped, insecure, childlike, frightened, anxious about the future, about becoming a parent, about the increased responsibility, about the financial burden as well as joy and excitement. These feelings and many, many others are all common and normal. They need to be expressed and worked through. If feelings surface that don't resolve, I suggest that you and/or your partner find a professional to talk them through with – a counsellor or psychotherapist.

You and your partner need to talk now, more than ever, to stay close. Remember that you *both* have rights and that it is important that you carry on making demands of each other, asking for what you need – reassurance, affection and so on. At times, you will both have to compromise. Be true to yourselves and keep finding ways to express who you are and what you need.

Pregnancy can be a time of going inwards, a glorious wrapped-in-cotton-wool sensation, a time where life slows down and nothing outside matters quite as much as it did before. There may be a sense of unreality – an I-can't-believe-there's-actually-a-baby-growing-inside-me feeling, or I'll-believe-it-when-I-see-it.

If you have never held a baby it can be difficult to visualise yourself as a mother with a small charge to look after. Many first-time mothers focus on the birth as a goal, as an end in itself, and are startled to find themselves on the other side of it, in motherhood, without any idea about 'what happens next'. It is rather like buying a business without planning on how you're going to run it.

I see birth rather like a station on the railroad of life: you get off the train to have your baby and then embark on the journey again. I encourage women to start seeing the birth as a (smallish) part of life's process to put it in perspective and to encourage them not to expect a particular type of birth. Far too many women have sacrificed themselves on the altar of natural childbirth and feel that they have failed when the birth didn't go as they wanted. If you want a natural birth then by all means aim to have one but be aware of other options to turn to without feeling sad or guilty. You may decide, anyway, that you want to take full advantage of the technical help available in hospital and have a completely pain-free birth.

However you decide to have your baby, it helps to realise that birth heralds the start of motherhood. Build pictures in your mind's eye of yourself as a mother. If you are pregnant or planning to be, start *now* by visualising or imagining yourself after the birth, as a mother. Your baby is a few hours old: is it a girl or a boy? How are you feeling? What are you doing? Are you at home or at the hospital? Your baby is a week or two old. You are at home now. How are you going about your life – with this new little person to care for? Imagine yourself as a mother in different situations, at home, walking in the park, shopping, visiting friends. Imagine yourself, your thoughts and feelings, your partner, your other children, your baby and the sort of life you are going to have together in your new family. Do you anticipate any difficulties? Do any negative images surface? You may come up against blocks, things you don't know about and this will help you to work out the areas you may be strong in and others where you may be weak.

Create a motherhood reality for yourself by making space and time every day to do this. Talk it through with your partner, your friends and, of course, with your baby – there is more and more evidence to suggest that the baby in the uterus is much more conscious than we can even imagine. This process will help you to look at your own attitudes to parenthood – what beliefs you hold, how many you carry from your own parents, areas of uncertainty or difficulty that date back to your own childhood.

You may decide to make a special space for your new baby, by preparing a room or a cradle, a corner in your bedroom, or to buy some clothes and equipment. On the other hand, you may not wish to get anything until after the birth. Do what is right for you. If you are living in a very small space, however, and are not able to give a room to your baby, at least plan where it will sleep – and think through how you will manage the nights when he or she arrives.

Once you can feel your baby moving – and that in itself is an extraordinary experience, like a bird or a butterfly fluttering its wings inside you – you know it's real. Be aware of the movements your baby makes, its own patterns of being awake and of sleeping. As it grows, see if you can notice the changes in position and tension that occur. During the last three months of pregnancy your abdomen will change shape frequently, bulging on one or both sides, or more in the middle. Ask your doctor or midwife to tell you how to feel for your baby's back or head or feet. When a small baby moves its hands or feet in the last weeks you can see little bulges. Talk to your baby, start including it in your daily life and make active links with it: start to understand your child's personality from how it moves inside you.

Others may want to communicate with your baby in ways that you find unacceptable. Ask people not to touch you if you don't like it. It's absolutely fine if you do – but if not, be clear and friendly in asking them to back off.

If you are scared of the birth itself, ask your mother, if possible, what your own birth was like. Some women have unconsciously repeated their own difficult birth in giving birth to their children. Ask your mother about her attitudes to childbirth – you may have taken on her beliefs unconsciously.

Do you have any fears or anxieties about being a parent? Voice them now: talk them through with people you trust, who will take you seriously and not dismiss your feelings as 'silly'. Try to identify what you are scared of. Your life *will* change – dramatically for some – and you can anticipate and prepare for some of the changes.

If you are to be the happy parent of two or more babies your extra baby may not be spotted until relatively late in your pregnancy (in the third trimester). You may have an increased susceptibility to anaemia and premature births are also common. The advice in this book still applies to you, and, because of your additional needs, *you* will need more of everything (not twice as much!) – more rest, more food, more support, more care – especially after the birth!

Pregnancy and birth are not always straight-forward – they may be complicated or even down-right difficult depending on your circumstances. The following women are all vulnerable in pregnancy either because they are physically or economically at a disadvantage or because they fall outside society's accepted norm: single parents, those over forty, ado-lescents, lesbians, those in poverty, those in deteriorating relationships, the disabled and chron-ically ill, ethnic minorities, isolated women or those who have multiple births.

It is beyond the scope of this book to go in great depth into all the ways that each of the above would best be helped, but most of the practical advice and homeopathic help outlined applies to any woman contemplating pregnancy and birth whatever her special needs or circumstances. (See also Organisa-tions, p. 305.) It is essential that you don't isolate yourself, that you get plenty of support if you fall into one of these categories. Having a baby is hard work – rewardingly hard work, but hard work nonetheless. Plan for it as you would a particularly difficult phase of your working life. Set up strategies for surviving it in one reasonably happy, healthy piece!

Women vary enormously in their capacity to work during pregnancy. I have known some women work literally up until the day before they gave birth while others stopped within a month of discovering they were pregnant. Do what feels right for you and what you want to do, if you can. If you choose to work up until the last minute you will have less time for your-self but if that is what you want, go ahead. If you have to carry on working from economic necessity, make as much of your free time as possible for your-self and your baby, your partner and any other chil-dren. Socialise only if you *really* want to and feel up to it. And remember that lunch hours at the office can be used for a nap, domestic chores can be delegated, and *ask* someone to drive you to the bus stop or station – or even into work!

Use the pre-natal classes run by the hospital, clinic, or community center for information and to learn relaxation and 'breathing' techniques and yoga exercises specifically designed for childbirth (mainly the Active Birth classes). You'll also begin to learn some of the practicalities of parentcraft, and, especially important, you'll meet other pregnant women and gain confidence from their experience. You'll learn a lot about babies and parenthood from chatting to other mothers and their partners. If you're new to the area, your health visitor (contactable through your GP) will let you know of local classes. Encourage your birth partner to come with you to these classes so that you can practise the exercises together afterwards.

Your partner may like to go to all ante-natal classes or none of them. Don't squash yourselves into an ideal of what you think you ought to be as prospec-tive parents.

Your pregnancy can begin to seem as though it will go on for ever – it may be the longest nine months of your life. *Don't* put your life on hold while you wait for the baby to arrive. Get on with the business of living. Everything in your life won't change – only some things!

YOUR FAMILY AND PREGNANCY

You may be fortunate in having loving family living close by. If so, cultivate them: encourage willing grandparents to become as involved as they want to be in your children's lives. Grandparents can be a marvellous source of nurture for grandchildren and support for parents.

If grandparents are not available, aunts and uncles are good alternatives, either real or 'adopted' ones. Close friends who have chosen not to have children of their own are often delighted to be asked to be a 'special' person in your child's life. If you have a relative or friend who would like to be that special person involve them from early in your baby's life. They may even be delighted to babysit every now and again.

Make friends with at least one other pregnant woman (whose baby is due at roughly the same time as yours if possible) so that you are not isolated after the birth. There is nothing worse than being the only one of a circle of friends to have a baby and to have no one to talk to about your new miracle.

If this is not your first baby, you may find yourself very stretched, especially if you are also working. Don't let the serious business of living, working, looking after everybody else and the house get on top of you. Make time to play cards or watch your favour-ite comedy video, gossip with a friend or play in the swimming pool.

Do have some fun, with friends, relatives and your partner, and make the most of the last months and weeks of spontaneous freedom. After the birth you will have to plan your outings more carefully.

The more children you have the more planning is involved!

Holidays are often stressful: they take us out of our familiar environment and highlight areas of difficulty in our relationships because there are fewer distractions. Go where you know that you have a good time. Now is not the time to experiment with a new type of holiday. If your health has been poor during your pregnancy go somewhere reasonably close to home just in case you decide to cut the holiday short. Check out the availability of good medical care if you decide to take a break abroad, especially towards the end of your pregnancy.

Sitting cramped for long periods of time is bad for your circulation. It is important that you stretch frequently during long journeys: make frequent stops if you're travelling by car and walk about. Get up and move around if you are travelling by train, coach or plane.

In the past mothers often chose not to tell their children that they were pregnant. I believe that children of any age, including barely verbal toddlers, can be informed about a pregnancy, unless there is a strong possibility of an early miscarriage. Our children know intuitively when something unusual is happening and if we choose not to talk to them their imaginations can run riot. You can start by saying the bare minimum, that you are pregnant, what that means, and how you are feeling about it, both physically and emotionally. Children respond to news of a pregnancy in many different ways. Some are delighted, some curious, some seem more or less unaffected, detached, others are openly furious, anxious about their future, sad about the loss of their position as the baby in the family. Support, acknowledge and therefore validate their feelings.

As the pregnancy progresses, talk frankly about how the family will change with a new member in language appropriate to the age of your child. Include your child or children in planning for the birth and for life after the birth. Take them to an occasional ante-natal appointment (with plenty of things for them to do and eat). Some hospitals will even tolerate well-behaved children when you are having a scan.

Don't ignore or try to hide the coming event. If you can't make yourself understood, there are many books for children on 'new arrivals' – you can use one to help you open the topic for discussion. I think it is important to state that the baby is growing in your womb (or uterus if you wish) and not in 'mummy's tummy'. Every child knows that it is food that goes into its tummy and this anatomical inaccuracy can lead to confusion, and even distress. There are mar-vellous books available that show clearly how the body is arranged inside, including photographs of the baby growing in the uterus – pay a visit to your local library or bookshop.

YOUR HEALTH AND PREGNANCY

BREATHING

Breathing is automatic: you cannot stop even if you try! During pregnancy you may notice that you are breathing more deeply than normal: this is due to hormonal changes.

Oxygen is vital to good health. Many of us develop poor but adequate breathing patterns, mostly due to bad posture or emotional stress. We hold our breath if frightened, sad, tense, anxious, angry or even excited. A physical shock or accident can also affect how we breathe. If those patterns of shallow breathing are repeated, breath-holding can become habitual. However, people who breathe shallowly tend to take a deep – or sighing – breath every now and again as a compensation.

Increase your awareness of your breathing, of how you breathe. When do you breathe deeply and when do you breathe shallowly? To get an adequate oxygen supply, it's important to breathe into the whole lung: if you breathe shallowly you may only be filling the top part.

Allow the air to come in through your nostrils and down into your lower back – your lungs reach up to your collarbone and down almost to your waist. Allow your ribs to expand outwards as you breathe in. Imagine that you have a couple of balloons in your chest that are filling fully with air each time you take a breath and emptying each time you breathe out. Allow this to happen rather than trying to make it happen and thereby causing a different tension pattern. Let your breath go on the outbreath – just let it go, without putting any effort into it.

If you find it difficult to breathe, if your chest is tight because you suffer or have suffered from a complaint like asthma, seek the advice of a physiotherapist, Alexander-technique teacher or cranial osteopath to retrain in breathing. If your breathing is shallow because of emotional tension then you may benefit from seeing a psychotherapist to release any suppressed feelings. Emotional tension can also lead to overbreathing, or hyperventilating, which can cause a drop in blood pressure and feelings of panic and dizziness.

Learn how to breathe in conjunction with your relaxation technique so that they work effectively together. (You will be taught how to do this at any ante-natal class you attend.) Practise letting go of physical tension as you breathe out.

CIGARETTES AND ALCOHOL (AND ALL OTHER DRUGS)

It is important to avoid alcohol while you are pregnant. Alcohol crosses the placenta and reaches the baby's brain within a very short time of your taking it. It's not worth the risk although the occasional glass of wine or beer is unlikely to do any harm. If you have a problem with stopping drinking, seek the help of AA (see p. 305).

Cigarettes can also affect your baby: if you continue to smoke, your baby may be smaller and possibly more vulnerable to infection. Homeopathy can help you stop smoking so see a homeopath for information as to how. There are also organisations (listed on pp. 305–8) which run short courses to help people give up, ask your GP about local groups.

Avoid all other drugs, whether prescribed, over the counter or illegal, while you are pregnant and breastfeeding. If you are on medication for a long-term complaint such as epilepsy, you must be guided by your doctor throughout your pregnancy as to the suitability of your medication.

DIET

What we eat is always an important factor in our general health and this is especially true during pregnancy when the body's requirement for essential nutrients increases. You will need to eat about 20 per cent more than usual, but your requirement for folic acid, vitamins B and C, calcium, zinc and magnesium will rise by 30–100 per cent.

Women whose supplies of stored nutrients may be low when they become pregnant should always take advice from a nutritionist (your GP will refer you): for example if you have had several pregnancies close together without time for recovery, or you are underweight (possibly anorexic), or you are on a restricted diet due to allergy or by choice. Some women have difficulty in absorbing nutrients, especially those who suffer from a chronic disease, women who smoke or drink heavily or who take drugs, and those who are taking prescribed medication regularly (such as steroids or anti-convulsants). Adolescents, who are still growing themselves, are also vulnerable, as are women who are overweight. It is important that you check with your GP or a nutritionist if you become pregnant *and* fall into one of these categories.

If you started your pregnancy with a good diet and are otherwise healthy then the most important advice I can give is that you enjoy your food and eat whatever you feel like eating. It is OK to incorporate a little junk food into your diet: your body will cope with it well as long as your basic diet is healthy. The following guidelines will help you build healthy eating patterns – for life, not just for pregnancy.

Do

- eat a varied diet. A diet with a little of everything is most likely to contain the wide variety of nutrients that you need. It is important that you include some of each of the main food groups every day, i.e. carbohydrate, protein, fat, fibre, vitamins and minerals. Make sure you eat plenty of pulses, wholegrains, fresh fruit and vegetables and if you are not vegetarian or vegan include dairy foods, eggs, fish (especially fatty fish like mackerel, herring and sardines) and meat, including kidneys, from organically reared animals only. Because of the highly concentrated levels of vitamin A in liver (thought to be the cause of a few isolated cases of abnormalities in babies, although not in the UK) doctors are presently recommending that women don't eat it in pregnancy. Hopefully research currently in progress will identify a safe quantity in the near future.
- eat plenty of carbohydrates, as they are your major source of energy.
- eat protein-rich foods every day, as they are responsible for the growth and repair of all the cells of your body (and therefore your baby's body too).
- eat a moderate amount of fat. Apart from providing energy, it also forms 'protective layers' which store vitamins A, D, E and K.
- eat plenty of fibre as it helps remove waste and toxins from the body.
- make sure you include plenty of vitamin- and mineral-rich foods. If you aren't sure of whether your diet includes the following essential ones, see a nutritionist or hospital dietician who will advise and reassure you. **Vitamin A** helps in the growth processes of the body; **B vitamins** contribute to energy levels and the formation and healthy

functioning of the brain and nervous system; **vitamin B$_{12}$** is especially important because it helps to form healthy blood and nerves); **vitamin C** builds resistance to disease, promotes speedy healing and the absorption of iron; **vitamin D** helps form strong bones, teeth and gums and aids in calcium absorption; **vitamin E** also promotes healing. Eat mineral-rich foods: **calcium** is essential for healthy bones, teeth, nerves, heart and blood; **chloride** is essential for the digestion of proteins and regulates the balance of sodium and potassium; **copper** aids the conversion of iron into haemoglobin and in the absorption of vitamin C; **iodine** helps with growth, energy and mental alertness; **iron** is responsible for healthy blood; **magnesium** helps form bones and the nervous system; **phosphorus** combines with calcium to make healthy bones and teeth; **potassium** unites with sodium to make healthy blood, body fluids and muscles; **sodium** works with potassium to balance the body's fluids; and **zinc** works with iron and copper to form and repair all the body tissues and keep the immune system strong and healthy.

- buy organic meat and free-range eggs. The flavour is better and there are none of the chemical residues which are present in the factory-farmed products.
- investigate soya beans and soya-bean products (tofu, tempeh and miso) as these all contain high levels of protein, iron, calcium, magnesium, potassium, phosphorus and B vitamins (not B$_{12}$).
- eat regularly, little and often, 4–6 smaller meals a day, unless you have a slow metabolism that thrives on eating larger meals at less frequent intervals.
- eat wholefood – well washed and scrubbed fruit and vegetables with the skins on, organically grown if possible.
- eat plenty of fresh foods in the ways that appeal to you. Some people prefer food to be cooked especially in the winter months while others like it raw the whole year round. Eat as much fruit, vegetables, especially green leafy ones, and/or salads as you can. Don't forget that you can use winter vegetables for winter salads such as finely chopped cabbage, celery, chicory, grated celeriac and carrot.
- buy fruit and vegetables in smaller quantities more often as vitamin C is destroyed by storage.
- eat green leafy vegetables every day as they are high in iron and essential vitamins such as vitamin K which helps the blood to clot.
- include nutritious snacks of nuts and seeds rather

than biscuits which are frighteningly high in refined flour, fat, salt *and* sugar.
- indulge any cravings during your pregnancy as long as they are reasonably healthy and as long as you are able also to eat a varied diet.
- avoid sugars (white, brown, treacle and even honey except in small quantities) as they have very little nutritional value. Substitute plenty of fruit, including dried fruits if you want something sweet – they contain essential minerals as well as tasting good!
- avoid all foods that contain additives, long-term effects are not known. The average Westerner is said to eat in the region of 4 pounds (2 kg) of additives a year.
- avoid refined carbohydrates as these provide 'empty' calories (carbohydrates without vitamins or minerals).
- avoid additional wheat bran and soft drinks as these can affect your ability to absorb essential vitamins and minerals.
- soak muesli overnight before you eat it as raw oats are difficult to digest.
- avoid anything you instinctively feel is 'bad' for you while you are pregnant or breastfeeding, even if it doesn't make logical sense.
- cut out stimulants – tea, coffee, chocolate, Coca-Cola and Diet Coke as these all contain caffeine. They prevent absorption of zinc and iron especially if you drink them with a meal.
- cut out all alcohol and be creative with your social drinking. Try drinking orange, grapefruit, tomato, apple or pineapple juice with or without soda water or sparkling mineral water; water! – cold, with or without ice, or hot, with or without a slice of lemon; blended iced drinks made with fresh fruit and ice; homemade lemonade; yoghurt shakes made with equal quantities of fresh yoghurt and water, with a sweet or savoury flavouring; grain coffees – a wide range is available in wholefood shops – vegetable broths.
- drink herb teas with caution as they are known to have a medicinal effect and can therefore be unintentionally 'proved' (see p. 10); raspberry leaf tea, taken in the last 3 months of pregnancy (2–3 cups a day) has been found effective at promoting a trouble-free labour. It is especially good for sedentary women with poor muscle tone or who have a history of gynaecological problems (or difficult births). Those who are fit and healthy should avoid it (or take it only on instruction from a herbalist) as it can cause the symptoms it was supposed to relieve (see Provings, p. 5).

Don't

- eat for two. If you put on too much weight during your pregnancy you may find labour more difficult, especially if you are unfit.
- worry if you put on up to 30 pounds (14 kg) during your pregnancy.
- diet. Your baby's health may be affected.
- eat soft cheeses like Brie, cheeses made from unpasteurised milk, hot dishes in canteens or pre-cooked meals from shops or supermarkets – they may have been inadequately chilled after cooking and contain bacteria (listeria) which can cross the placenta and harm your baby.
- eat muesli without soaking it first.
- eat vast quantities of spinach, rhubarb, parsley, watercress or chocolate as the oxalic acid they contain hinders the absorption of calcium.
- substitute beer and wine with those that are alcohol-free or low in alcohol as some contain high levels of additives and chemicals, the effects of which on your baby are not known.
- take vitamin or mineral supplements during your pregnancy without taking professional advice from a nutritionist, who will advise you on how to alter your diet to get the extra nutrients you need rather than taking supplements.
- become fanatical about eating only 'pure' foods. Your body *can* recognise junk and deal with it.
- take antacids for heartburn (see p. 91) as they prevent iron from being absorbed.

Seek help if

- you are not able to maintain a healthy diet.
- you are not putting on weight or are putting on too much weight.
- you are a vegetarian or a vegan and are worried that you might not be getting enough B_{12}, iron or calcium from your diet.
- your cravings are peculiar (see p. 90) or uncontrollable.

EXERCISE

Exercise increases strength, stamina and flexibility, all vital during pregnancy, birth and the post-natal period where you will want your body to return to a good shape.

Do exercise regularly – the more physically fit you are the better. Even if childbirth lasts for 'only' 8 hours it can be very arduous and therefore the single most important aspect in preparing for birth is the physical one. It has been compared with climbing a mountain or running a marathon. In my practice I have observed that it is women who exercise who have relatively easier births and recover faster. If you don't enjoy exercise, you could consider going to classes or finding someone to come to your home. Walking, cycling (if you're experienced and confident), dancing and swimming are good for building strength and stamina, yoga and gentle exercise programmes for pregnancy will help build up flexibility and suppleness.

Don't carry on exercising if you become breathless, exhausted, overheated or in pain. These symptoms are telling you that you have reached your limit and you need to stop and recover before you go on. And pregnancy is *not* a good time to take up a new and physically demanding form of exercise! Avoid weight-training as the ligaments in your body soften and may easily be overstretched. Don't have a sauna or a very long, hot bath after vigorous exercise as recent studies have shown that your baby may have difficulty in regulating its own temperature, in cooling down. After the birth, keep up the exercise and don't forget that walking with a pram is good for you *and* your baby!

Exercise for Pelvic-floor Muscles

Even if you take no other exercise, this one is vital to prevent stress incontinence, prolapses and piles, among other things. The pelvic-floor muscles support all the organs in your pelvis; they lie in a figure of eight around your anus and vagina. Be aware of where they are by waiting to go to the loo until your bladder is full, start to pee then stop the flow of urine and hold it for a few seconds without dribbling. Start and stop several times. If you can do this easily your pelvic-floor muscles are in good shape. Do this from time to time when you pee to check them. The following exercise will build strong pelvic-floor muscles: imagine you are lifting these muscles upwards in stages – like a lift – up to the first floor and then the second and the third, holding them at each stage for a few seconds. Do it daily and frequently – anywhere! You can do it in the supermarket queue or while you're waiting for a bus. When you are in the bath or shower you can check this by holding a finger inside your vagina, as you contract the muscles you should be able to feel them.

POSTURE – CARRY YOUR BABY ACTIVELY

Some women carry their babies with their whole bodies – accommodating and adapting to the change in shape and the extra weight. Others find the extra weight difficult to cope with and waddle, with their babies pulling them forward, forcing them to shift their centre of gravity which causes many aches and pains. Carrying your baby actively will be strengthening and lessen your chances of developing backache; you will feel more supple, less collapsed, less heavy – more in charge of your body.

Seek the help of an Alexander-technique teacher if you feel that you are collapsing forward as your baby grows – if you find it increasingly difficult to get up out of chairs for example. An Alexander teacher will help you to be more aware of how you use your body, where tension exists, and will suggest less stressful ways of moving in everyday situations such as standing, sitting, lifting, walking, etc.

Your imagination can be a strong healing force in your life: your mind and body are closely linked. The shape our bodies take can reflect our feelings: people who are depressed tend to slump. You can try this now: remember a recent situation in which you felt very angry and relive it in your imagination. Which muscles tense? How are you breathing? Now, remember a happy time, one which made you feel warm and contented. What happens to your body?

To carry a baby we need to expand: some women are frightened they won't stretch enough. Don't be. Imagine your body widening, lengthening and expanding, growing with your baby. If you feel tense and contracted or find it difficult to feel expansive then accept it, be compassionate towards your body, but keep trying – gently and persistently. Practise 'widening' or 'softening' to give room to your baby: actively imagine a space opening up inside you and giving your baby the room it needs. Tell yourself that you are capable of doing this, your body has been built to do it.

Try not to allow the weight of your baby to pull you forward: imagine a heavy tail attached at your coccyx (tail bone) dangling between your legs, let it pull down, naturally tucking your bottom in. Don't lock your legs when standing: imagine them being soft and warm. Imagine that feeling in your knees and buttocks, whether standing, stooping or sitting, or anywhere in your body where you feel tension building up. Don't let your body collapse into inactivity. Most important of all is to imagine these things

happening and then to let them happen. Trust your body to do what it knows best.

RELAXATION

It is important that you build some good relaxation time into your life, time to unwind and recharge. It is possible to enjoy yourself and relax at the same time by walking, sitting outside and daydreaming, taking a long bath, massaging yourself with a body lotion or oil after the bath, reading a good book, talking to a good friend, playing in the sandpit with your toddler, reading to an older child and so on.

Specific techniques for relaxing such as autogenic training, biofeedback, guided visualisation and meditation, have been found to be enormously beneficial – experiment to find one that suits you, especially if you find it difficult to relax.

A simple relaxation exercise that you can do anywhere is to lie on the floor, with a cushion under your head and one under your knees, or sit with both feet flat on the floor. Close your eyes and listen to your breathing. Allow it to become even and a little deeper. Feel your body 'sink' into the floor or the chair, let it become heavy and soft. Breathe out any tension. Imagine something really nice, walking in a sunny flower-filled meadow, skiing on your own private ski slope in the Alps, swimming in a warm tropical ocean, lying on warm sands, boating on a highland lake or walking in the forest. Spend as long as you like in your chosen place – a minute if that is all you have or longer if you are sitting on the tube or relaxing on your bedroom floor when you come home. You can repeat this any time you like if it works for you – you'll find it helpful last thing at night as it will help you sleep well.

REST

Rest as much as you need to – your body will let you know just how much – especially at the beginning of your pregnancy. A nap in the afternoon and a longer sleep at night are fine, especially if you are working. Your energy should increase after the first few months, but if it doesn't and the advice in this book doesn't help (see Exhaustion, p. 89) seek professional help. You shouldn't have to drag yourself around for your entire pregnancy.

As a general rule don't stand if you can sit, or sit if you can lie down. If you are a first-time mother, depending on your job, you will have more freedom to rest when you like. If this isn't your first baby, be creative about resting as you care for your family: I know a woman who spent a large part of each day in the bath because it was relaxing for her and fun for her boisterous eighteen-month-old. Entertain your young charges with activities that are restful for you like reading, watching television or a video, playing with Lego or Playdo, drawing or painting. Some children are like puppies and need a long run each day in the fresh air otherwise they become uncontrollable indoors. Time their outings so that you take them out when you are feeling energetic and can benefit from the exercise.

Invest in a tall stool so that you can take the weight off your feet when ironing, washing up or cooking. Squat instead of bending down to pick up weights, like shopping or children. Sit on the bed, a small stool or chair to dress small children or do things with them at their level.

SEX IN PREGNANCY

Some women feel wonderfully sexual when pregnant – they love feeling rounded and full and womanly – and enjoy not having to worry about contraception. Many couples grow closer during pregnancy, and are able more easily to express tenderness, affection and love. Others experience a loss of libido. This may be due to having difficulty in getting used to a constantly expanding body or perhaps to emotional difficulties in the relationship. Some partners find their pregnant woman incredibly sexy and others quite the opposite. It's essential that you communicate honestly and openly with each other about your feelings and sexuality. (See also Loss of Libido, p. 94.)

STRESS AND TENSION

Be aware of stress, both physical and emotional, when you are pregnant and reduce it, if necessary, by sorting out your priorities. Pregnancy is a good time to decide what is important and what can be temporarily shelved. Make a list of what really counts in your life and needs attention to survive, and another of what isn't so necessary. You will find that cooking and housework can go quite low down on your list and that you and your family go to the top. Any time you start feeling that items lower down the list are getting too much attention and draining you, ask yourself what you would do if you caught flu and couldn't cook, clean or even go to work. Keep things

in perspective by constantly checking what *really* matters and what could go if it *had* to!

Take with a fistful of salt any advice, unsolicited or otherwise from relatives or friends! This is one of the few times in your life when you will be overwhelmed with it, even from people you barely know. Select and accept what feels right to you. Don't listen to other women's horror stories of their or their friends' babies' births; some feel a strange compulsion to repeat them to newly pregnant first-time mothers. Ask them to stop, repeatedly if necessary, until they do! Don't read too many books on childbirth or parenthood. Choose one or two and read the parts that seem relevant to you. If you are reading compulsively to make sense of something that's confusing you, ask a professional for the advice you seek.

If you feel tension or pain building up in your body at any time, breathe gently into the tense or sore muscles and allow them to soften and expand – imagine this happening. (See also Breathing, p. 40.) Contract any muscles which are still tense, and stretch them, then gently move your body, twisting and turning. See if you can find a more comfortable position, whether you are sitting, lying or standing. Stiffening into one position is bad for you – keep moving! Find a comfortable position to sleep in at night.

Feel your body moving as you go about your daily life. Let your hips swing gently, stop to rotate them when you are walking the dog or watching your older child play in the park. Slow belly-dancing is a marvellous form of exercise, created specifically to help women prepare for childbirth. In pregnancy (especially the later months) it promotes suppleness and strength. Dance to music: children of all ages will join you in this. Bend and stretch and lift, using your whole body without stressing or straining it or making sudden, jerky movements.

If your baby is pressing uncomfortably in one place, try moving your body and imagining that your pelvic area is widening. Breathe deeply and slowly and talk to your baby – asking it to move.

Wear comfortable clothing that enhances your feeling of well-being, and colours that make you feel good.

TOXINS

Avoid unnecessary toxins such as hairsprays, hair dyes, perms, head-lice treatments, garden pesticides, household sprays or any heavy duty (chemical) cleaning products, paint fumes (especially gloss paint), varnish fumes (including paint and varnish stripping chemicals), glue and typing correction fluid fumes, smoking (including other people's smoke), aluminium pans in the kitchen, excessive car pollution (unnecessary journeys entailing traffic jams). These can all cross the placenta and be absorbed by your baby. It is sensible to avoid extensive dental treatment, except to have your teeth cleaned and checked (see also Teeth, p. 102).

Wear gloves when gardening or changing the cat-litter tray to avoid the risk of toxoplasmosis: relatively common in adults it can cause severe health problems for your baby. For the same reasons, wash your hands after handling raw meat and don't eat raw or undercooked meat. Reheated meals must be cooked to a high temperature to avoid food poisoning. Avoid raw eggs, unpasteurised milk, shellfish, pâtés, blue-veined cheeses and soft cheeses like Brie and Camembert.

PREPARING FOR BIRTH

Although much of the following relates to birth or the post-natal period, you will need to read it when you are pregnant and think through the issues raised so that you can make your birth plan.

HOSPITAL OR HOME BIRTH

Start by exploring your options. What is available to you in the area in which you live? Try to work out what you really want and what might suit you. Check out the choices and don't make a decision until you are sure. Remember that you *can* change your mind.

Is your home important to you? Is it where you feel most relaxed? Were *you* born at home? Do hospitals make you nervous? Do you know in your heart of hearts that home is where you'd like to give birth? Home may represent all that is normal, familiar, healthy and where you feel at ease. You will have more freedom at home to do largely what you want in your own time. You won't have to worry about hospital routine or procedures, and won't be disturbed by other labouring women and/or their families, or student doctors and midwives in, say, a teaching hospital. Your other children will be there and afterwards you can tuck yourself into bed with your whole family around you. You won't be separated from your partner after the birth. If you want a home

birth then ask your GP. If he or she is not supportive, contact your local independent midwives, health authority or a childbirth organization.

Is full medical support vital to you? Are you comfortable and at ease in a hospital environment? Have you had good, positive experiences in hospitals? Are you good at dealing with hospital staff, at getting what you want? Do you want a break after the birth – a time for just you and your baby, where your meals are delivered at regular intervals, where the demands of your other children are being met by someone else? Do you feel anxious at the thought of having a baby at home because of the risks, because your home is too small or too crowded, or because you know in your heart of hearts that hospital is best for you? More importantly, do you have a medical condition that may need expert help at the birth itself such as twins who present themselves prematurely, or pre-eclampsia?

PRE-NATAL VISITS

These are booked once a month from 12 weeks onwards up until the 28th week and then every two weeks until the 34th week, then weekly until the birth. They will help you to form links with your doctor, consultant and/or your midwife, hopefully, but not necessarily, the ones who will attend your labour. Visits are more frequent towards the end of your pregnancy as complications are more likely to arise then if at all. You'll only have to undress for the first one. The following are all checked at each visit: your blood (see p. 49) and urine (for infection); your weight and blood pressure; the baby's position and heartbeat.

You can take your partner or a good friend with you to ante-natal visits as support and also to make the boring bits pass quickly – like waiting for your appointment! As queues in hospital ante-natal clinics can be long and slow-moving, at least take a book or something to occupy you.

Take an active interest in what is happening to your body during your pregnancy and avoid becoming a passive consumer of health care by asking questions at every stage. Make a list before your appointments of the information you need as well as any points you wish to make to the clinic staff.

Seek professionals with whom you feel comfortable and can trust. If you are frightened or anxious then say so, otherwise, in trying to hide your feelings, you may come across as 'prickly' or 'difficult'. Ask for support and help. Be as honest and open as you can.

TESTS

Medical tests pose a dilemma: you may believe in minimal medical interference but want to do the best for your baby so when the doctor offers a particular test you may feel obliged to have it. Doctors may pressure women to have the favourite test of the moment although rising costs have meant that tests (especially expensive ones) are not pushed routinely now. Most doctors now only advise having a test if the result will cause the parents to take action. Tests and procedures are constantly being improved: check out the up-to-date information with your doctor, consultant, or childbirth organization (see Organizations, p. 305).

Tests are often stressful and I have provided guidelines for how to approach and deal with them to minimise stress and to make the most of what is offered by the medical profession, whose aim is to help you stay healthy and produce a healthy baby.

Some of the following tests carry the minor risk of bruising from needles or rough examinations, and of feeling emotionally 'abused'. Take Rescue Remedy (see p. 165) with you on every hospital visit and take frequent 2-drop doses if you are feeling edgy or panicky. You can take *Argentum nitricum*, *Lycopodium* or *Gelsemium* before the visit if you are in a particularly nervous state.

Afterwards, take *Arnica* routinely for bruising and/or shock; *Staphysagria* if you feel 'abused' or 'violated', even if you were in the hands of kind and sympathetic doctors and nurses, and are suffering from more severe pains (not just soreness). Some women are very sensitive to having their body examined – dislike internal examinations, having needles stuck into them, cervical smears: *Staphysagria* will deal with both the physical and the emotional effects. Take *Hypericum* if you have shooting pains anywhere after one of the tests, for example, if a needle hit a nerve.

Use the following Dos and Don'ts to help you decide whether and/or when to have each test.

Do

- weigh up whether the benefits of a test will exceed its risks. The results can mean that further tests, or action, need to be taken. The following questions may help: What will I learn from the test? How accurate is it? What are the risks to me and/or my baby if I have it? How long will I have to wait for the results? What procedures (or tests) will be needed if it is positive? How far am I prepared to go if the test is positive? Where would I be happy to go for this test (hospital/GP's surgery, etc.)? Think carefully and listen to your instincts about whether you want or need each separate test.
- talk it over with your doctor and try to find out if he or she performs tests routinely. Be sure you understand what is happening and why. If in doubt get a second opinion. Talk to your partner and to other women who have had the test.
- get as much information as you can about each test that is suggested. Ask your doctor to describe *exactly* what will happen for each one. Ask a childbirth organization or your library for up-to-date detailed information.
- ask whether the results of a particular test will affect your doctor's plan for your care or will necessitate treatment. If it won't, the test may not be necessary.
- weigh up the options and the possible outcomes carefully. Ask yourself what is the worst that can happen, if you have a test or if you don't.
- question the necessity of taking all your clothes off if, for example, you are just having a blood test.
- take a partner or friend to a pre-natal visit that involves the discussion of a test. Ask that they write down information given by doctors, nurses, consultants or midwives. Studies have shown that patients remember remarkably little of what doctors tell them. Your partner can ask the medical professionals to spell unfamiliar terms so that you can look them up later.
- ask questions whenever you feel confused. Some pressurised doctors forget to tell you what they are going to do next, and don't answer patients' questions satisfactorily. They may even leave the room without saying if or when they will return. Be persistent and assertive, without being aggressive, and ask for as much reassurance as you need as often as you need it.
- be friendly, firm, clear and persistent about your own needs and preferences at each stage.
- let your doctor, consultant or midwife know if you are finding the ante-natal visits and tests stressful. Some women mask their anxiety or fear or distress with a hardness that comes across as aggression, which can put up the backs of medical professionals. Talking will help.
- ask your partner or friend to ask the questions if you find yourself drying up once your clothes are off.

Don't

- accept that because the doctor has said you need it that they are right. Try to understand why you are being tested. This will be empowering.
- let yourself be separated from your partner during a test procedure that you have agreed to *whatever happens*. He or she *can* go to the toilet with you – and wait outside if necessary – unless you feel happy to go on your own.
- put up with a hostile and unsympathetic doctor, consultant or midwife, *whatever the reason*. Ask to see someone else or get dressed, if necessary, and leave.

Alphafetoprotein

This blood test is performed between 16 and 22 weeks of pregnancy to measure the levels of alphafetoprotein being passed by the baby's liver back into the mother's bloodstream via the placenta. The AFP test, as it is known, is used to detect the *possibility* of one of a number of common defects in the development of the foetus. Altered AFP levels can indicate that:

- the baby has a so-called neural tube defect, including spina bifida, Down's syndrome or anencephaly.
- the baby has an abnormality of the kidneys or intestines.
- a miscarriage is threatened.
- you are carrying more than one baby.
- your dates are wrong: the AFP levels double every five weeks in the fourth, fifth and sixth month of pregnancy.

  It is important to be aware that this test has an approximately 20 per cent false-positive rate. If you test positive then you have a one-in-five chance of being alarmed unnecessarily.

Do

- have a second AFP test before you consider a scan (if your levels were high) if the first one was positive; or have a scan before a second AFP test if you're anxious and want to reassure yourself that you're not carrying twins or a baby with a defect.

Amniocentesis

Used to test for certain chromosomal/genetic disorders. The sex of the baby can also be determined. This test is offered to all pregnant women in their late thirties and early forties because the risk of conceiving a Downs' syndrome baby increases with age.

At 35 the risk is 1 in 365, but at 40 it is 1 in 100. It is also offered to younger women who have a family history of genetic weakness.

Amniocentesis carries a slight risk of miscarriage or damage to the placenta or baby. It cannot be performed until the 16th week of pregnancy because it is not possible to obtain enough amniotic fluid before then. Because the tests take up to three weeks to be processed, a woman can be 4½ months pregnant before she has the results. To contemplate an abortion at that stage in a pregnancy is a very painful decision not least because it involves an induced labour rather than a suction abortion under a general anaesthetic. Counselling is essential.

The procedure for amniocentesis is:

1 An ultrasound is used to locate the baby (see p. 50) to avoid disturbing it or piercing the placenta and a cross marked on the spot where the needle will enter.
2 A long, very fine needle is inserted and about 4 teaspoons of amniotic fluid are drawn off. The procedure may need to be repeated more than once to get enough fluid, or again if there is blood in the sample, or if the doctor can't get the needle in in the right place.

  Although the needle is not usually felt as it passes through the fat and muscles of the abdomen it may sting, prick, cramp or feel like a pressure as it pierces the wall of the uterus. Afterwards more intense pains, including strong cramps, are common; spotting of blood or leaking of amniotic fluid from the vagina occur rarely. The site where the needle is inserted may feel bruised.

Do

- take a loving partner or friend.
- breathe (see p. 40) into your abdomen. Use any relaxation routine you know.
- feel yourself slowly sinking into the couch.
- tell your baby what's happening reassuringly.
- ask your partner to talk to you reassuringly.
- take time afterwards to recover fully. If it has been at all traumatic for you take it easy until the shock passes.
- take the homeopathic remedies suggested on p. 47.

Don't

- look, even if you are curious – at least until *afterwards*. Either shut your eyes or ask for a sheet to be put up to protect you from seeing it done.
- let your partner be separated from you for a moment.

Blood Tests

These are straightforward and usually performed by your doctor (or at the hospital). A small amount of blood is taken from your arm. If you have never had blood taken before or if you find it a difficult procedure, ask your doctor to go slowly and explain everything to you. Lie down to have it taken if you are inclined to faint at the sight of blood and/or a needle.

Blood is routinely taken to test for blood group, Rhesus factor (see p. 50), anaemia (see p. 80), rubella antibodies, sometimes for venereal diseases/herpes virus or hepatitis, sometimes for sickle-cell disease/thalassaemia, or glucose tolerance (if there is a family history of diabetes or large babies) and alphafeto-protein (AFP) (see p. 48).

Chorionic Villi Sampling (CVS)

Sometimes known as chorion biopsy, this tests for Down's Syndrome and has the advantage that it can be performed when you are nine weeks' pregnant instead of waiting until 16 weeks for amniocentesis. The results take two to three weeks to come through. The placenta is formed from chorionic tissue; a sample is taken by inserting a tube into the cervix or a needle into the abdomen.

1　Your vagina is swabbed with an antiseptic if the sample is taken through the cervix.
2　The whereabouts of your placenta is located by ultrasound.
3　Either a thin tube is passed through the cervix and guided to the placenta using the ultrasound, or a needle is passed through your abdomen (see Amniocentesis, p. 48).
4　A tiny fragment of chorionic tissue, the size of a few grains of rice, is sucked into the tube or needle.

There is a greater risk of miscarriage from this test and its accuracy is not precisely known. If the foetus is discovered to be abnormal then a straightforward abortion (vaginal termination under general anaesthetic) can be performed instead of the induction of labour after amniocentesis.

See Amniocentesis (p. 48) and follow the advice given there as this procedure can also be traumatic, either emotionally, physically or both.

Electronic Fetal-Heart Monitoring

The monitoring of the baby's heartbeat in pregnancy is traditionally carried out by a midwife who uses a special stethoscope which looks like a small ear trumpet. Recently, however, the use of electronic or ultrasound monitoring using small, hand-held monitors has begun to increase. No evidence as yet supports the use of these types of monitoring in pregnancy.

Do

• question your doctor or midwife thoroughly as to why they wish to do it and what effects, if any, it will have on your baby.
• refuse to be monitored in this way if you are unhappy with their explanations.

Fetal Lung Maturity

Various tests can be performed on the amniotic fluid which give information about how well the lungs of the foetus have matured, especially important in a woman whose baby must be delivered before term because of complications towards the end of her pregnancy. It is recommended that any woman who chooses to have an induction or a Caesarean should take advantage of these tests to avoid an unnecessary premature delivery and subsequent intensive care of the baby.

Internal Examinations

An internal vaginal/pelvic examination is carried out at your first ante-natal visit after a positive pregnancy test, usually about 6 weeks after your last period, to confirm the pregnancy by noting the changes to your cervix and uterus. Your doctor will take a smear, investigate the health of your vagina and cervix, check for fibroids and any other problems such as thrush.

An internal examination may be absolutely fine or it can feel intrusive and painful.

Do

• tell your doctor if you have difficulties with internals.
• ask your doctor to be gentle and to warm the speculum (if one is to be used) and to proceed very slowly.
• consciously relax your pelvic-floor muscles.
• breathe slowly and deeply and imagine yourself becoming very heavy on the couch. Breathe down

into your belly and close your eyes if necessary.

- ask your partner (if present) to hold your hand and give you whatever reassurance you need.
- ask your doctor to stop if you become tense or feel pain and to start again when you are ready.

Kick Chart (Fetal Movement Counting)

Towards the end of your pregnancy (commonly between the 30th and the 40th weeks) you may be asked to keep a 'kick chart' to record your baby's kicking episodes over a 12-hour period. In some areas a one-hour period is charted. This test verifies that your baby is continuing to thrive or acts as an early warning that there may be problems. Unfortunately, this test does not take into account the individual baby – some babies are naturally less active than others.

Do

- refuse this test if you don't want to do it. It has been found to induce unnecessary anxiety and stress.

Placental Function Tests

The placenta acts as lung and digestive tract, ferrying oxygen and nutrients to the foetus and removing carbon dioxide and waste products. Its health is verified by testing the levels of hormones, either by measuring the urine over a 24-hour period or by a blood test. These tests on their own are notoriously inaccurate with unnecessary inductions being the unfortunate result.

Do

- thoroughly question the value of these tests *in your case*.
- think before you agree to have a placental function test and if necessary get a second opinion.

Rhesus Factor

At your first pre-natal visit your blood will be tested to identify its group (A, B, AB or O) and for the presence of Rhesus factor, a protein which attaches itself to the red blood cells, which determines whether you are Rhesus negative (Rh−) or Rhesus positive (Rh+). Eighty-five per cent of women are Rh+.

If you are Rh−, the baby's father is Rh+ *and* the baby is Rh+ and some of your baby's red blood cells 'leak' into your bloodstream in late pregnancy or during or after the birth, your immune system pro-

duces antibodies to fight the invaders. This isn't a problem in a first pregnancy. In a subsequent pregnancy where the baby is Rh+, if the antibodies pass back into the baby's bloodstream, they can cause severe anaemia.

If you are identified as Rh−, another test is automatically performed to check for Rhesus antibodies. If this is your first pregnancy and there are no antibodies, an injection of serum (anti-D) will be given up to 72 hours after the birth to halt the production of antibodies so that a subsequent pregnancy will not be in jeopardy. This injection will be repeated as a preventive measure after all births, and also after an abortion or miscarriage.

If you do produce antibodies in your first pregnancy (perhaps you had an earlier miscarriage) then you and your baby will need regular checks throughout the pregnancy. Ultrasound scans will check the baby's development; amniocentesis (see p. 48) or CVS (see p. 49) will check for anaemia. In an emergency, a blood transfusion can be carried out on a baby *in utero* from 22 weeks on or immediately after the birth if a baby is induced early. You can self-prescribe if you find any of the tests distressing.

Do

- tell your doctor of any abortion and also any suspected miscarriage(s) especially if you are Rh−.

Ultrasound

This is usually first performed at about 16 weeks. High-frequency sound waves bounce off your inner organs to make pictures which can be recorded on a monitor. It is still a slightly controversial procedure because as it is relatively new no long-term effects are known. Experiments on animals have shown ultrasound to have an adverse effect on their immune system, giving reduced resistance to disease. Different levels are used on humans, however, which are thought to be perfectly safe. In any case its use in the first three months of pregnancy is not advised, nor repeated use of it later on unless absolutely necessary.

For some women the great benefit of being able to see that they are carrying a real baby, before movements are felt, helps to make the pregnancy seem more real. It is used to check where the placenta is lying; to confirm that a foetus is present and that the ovum hasn't 'blighted' or a (very rare) hydatiform mole developed; to check for ectopic pregnancy (one that has implanted in the fallopian tube), twins, fibroids, some abnormalities; to determine the sex of the baby (if required); to confirm dates, by measuring the size of the head. The procedure is:

1 You are asked to drink 2 pints (1 litre) of water. Then you wait, bursting to pee. A full bladder pushes your intestines out of the way and provides a point of reference for the technician.
2 You lie flat on a couch and your abdomen is oiled or gelled so that the probe – a 'box' about the size of a video cassette – can make good contact.
3 The technician guides the probe to and fro over your abdomen to build up a picture of your baby. If your baby is active this will have to be repeated until a satisfactory picture is obtained. The accuracy of the picture and its interpretation depends on the skill of the technician.

Do
- ask yourself whether this test is necessary – whether its results will determine the management of your pregnancy.
- make sure you take your partner or a friend. Although they have no legal right to be present, you can refuse to have the test unless they are.
- ask the operator to describe what you are seeing.
- ask if a photo can be taken: some hospitals will do this.
- consider refusing this test if you are a healthy woman with no medical complications.

Urine Tests

Urine is tested at your first and all subsequent antenatal visits for the presence of protein (kidney problems); sugar (diabetes); ketones (undernourishment); bacteria (infection). Giving a clean urine sample is a bit fiddly but well worth the effort as it is common for bacteria that are lurking externally to be washed into the urine and a false diagnosis of infection made. If you test positive for bacterial infection *and* you have no symptoms (pain/discomfort on urination or frequent urination) then ask for a re-test paying special attention to giving a clean sample as outlined below.

1 Wash your whole external genital area well with water (not soap) – you can use a bottle of warm water if you are at home (see p. 85). If you are at the hospital you will have to improvise with a paper cup or with wetting some toilet paper.
2 Hold both your labia apart before you start to pee.
3 Take a mid-stream sample of urine which has not come into contact with your skin.

X-rays

Performed routinely in pregnancy until ultrasound became freely available, X-rays should be avoided. There is a case for women with a small pelvis to be X-rayed to confirm that a vaginal birth is not possible.

Do
- avoid X-rays when pregnant.
- ask for a second opinion if your consultant diagnoses a small pelvis and suggests an X-ray.
- ask your dentist for a lead apron if you need dental X-rays during your pregnancy (but see also p. 102 on dentistry in pregnancy).

The following general guidelines are to help you think through what you may need or what may help you in labour. Pick and choose the things that appeal to you.

PLANNING FOR BIRTH

You'll need to think about the things and the people you want around you during labour – *when* you are pregnant. Some women pack their 'birth' bag months ahead of the birth – whether they are having a home or a hospital delivery – others leave it until the last minute.

It is advisable to check with hospital staff/ midwives that your plans for taking in anything from bean bags to two birth partners are acceptable. And that includes finding out their attitudes to your eating or drinking in labour – to your bringing snacks in to the hospital (or having fry-ups at home!). And then don't forget to write it in your birth plan (and in your hospital notes if necessary).

Create an Environment

It is easier to create an environment if you're having your baby at home but it is quite possible to feel at home in a hospital labour ward with a little planning. First, go to see the labour ward at the hospital and think about things you could take with you to help you relax and feel secure. For example, hospital smells can be off-putting, so take a favourite 'scent' with you, a perfume, aromatherapy oil, incense or favourite pot-pourri. If you are superstitious, take a lucky mascot. Here are some ideas of things to have around, which can all be helpful, whether you are at home or in hospital: flowers; a light scarf to drape over bright lights; a special photo, a crystal, a cross, a stone, a teddy bear – something that gives you a special strength when you look at or hold it; a personal stereo or cassette deck: if you like music make a compilation tape of your favourite pieces of music, or take a varied selection of tapes to suit your moods; hair combs or hair bands to keep your hair from bugging you; lip salve or balm in case your lips become uncomfortably dry; a favourite oil or talcum powder for massage; a toothbrush and toothpaste to refresh your mouth from time to time; a small sponge and a flannel; a delicious soap and a soft towel; some pillows or cushions and/or a bean bag – they'll smell like home and won't slip and slide around like hospital ones which are covered in plastic; a comfortable nightie or big nightshirt; if you haven't got one with you ask for two hospital gowns and wear the second one as a dressing gown; two pairs of woollen socks – your feet can become unexpectedly cold in the later stages of labour; a hot-water bottle – essential if you know yourself to be a chilly person, or chilly under stress; card or board games and some books, magazines or comics; a camera *and* enough film (a fast film so you don't need a flash) – some people take videos; change for pay telephones if you are in hospital, plus, of course, your address book or a list of telephone numbers; your homeopathic remedies; a copy of your birth plan (see p. 65) – use this as reassurance if necessary – to remind you of your personal goals.

Go with the Flow

Don't go into labour with a fixed idea of how you want it to be. Put your faith in yourself, God, Mother Earth, the Goddess of Creation, whoever, and be prepared to let yourself go, to relax and move along with whatever happens in an active, participative way. 'Go with the flow' means accepting that your experience will be different from anyone else's. *You* are not in control, your body takes over as birth involves a complex series of involuntary physical processes which will mostly just 'happen'.

Be Creative

You'll be surprised by what you want in labour: don't ignore an 'inner voice', however crazy and funny it might seem. Allow yourself to respond – it's a great opportunity to step outside your ordinary, everyday self. I know one woman who spent most of her labour on the loo and another who danced through every contraction. Your intuition, gut feeling, instinct

– call it what you may – is your most reliable guide. No one knows better than you what you need. You may feel like grunting, groaning and moving in ways that may have been unfamiliar to you before. Don't feel self-conscious, critical or judgemental – trust yourself now, more than ever before.

Get Good Support

It is important that you feel supported in labour by your partner, friend, midwife, doctor, so that you *can* let go of being in control and allow your body to do its job. Think *carefully* about who you want at the birth: they should be people who aren't going to take it personally if you feel like being alone, or if you let it all hang out if the pain becomes intense, people you can lean on and rely on, who will not bring with them fears or anxieties of their own. *Don't* invite a friend who wants to be reassured that birth isn't as bad as everyone says it is: she may inhibit you by making you constantly censor your behaviour.

It is essential that you make and maintain a good working relationship with your midwife, doctor or consultant. Be polite, friendly, reasonable and persistent if necessary with your requests. Ask for their understanding, support and help and be prepared to compromise to maintain goodwill. You can reasonably expect support from your medical practitioners: ideally, you want to feel good after every pre-natal and post-natal visit. Their quality of care 'should educate and empower, should enhance every woman's feeling of *her* ability to do what she's doing well'. (*Our Bodies Our Selves*, Boston Women's Health Collective, 1984)

Make Demands

Give yourself permission to ask for what you need when you need it. This is not a time to hold back. If you have trouble asking for what you want ordinarily then practise in your pregnancy. Make a simple demand every day – 'Please will you run my bath for me?' – to get used to the idea! During labour ask yourself from time to time 'What do I really want right now?' and then ask for it, however small, large or unusual.

Express Your Feelings

Laugh if happy, cry if sad, shout if angry – this is the one time in your life when you can really let go. Don't hold on to your feelings. They can be tremendously empowering during labour.

Make Positive Affirmations

This can provide a lifeline in labour, an important source of encouragement that will help you access your innermost resources of emotional energy. Tell yourself out loud 'I can do it – I'm brilliant – I'm so clever – I'm doing great/my best – I'm going to have a baby.' Partners can also run a barrage of positive, encouraging statements, 'Great, good – you're doing really well – keep it up – let yourself go – that's right – well done – let yourself open up – marvellous – excellent – you're doing so well – just relax – you're the best – I love you.' These are especially effective if your partner looks into your eyes and says them during and after each contraction.

Use Visualisations

Visualisation is useful for helping your body do what it has to do – to relax and to open up. In the early stages of labour imagine yourself on a sun-drenched beach, swimming in a magical river or pond, playing in a meadow – just close your eyes and let your imagination run wild. Imagine your cervix is a flower that is slowly opening. Imagine your body softening and melting. Let your mind's eye come up with images that are important and meaningful to you and use them.

Use Distractions

Play games – simple card games, crosswords or even chess . . .

Laughter is a marvellous distraction from pain. Have fun, especially in the early stages, if you can and if you feel like it. Listen to funny tapes or records, read a book that makes you laugh out loud or get someone else to read it to you. Remember funny/ridiculous times in your life. Tell jokes.

Watch television if you're at home. You can video a favourite series, a comedy or a soap, and save it all up for your labour. You could watch it in the early stages, before you go to the hospital.

Keep Your Energy Up

It is vital that you keep your energy up during labour so the following are all important:

Breathe Oxygen is an essential component of any hard physical exertion. Pain makes us tense up and breathe shallowly – that is why breathing techniques are taught in pre-natal classes as a lack of oxygen in labour can make it more difficult than it need be. However, you may find that the method you learnt becomes just another 'thing to do' and doesn't work for you in labour: use it as a starting point to follow your instincts and breathe in a way that suits you. (See also p. 40.)

Drink You must keep up an intake of fluid in labour to prevent dehydration or you may need a drip (see p. 61), which is usually preventable. Try using a bendy straw or sucking on a sponge or flannel or ice cubes if you don't feel like drinking. If you vomit all fluids then you will have to accept them intravenously (try prescribing on the vomiting first though – see p. 114).

Nourishing fluids will help your labour along: if you are at home you can make milk shakes – with banana and wheatgerm for added energy. You can drink milk hot or cold, with honey or sugar, watered down or put in the liquidiser with ice cubes. Vegetable or meat stocks are also good as are soups which have been puréed and thinned with milk. Drink plenty of freshly squeezed fruit juices (lemon, orange or grapefruit), hot or cold. Add honey or sugar to your juices and you have an energy-rich drink. Drink herb teas, ordinary tea or even a little coffee. If you are going to hospital take a Thermos flask of your favourite drink or soup and bottles of juices.

Eat Blood sugar levels must be kept high, especially during early labour. Remember, you are taking the equivalent physical exercise of climbing a mountain. Eat what you fancy in the early stages. Later on, try to have at least some small, easily digestible morsels at frequent intervals. Toast or crackers, fruit dipped in honey; porridge; stewed dried fruit; some egg custard. Many hospitals won't approve of you eating in labour in case you need a general anaesthetic but take in some crackers, a bag of fruit, a jar of honey and a sharp knife. If you don't eat you may *need* medical intervention because you will run out of energy. You *must* have something even if it is juices and lots of honey/sugar.

Rest Balance the hard physical exertion of labour with rest so that you can 'stay the course'. Spread yourself between contractions: in a long labour you might be able to sleep. Drape yourself over a bean bag or a pile of cushions. Ask your partner or midwife to rest a hand on your belly and to wake you as soon as it tightens when the next contraction begins so that you can easily find your rhythm and go with the flow of each contraction, as they climb in intensity, peak and gradually fall away. You can sleep between as many contractions as you need to, to get a good rest. Midwives and doctors may not approve of this as it has been known to slow down the contractions, but this will only be temporary.

Urinate It is essential that you pee every 1–1½ hours throughout your labour: the baby's head descending can damage a full bladder. The sensation of needing to pee may not be as noticeable as normal, but keep trying anyway as a full bladder can slow down labour. It also provides you with a distraction – something to do at regular intervals. You don't have to pee on the toilet – although walking to and from it can be beneficial it can also be a nuisance. Squat over a bucket, washing-up bowl, potty or bedpan. (See Labour pains, p. 288.) If you have difficulty in peeing, tensing and relaxing the pelvic-floor muscles a few times can start the flow.

PAIN RELIEF IN LABOUR

It is as important to know what is on offer and think about it in pregnancy as it is to decide whether to take music, flowers or a homeopathic first-aid kit into hospital with you. 'Again and again, women are grateful that they were told what might happen because, generally, it didn't. But when it did, they had only the problem itself to cope with, not their own shock and surprise as well.' (*Drugs in Pregnancy and Childbirth*, Judy Priest, Pandora, 1990)

Some women find that, uncharacteristically, they can cope with extraordinary pain in labour, while others crumble at the first contraction. *Don't try to bear more than you can.* If you need drugs, take them. Don't feel guilty. You are not a failure. You have a right to ask for pain relief. You deserve *not* to suffer. An 'active' labour is one in which you are actively involved at each stage: you can be active in deciding to ask for pain relief. Ask your hospital which drugs they prefer and which they don't offer.

The differences between women and their desires for labour are eternally fascinating. I remember well two women I delivered five years ago, both on the same day, with the same student midwife. The first was very glamorous and very neat, taking enormous trouble with her hair and make-up. She looked like a film star. She opted for an epidural and had a syntocinon drip, and I remember that as the baby's head emerged over the perineum she literally laughed the baby out. Each time she laughed, a little bit more of the baby's head emerged. It was a beautiful labour and delivery, enjoyed by her, by her husband and by me and the student. When that labour had finished, the telephone rang. It was a woman who I had booked in for a home delivery and who was now in labour. The baby was born after about four hours with no analgesia. It was a beautiful delivery and a very happy experience for us all – woman, husband, big brother (aged six), student midwife and me. In fact, the GP arrived soon after the delivery and made me giggle by asking me if I had been 'taking anything' because I was so 'high'. I reassured him that I had not, but that it had been my privilege to have been present in one day at both ends of the spectrum of obstetric care, and both had been wonderful and exciting.

(Caroline Flint, *Sensitive Midwifery*, Heinemann, 1986)

Most orthodox drugs taken in labour will cross the placenta into the baby's bloodstream and affect the baby in a similar way to the mother, but you must ask yourself what would be the value of experiencing pain above your own personal threshold when this would be so stressful that your tension and distress would also be felt by your baby. Weigh up what would be best for you *as an individual*, rather than working towards an ideal set by someone else.

A synopsis of drugs and techniques for pain relief in labour follows.

Acupuncture

Like hypnosis, acupuncture works better for some than others. There are two types: *acupuncture analgesia*, where you lie down and the needles are attached to machines which keep the points stimulated, and the pain at bay; and *therapeutic acupuncture*, which works more like homeopathy – specific points are used, the needle is not left in, to alleviate emotional and physical symptoms and help a woman cope with her relationship to the pain and stimulate the body to work more effectively.

Pros
- you have additional support.
- it won't affect you or your baby adversely.

Cons
- there is an extra person in the room.
- you may have to be immobile depending on the type of acupuncture used.
- you may not feel like having needles stuck into you (it may feel invasive).

Caudal Anaesthesia

A local anaesthetic is injected into the base of the spine to anaesthetise the vagina and the perineum. The area that is anaesthetised is more restricted than with an epidural; this technique is rarely used because it has a tendency to slow down labour. It is sometimes appropriate in the second stage where a forceps delivery is needed.

Entonox (Gas and Air)

This is a mixture of half nitrous oxide (laughing gas) and half oxygen, which is inhaled through a rubber mask. The mask has a valve which opens only when you breathe in. It takes the edge off the pain rather than providing complete relief. It is said to be of most use towards the end of the first stage especially if the contractions are severe, but also if it is too late to give pethidine or an epidural. Some women swear by it, others have found it totally useless.

It is important to start using it before a contraction begins as the effects build up slowly. The effect starts 10–20 seconds after you start to inhale it and reaches its peak after about 45–60 seconds. It then decreases in effect very quickly.

Pros

- you can control how much you use and when you use it.
- it gives fairly good pain relief, especially towards the end of the first stage, in transition and/or also if you need stitches.
- it provides extra oxygen for you and your baby.
- you can move around, as far as the rubber tube will reach.
- it is quickly exhaled and has a minimal effect on the baby.

Cons

- it doesn't work for every woman.
- it doesn't work for contractions that begin with intense pain.
- it doesn't provide effective pain relief and is therefore not good for very strong pains.
- it makes many women feel out of control and confused because of feeling slightly 'high'.
- some find the smell of the rubber tube unpleasant.
- some women hate having a mask over their face – it makes them feel trapped.
- some women feel sick or dizzy.
- it can stop working after a while.
- it takes a while to get the hang of it.

Do

- get some instruction early in your labour and practise using it when your contractions are manageable.
- try it out if you are in pain in the first stage because it is worth using if it works.
- breathe deeply but at a normal rate as it is not as effective with shallow breathing.
- start using it at the first sign of a contraction. Ask your partner or midwife to place a hand on the underneath bit of your 'bump' just above your pubic bone if you have difficulty feeling when the contraction first starts.
- take a few deep breaths, between 3 and 6, put the mask down and carry on dealing with your contraction in the ways that have been working for you. The effect of the gas will build up of its own accord and hopefully peak as your contraction peaks. (If you continue to breathe in the gas and air during a contraction then you will feel dozy and unable to judge when the next one begins.)
- suck a sponge between contractions if your mouth gets dry.

Epidural Anaesthesia

Although a local anaesthetic is injected into the spine, it is not a spinal anaesthetic and only affects the nerves that supply the pelvic cavity with sensation (pain!). It doesn't affect mobility. This means that most women have control of their legs even when the pain is gone. There are no side effects to the baby.

A needle is inserted between two vertebrae in the lower back into a canal called the epidural space. A very fine tube is threaded through the needle, which is then withdrawn, the tube is taped in place and a local anaesthetic injected into the tube. This numbs the nerves from the waist down. 'Top-ups' can be given if the pain returns.

Pros

- you are fully conscious.
- it is an effective painkiller and is therefore good for a forceps or Caesarean delivery.
- because it deals with pain, emotional distress is also relieved.

Cons

- partners are sometimes asked to leave the room whilst the anaesthetist inserts the epidural. This can take up to 20 minutes, perhaps more if insertion is difficult during which you will be asked to lie perfectly still (on your side). The combination of having to be still, contractions coming regularly and painfully, and lacking your primary support can be distressing.

- it may work on only one side of the body.
- it doesn't always take effect, which can be very distressing – the pain can seem overwhelming if you had thought you would soon be pain-free and were let down.
- it lowers the blood pressure, which can cause dizziness, nausea and even fear.
- some women feel cold and shivery immediately after the anaesthetic is injected.
- it is difficult to push in the second stage because the area is numb and the likelihood of a forceps delivery is higher.
- you can't move around.
- one intervention begets at least three others. You are likely to have to put up with three or more of the following: breaking of your waters (see p. 63); an electrode may be attached to your baby's head (see p. 62); you may be connected to an external monitor to record your contractions (see p. 62) and/or an intravenous drip (see p. 60); you may be given syntocinon (see p. 63), and/or a catheter (see p. 60).

The after-effects of an epidural vary: women have experienced back pain, headache, general soreness, numbness and/or aching legs, and, very rarely, complete numbness from the waist down, which can take up to 72 hours to clear.

General Anaesthetic

A general anaesthetic is sometimes administered for a Caesarean section, usually only in an emergency. Some hospitals will agree to your partner being present to receive your baby, others will want your partner to wait outside and will bring the baby out when they are sure all is well.

Pros

- If there are complications, especially if the baby is in distress, a Caesarean can be performed very quickly.

Cons

- you are not conscious for the birth of your baby.
- although the art of anaesthesia is much improved these days and the risk to your health less than it used to be, it is physically stressful.
- you may take a while to recover from the anaesthetic: some people vomit or feel nauseous and

others feel high and take a long time to feel fully themselves again.

- bonding with your baby can take longer.
- afterpains can feel worse because you were not accustomed to the intensity of contractions during labour.

Homeopathy

Like therapeutic acupuncture, homeopathy works by treating the psychological state of a woman in labour, her fear, anxiety, rage, disappointment, etc., and also by easing the minor physical complications like exhaustion, a cervix that isn't dilated, or tired muscles. If you have chosen to have a labour kit (see p. 302) and don't have a homeopath present, your partner can take charge of prescribing so you don't have yet another thing to think about.

Pros

- it's gentle and doesn't have side effects.
- you have the additional support of a person you trust if you have chosen to have your homeopath present.
- your homeopath can put together a selection of remedies (your labour kit) specifically for you if you don't want an extra person at the birth.

Cons

- you may be too busy to work out which remedy to take when.
- you have an additional person at the birth if your homeopath is present.
- you may get fed up with the sugary taste of the tablets.

Hypnosis

When hypnosis works, a person is fully conscious but is not aware of pain. Like acupuncture, some surgical operations have been carried out on people who respond particularly well to hypnosis, without them feeling any pain. Some people are easily hypnotised and some need several sessions for it to work. It is important to begin your 'training' during your pregnancy with a hypnotist who is willing to attend the birth.

Pros

- you have additional support in labour.
- it won't affect you or your baby adversely.

Cons
- there is an extra person in the room.

Paracervical Block

A local anaesthesia which is used in the first stage. Local anaesthetic is injected into the groin area where the nerves that feed the uterus collect, providing pain relief in the uterus without affecting the contractions. It is easy to administer and effective in a large percentage of cases for up to 4 hours. It is more widely used in the US and in Scandinavia but has not as yet gained acceptance in this country.

Perineal Block

Local anaesthetic is injected into the perineum to anaesthetise the area where an episiotomy is to be performed, or a tear repaired. The effect lasts about an hour and a half, provides complete pain relief during stitching and can be repeated if necessary. Sometimes it doesn't work well or for very long in which case more can be injected. Very occasionally it doesn't work in which case another method of local anaesthesia can be used.

Do
- complain loudly if it hurts when you are being stitched up.

Pethidine

An analgesic drug derived from morphine. It is used after labour is established and administered by intramuscular injection. The digestive system has slowed down and the stomach will not now efficiently absorb drugs taken orally. Pethidine relieves pain as well as producing a sense of well-being and even euphoria. It takes about 15 minutes to work and the effect lasts about four hours.

Pros
- it works well at relieving pain for many women even in small doses.
- it gives women a break; many women sleep for some time after a pethidine injection, sleeping through contractions and waking feeling more refreshed.
- it has a softening effect on the cervix which will help it to dilate.

Cons
- it may have no effect whatsoever.

- some women feel 'high' and can still feel the pain through a drugged haze.
- it crosses the placenta, relaxing the baby so that its breathing may be affected after birth.
- it can cause temporary amnesia: some women have difficulty in remembering their labour, which can be distressing.

Pethidine plus Phenergan or Sparine

Phenergan and Sparine are both tranquillisers which help relieve anxiety, nausea and vomiting. They can be useful early in labour: if it is a long one, and sleep is needed but not possible because of pain.

They accentuate all the pros and cons of Pethidine alone.

Pudendal Block

Local anaesthetic is injected into the side wall of the vagina to anaesthetise the nerves that feed the vagina, perineum and labia. This is used in some instances before a forceps delivery, especially a low forceps. It is a good alternative to a general anaesthetic but has been largely replaced by epidural anaesthesia.

Cons
- one side only is free of pain.
- the injection itself can cause bruising.

T(E)NS (transcutaneous nerve stimulation)

This is a safe method of pain relief that has not proved very effective in trials conducted so far. Two pads are attached with plasters to the back, one on either side of the spine, and are connected to a small hand-held generator. This conducts a low electric current to the nerves that feed the uterus. The generator can be switched on during contractions to block the pain.

Pros
- there are no side effects.
- you can be mobile.

Cons
- it has not been found very effective so far.
- it has to be used from the beginning of labour to be of any use.
- if it helps in early labour, its effectiveness with strong labour is limited.

Tranquillisers

These are sometimes offered early in the first stage if labour starts in the evening, if it is progressing slowly and the woman is anxious or exhausted. It is hoped that she will rest and/or sleep for a while to build up some reserves of energy to carry on with her labour. She might do just as well to pour herself a glass of wine or whisky. (See Slow Labour, p. 113.)

MEDICAL INTERVENTIONS IN LABOUR

The major interventions are internal examinations, enemas, inductions, drips, breaking of the waters, blood-pressure monitoring, catheterisation, fetal heart monitoring, episiotomies, forceps deliveries and Caesarean sections. The shaving of pubic hair is now rare.

Interventions can be and are life-saving. However, some women feel that the experience of birth has been taken away from them; that one intervention leads to another; that they feel increasingly powerless and passive; and the emotional trauma of some interventions can lead to post-natal depression.

It is important to question all interventions thoroughly. The routine administration of anything for the convenience of a system (the hospital) or a person other than the woman in labour (such as the obstetrician) is wrong. If it is appropriate and necessary you may feel disappointed that you have had to resort to it. Try to 'go with the flow' if you find yourself in this situation – the intervention may save your life and that of your baby. Here are some suggestions to help you minimise or heal the trauma.

Do
- understand each intervention as fully as possible during your pregnancy. Discuss them with your doctor and midwife in as much detail as you need to.
- make a good birth plan (see p. 65). Decide ahead of time what you are prepared to fight against unless a crisis demands that it be done. Ask that you be consulted fully and at each stage if an intervention is required but not stated on your birth plan.
- use homeopathic treatment and/or the self-help measures outlined below for each intervention if it is necessary.
- build a co-operative relationship with midwives,

doctors and other hospital staff so that you feel part of what is happening, not a victim to it.

Blood-pressure Monitoring

If you are having a hospital birth your blood pressure will be taken at regular intervals. Some women find this distracting, that it breaks their concentration, others hardly notice.

Do
- make sure you don't have to change position to have it done.
- ask that verbal reassurance be given each time it is taken. The well-intentioned but misguided habit of not talking to women in labour can create an undertow of anxiety. Partners can ask the midwife to confirm that all is well if he or she forgets.

Breaking of the Waters

See Inductions, p. 63.

Caesarean Section

Caesarean section has only recently become a safe operation and due to the increasing effectiveness of the technique has become a routine intervention in some countries. The major reasons for performing a Caesarean are: a small or malformed pelvis; fibroids or ovarian cysts lying below the baby; placenta praevia, where the placenta is lying over the neck of the uterus; the baby is too large to pass through the pelvis or is in an exceptionally awkward position, especially if the shoulder is presenting and in some instances of breech presentation; the first stage is long and arduous and the cervix is not dilating; labour is induced and the induction doesn't work; the baby is in distress in the first stage as there is a danger of it suffering from lack of oxygen, which can cause brain damage or even death; the mother has pre-eclampsia, eclampsia, an active attack of genital herpes, diabetes, kidney disease or chronic hypertension; the mother haemorrhages; and if there is a known history of difficulty with vaginal births. An 'elective' Caesarean is one that is planned and agreed to before the birth, because the mother's pelvis is small for example. A date is set before the birth is due for admission to hospital. An 'emergency' Caesarean is decided on after the labour has started because of an unanticipated complication such as a badly positioned baby or a very long labour.

Caesareans are performed under epidural or

general anaesthesia. With an epidural you are conscious and can watch your baby being lifted out and hold the baby immediately. It is safer for the baby (because the drugs used in general anaesthesia can affect it) and recovery is usually quicker. (See Epidural Anaesthesia, p. 55.) With a general anaesthetic you are unconscious throughout the birth and for some time afterwards. It can be administered quickly and is always the preferred method in an emergency.

In an emergency it is very important that your midwife or partner keeps up a comforting 'banter' of reassurance and information, both physically and verbally.

> If you are the midwife who has been with the woman during labour or prior to her elective section, your main duty is to explain over and over again exactly what is going to happen. . . . having an operation is the nearest brush with death that most of us experience in our lives. We are literally giving our body up to the care of another. Most people feel that they will never wake up after an operation, that the end has come. To have the physical comforting of another at this time can make all the difference in the world.
> (Caroline Flint, *Sensitive Midwifery*,
> Heinemann, 1986)

If you have a general anaesthetic you will not be given a 'premed', an injection to relax you and make you sleepy before you go to the operating theatre, as it contains morphine or a morphine-based drug which can cross the placenta and affect the baby, but you will be given atropine to reduce the secretions from the mucous membranes of the chest, nose and throat. You may be asked to breathe oxygen for a few minutes to give your baby an extra boost immediately before the anaesthetic is given. An intravenous drip is inserted into a vein in your arm and a small amount of anaesthetic is injected.

If you are having an epidural Caesarean, see p. 58 for a full description of the procedure. A screen is erected at shoulder or waist level so that you can't see the operation itself. You can ask for it to be lowered when your baby is actually being lifted out – the excitement of seeing your baby emerging will divert your attention from the operation and in any case at this time there won't be anything gory to see.

With both types of Caesarean your pubic area is shaved and a catheter inserted into the urethra to drain urine from your bladder. The incision in the abdomen is either vertical (in the middle below the navel) or more usually transverse, known as the bikini cut, running just below the top of the pubic hair and above the pubic bone. When the hair grows back the scar is virtually invisible.

The muscles of the abdomen are gently separated and the organs inspected. The bladder is cut free from the uterus and a small incision made in the lower part of the uterus. The amniotic sac bulges out, if still intact, and makes quite a noise on being cut. The baby is then lifted out, sometimes with the help of forceps, and any fluid or mucus removed from the mouth, nose or eyes. The cord is clamped and the baby then handed to the midwife or the mother, if she is conscious and the baby is breathing well, or the partner if present.

An injection of ergometrine or syntometrine is given to contract the uterus and about 40 seconds later the placenta is delivered. The organs and muscles are stitched back into place with two or three layers of stitches; the bladder is reattached to the uterus and the four layers of abdominal muscles sewn up one by one with fine, dissolving stitches. The skin is either stitched or closed with metal clips which are removed when the scar has healed. The operation takes under an hour from start to finish. A Caesarean scar takes about three months to heal completely.

A midwife will be present to care for the baby immediately after the birth. Hospital policies vary with regard to partners being present and although most will allow partners if an epidural has been administered, they may not if you have a general anaesthetic. Check this at your ante-natal visits and specify in your birth plan (p. 65) and/or on your hospital notes that your partner's presence has been agreed to (if it has). Ask your midwife to take photos of the baby emerging, and also that your partner and baby will be with you when you come round. Ask for your midwife to be on hand to take a photo of your first meeting with your baby – your wooziness from the anaesthetic will mean you won't remember this moment and it's wonderful to have it recorded.

Complications include haemorrhaging (loss of blood); injury to organs close to the uterus (the bladder, bowel or ovaries); post-operative infection or blood clots; and emotional distress. Many, if not most, women have an overwhelming desire to push out their babies themselves and a Caesarean, or even a forceps delivery, can cause distress or feelings of failure.

You may feel that you have given over the birth of your baby to somebody else. Afterwards, it is no solace to be told that in another age you would have died. Feelings can range from distress to rage, and it is important to talk and talk to heal emotional wounds, to prevent depression and isolation. Knowing other women who have been through the same experience is helpful.

With subsequent pregnancies the scar may feel sore as the uterus grows – as it stretches so does the scar. Repeat Caesareans will be performed in the same scar, but more and more women are successfully delivering subsequent babies vaginally. You need reassurance, information, encouragement and support to give you the self-confidence to do so if you want a vaginal delivery after you've had a Caesarean.

The following advice applies to when you are conscious before a general anaesthetic if you are having one.

If you are having a general anaesthetic you will not be allowed to take anything by mouth. A few drops of Rescue Remedy rubbed into the forehead works wonders for anxiety and fear. If you are having an epidural and are allowed to take homeopathic remedies then you may need one for emotional distress. Try *Lycopodium* for anxiety, *Argentum nitricum* for anxiety with a strong feeling of failure, *Aconite* for fear or *Pulsatilla* for the weeps. (For information about the post-natal recovery period after a Caesarean see p. 127.)

Do

- prepare yourself adequately if you are having an elective Caesarean.
- go with the flow if you are unprepared for it. If you have been trying for a natural birth remember that you have done your best: you did what you could and now it's time for modern medicine to make things easy, to do its best for you and your baby.
- breathe steadily, slowly and deeply.
- relax. You can let go now, you are being taken care of, there is nothing more that you have actively to do and your baby will soon be with you.
- ask for support, information, for the people with you to talk to you, to hold your hand, to stroke your head. Whatever it is that you need, ask for it now.
- allow your feelings to surface, especially if your partner is with you.
- ask your partner or midwife to talk to you continuously – encouraging, soothing, reassuring, loving words – the silences in an operating theatre can be especially hard to take.
- let the medical staff know what you are feeling if you are finding it difficult to cope and ask for reassurance if you need it.

- use affirmations or guided visualisations (see p. 54) to take your mind off what is happening to your body. Ask your partner or midwife to hold your hand and talk you through something pleasant in your past or your imagination!

Catheterisation

A catheter is used with both forceps and Caesarean section deliveries (and with an epidural) to minimise the risk of injury to the bladder as a full bladder is vulnerable to being damaged during birth (especially during the second stage). A fine tube is inserted into the urethra up into the bladder to draw off urine as it gathers. If you have had an epidural you won't feel anything. If you haven't you may feel a strange pulling or drawing sensation as it is inserted. Some women find them painful on insertion and uncomfortable once they are in place. After a Caesarean section the catheter may be left in place for up to 48 hours. If you are unable to urinate after the birth a catheter is used to drain the bladder (see Retention of Urine, p. 115).

A catheter can leave the urethra feeling sore and sensitive, rather like mild cystitis.

Staphysagria may help if the urinary tract is painful or *Arnica* if it feels sore and bruised. You may need to alternate these two remedies if both are indicated.

Do

- relax your pelvic-floor muscles (p. 43) when the catheter is being inserted.
- ask the midwife or doctor to stop and proceed slowly if it is uncomfortable.
- urinate frequently after the birth even if it hurts. 'Bottle wash' (p. 85) or pee in a warm bath until it ceases to be painful.

Drips

An intravenous drip is used to give glucose to women who have become dehydrated, or salt to keep blood pressure steady or oxytocin to speed up labour. You can avoid a glucose drip by keeping up a regular intake of fluids, especially if they contain honey or sugar. If you are vomiting and unable to keep anything down you will need a glucose drip. The disadvantages are that it makes mobility difficult and can feel uncomfortable.

Do

- carry on being as active as you can: ask for the drip to be attached to a mobile pole. Ask your partner to move it around after you.

- ask that the drip be put into the arm or hand you use least.

Don't

- forget to urinate frequently, even if you don't feel like it, every 1–1½ hours.

Enemas

Enemas were an aberration of hospital routine that are almost never administered now. A tube is inserted into the anus and half a pint of soapy water runs into the rectum from a bag held above the body. The liquid is held in the rectum for a short time and then evacuated along with the contents of the rectum. Enemas were performed from good intentions, with the idea that an empty bowel is desirable in labour, but this is virtually impossible. If you clear the rectum, as an enema will, then the contents of the large bowel and small intestine simply move down. Enemas can be uncomfortable and sometimes painful – nature works well enough as most women have a bout of diarrhoea before labour starts. Others find they empty their bowels during the first stage.

In any event most women pass some faeces during the second stage (the delivery) and this is usually dealt with kindly and considerately. Your midwife will protect your emerging baby by holding a pad against your anus.

Do

- empty your bowels as frequently as you need to during your labour.
- ask for reassurance and support from your partner, friend or supportive midwife if you feel ashamed, embarrassed or disgusted.
- try to see the funny side of it.

Don't

- worry or be ashamed if you pass faeces during birth. It is a normal, healthy function of the body. You are not alone.

Episiotomy

The routine snipping of the perineum during childbirth is now being questioned. It is a necessary intervention with a forceps delivery and to hasten delivery if the baby is distressed, but there are many experienced midwives who have delivered hundreds of babies, whose 'mothers' have not even torn, save for minor, first-degree tears that heal of their own accord.

A woman whose birth is managed well by a competent midwife rarely tears and rarely needs an episiotomy. A tear is more difficult to stitch than an episiotomy but it is easier to heal and therefore many women are preferring now to risk a tear than to be cut.

Things often happen so fast it isn't easy to think of taking a remedy. *Aconite* will help you to regain control if everything is going too fast and you are feeling panicked. One dose of any potency will be enough to slow things down a little and prevent a tear.

Do

- prepare the perineum during the last month of pregnancy by massaging almond or olive oil into it, by visualising it becoming supple and stretchy, by sitting in the 'tailor pose' to encourage your pelvic-floor muscles to stretch and become more supple.
- maintain an upright posture during labour especially during second stage (supported standing or squatting, kneeling on all fours, etc.) as an episiotomy is rarely needed in this position.
- massage oil into the perineum as your baby crowns. Some women have found *Calendula* oil especially effective.
- apply hot pads to the perineum once the head is crowning, sanitary pads or flannels wrung out in very hot water to which 7 drops of Rescue Remedy and a squirt of *Calendula* tincture have been added. This is soothing and encourages blood to flood into the area, which will further relax and stretch the tissues.
- visualise your perineum opening like a flower.
- open your mouth wide to assist it – there's an important link between your mouth and your vagina.
- make 'raspberry' noises with your lips flapping as this helps the perineum to relax.
- take your time – there's no great hurry.
- rather than trying to push, let your body do the work.
- ask for constant reassurance that you are doing fine, that your body is coping brilliantly, that your baby is nearly with you.
- laugh or cry if you feel like it, you are about to meet your baby.

Don't

- tense up in fear that you will tear or be cut.

Fetal-Heart Monitoring

The baby's heartbeat is monitored regularly through labour because a deviation from its regular pattern can indicate that it is in distress. The heartbeat can be heard by placing an ear, a stethoscope or ear trumpet on the abdomen near where the baby's heart is lying. Portable electronic monitors are now often used and can be applied whatever position you choose to labour in.

Sophisticated, electronic fetal-heart monitors that also print out a graph of the heartbeat are valuable in high-risk births where they can be life-saving but their use in low-risk births is questionable, especially if everything is going well. There are two types of monitor, both of which are hooked up to a machine that 'prints out' the contractions in a graph. One is attached by a strap to your abdomen – the strap itself can be uncomfortable, even painful at times when the contractions peak, and the strap tightens. You can't be fully mobile although the monitor can be attached if you are on all fours. The other type of monitor involves clipping or screwing an electrode to the baby's head. This is attached by a wire to the machine. The waters will have to be broken if they haven't already done so. The disadvantages are that it may be painful for the baby and can cause a sore spot on the scalp. It is not possible to be mobile. In both cases the machine becomes a hypnotic focus of attention and the woman in labour can be inadvertently ignored.

Different remedies will help depending on how you feel: *Aconite* if you are shocked or afraid; *Staphysagria* if your body feels 'invaded' – especially if your baby has an electrode on its scalp; *Pulsatilla* if you feel despairing and miserable. Take *Arnica* from time to time to help minimise any bruising to your baby's scalp.

Do
- negotiate for a hand-held monitor to be used to check your baby's heartbeat unless you are in a high-risk group and you trust your doctor's advice. Seek a second opinion if you want to be absolutely sure.
- ask that the monitoring be incorporated into your rhythm of labour.
- ask that you be verbally reassured every time that it is done. Make sure your partner asks for this reassurance if the midwife or doctor forgets.
- ask that the machine be turned so you can't see it, or draped with a cloth (if you are connected to the full works) so that you are not mesmerised by its every quiver.

- ask to be put in any position other than lying on your back if you are uncomfortable.

Don't
- let this test distract you from the rhythm of your labour as it can create unnecessary tension.

Forceps Deliveries

Forceps are used once the baby is at least two-thirds of the way down the vagina and stuck (if they become stuck higher up a Caesarean will be performed instead). Sometimes they are used simply to turn the baby's head if it is poorly positioned, or to turn it and then 'lift' or guide it out.

You will have to lie down on a hospital bed with your feet resting in stirrups. A catheter is inserted (see p. 60) and a local anaesthetic injected into the vagina to numb it. The forceps – Wrigleys or Keillands – look like a pair of salad servers. They are gently placed, a blade at a time, up and around the head of your baby and the handles locked together. Your doctor will then guide the baby out with each contraction. It can feel as if your insides are being dragged out – they aren't – but it is only for a very short time. It usually takes no longer than a couple of minutes.

A suction or vacuum delivery (also known as ventouse) is not as physically, and therefore emotionally, traumatic but it can take longer to insert. A cup is fitted to the baby's head and the suction takes about five minutes to build up to full strength. This type of forceps delivery is increasing in popularity because it is much kinder to mothers and babies: it is less painful because an episiotomy isn't needed and although your baby's scalp may swell where the cup was applied there is no risk of the bruising to face or head which is common with Wrigleys' or Keillands' deliveries.

Hospital staff need to be sympathetic and give lots of information while a forceps delivery is being carried out. Good pain relief is also essential. A forceps delivery is more common if your baby is premature; if its head is big; if it is badly positioned (for example, breech); if it is posterior and needs turning round to come out; if you have had an epidural (because the loss of sensation means you won't feel the urge to push); if you've become tired; if the second stage has gone on for too long – typically for two hours with no results because you and/or the uterus are exhausted; if your baby is suffering distress in the second stage with the contents of its bowel (meconium) in the amniotic fluid.

Take Rescue Remedy throughout, either in sips of water, or by sucking on a sponge that has been dipped in the water containing Rescue Remedy, or by sponging your forehead with the water. (See Healing after Labour, p. 127, or Emotional Distress, p. 123, for remedies to help with healing after a forceps delivery.)

Do

- prepare yourself before the birth **not** to have an overwhelming expectation of pushing the baby out yourself.
- tell your consultant or hospital registrar that if you need forceps you would prefer a suction delivery and check that staff trained and experienced in performing this will be available. State your preference on your birth plan (see p. 65).
- go with the flow.
- relax your legs – consciously and repeatedly.
- remember that it is for the best and that your baby will soon be born.
- ask your partner or midwife to hold your hand or cradle or hug you.
- be reassured by your birth partner. It can help if he or she looks into your eyes (partly to distract) and says soothing, repetitive things to you.
- count to 100 slowly, with the aid of your partner, and the baby should be out before you have finished.

Inductions

Inductions are carried out if there is more than one baby, if you have diabetes or high blood pressure, if there is an abnormality in the baby or if the baby is too large or too small – and are far too common in babies that are 'late', an unnecessary intervention because the accurate calculation of dates is so difficult and most women go into labour at their own right time. Inductions can also be carried out for the convenience of the hospital or obstetrician, or even the parents, and are then of even more dubious value.

Synthetic hormones are used to bring on labour. Prostaglandin is given in the form of pessaries or cream, inserted into the vagina every 6–12 hours, which usually brings on labour after two doses; Syntocinon is given intravenously (via a drip, see p. 60) either to instigate labour or to speed it up. The possible side effects of these drugs are vomiting, diarrhoea, migraine or vaginal irritation from prostaglandin and oedema and high blood pressure from Syntocinon, and jaundice in your baby. 'Induced' contractions are always more violent and prolonged

than natural ones and can contribute to you feeling powerless and out of control. The contractions don't follow a wave-like course but become intense quickly and remain intense for a longer period. Women who are induced are more likely to ask for an epidural to reduce the pain.

'Breaking the waters' is another method of induction. Also known as artificial rupture of the membranes, it is performed by puncturing the bag of waters with an instrument similar in shape to a crochet hook. The disadvantages are that it can feel uncomfortable; it increases the risk of infection, especially if it is done in hospital; the baby's head and your cervix are no longer cushioned by the amniotic fluid and the stronger contractions that ensue can be harder to cope with. The waters are also sometimes broken when labour is well under way to speed up the last of the cervical dilation and to check the amniotic fluid for meconium if the heartbeat shows some distress. If induction is proposed:

Do

- have sexual intercourse. Semen contains prostaglandin which can start labour.
- consult an acupuncturist.
- try homeopathy. Take *Caulophyllum 30* every 2 hours for up to 6 doses over the course of a day. Wait for three days and repeat. If labour still hasn't started, your baby may not be ready yet to be born.
- eat a strong curry. Spicy food can speed things up!
- take some vigorous exercise – a long, brisk walk can bring labour on.
- See also False Labour, p. 111, and Late Labour, p. 112.

NB If none of the above has any effect the chances are that your dates aren't quite right or you and your baby aren't quite ready.

Don't

- be frightened of having a 'dry' birth if your waters rupture (naturally or otherwise). Your amniotic waters are constantly being replenished, and will continue to be throughout your labour.

Internal Examinations

Vaginal examinations are necessary at various points during labour to monitor progress. They can be painful partly because women are often asked to lie on their backs while they are carried out. Some midwives are happy to do internals while women are in their favourite positions – lying on a bean bag, leaning against the bed or even standing or squatting but they may still be painful.

The following remedies will all help after an 'internal': *Aconite*, if you are in a lot of pain and very shocked; *Chamomilla*, if you are in a lot of pain and very angry; *Staphysagria*, if you are very angry and indignant and resentful; or *Arnica*, if you feel sore and bruised.

Do

- check with the midwife when you make your birth plan (p. 65) what the procedure is and whether it can be adapted if necessary.
- relax, breathe slowly and evenly and count slowly to 100.
- ask for a breathing space if the midwife can't find what she is looking for and you have been prone for too long. Get up and walk around and then let her try again.
- ask for your midwife to remove her hand during contractions.

Shaving of Pubic Hair

Shaving of pubic hair is rare nowadays but some women are still shaved routinely on admission to hospital. This is a pointless practice that should be resisted by all women in labour. There is no evidence to support its usefulness and it can be painful, especially if the skin is inadvertently 'nicked'. When the hairs grow back after the birth the itching is intolerable as the hairs grow through and the stubble scrapes the delicate skin on the inner thighs.

Don't
- agree to having this done – unless, of course, you are having a Caesarean, in which case ask if the shaving can be restricted to the area over the pubic bone only.

POST-NATAL TESTS (INTERVENTIONS) FOR THE BABY

Immediately after the birth, and again five minutes later, your baby is tested for its general vitality. This is the Apgar test and points are given for heart rate: 0 = absent, 1 = less than 100 beats per minute, 2 = more than 100 beats per minute; breathing: 0 = absent, 1 = slow or irregular, 2 = regular; skin colour: 0 = blue, 1 = body pink and extremities blue, 2 = pink all over; muscle tone: 0 = limp, 1 = some

movements, 2 = active movements; and reflex response: 0 = absent, 1 = grimacing only, 2 = crying. Most babies score between 7 and 10 points at birth and those who score low immediately after the birth usually score 9 or 10 after five minutes.

After the birth your baby will be measured, checked and tested for the following: weight; length from head to toe; the circumference of the head; the genitals – to make sure they are all in order; the anus – to make sure it is not blocked; the heart and lungs – to make sure they are strong and healthy; the pulse; the palate of the mouth – for cleft palate; the jaw – for dislocation; the joints – especially the legs and hips for dislocation; the legs and feet – for clubfoot and to make sure the legs are the same length; the spine – to make sure the bones are in the right place; the liver and spleen – to make sure they are the correct size; the bones of the skull and the fontanelles; the chest and breathing.

A Guthrie test is performed on babies when they are about a week old: some blood is taken from the heel by pricking it with a needle – this is commonly called a 'heel prick'. The blood is checked for phenyl-ketonuria (a form of mental handicap) and for thyroid function, both of which are treatable if detected early enough. Heel pricks are sometimes repeated in babies where the blood-sugar levels are being checked at regular intervals after the birth if diabetes is suspected. Vitamin K is given to help the clotting of blood, either as drops orally, or by injection. Recent research has shown that it may save lives. Although an oral dose (by mouth) may be kinder to your baby than an intramuscular injection it is not as effective. Talk this issue through with your GP or consultant.

Occasionally babies are shocked or distressed by some of the post-natal checks especially the heel prick. As you will probably be taking *Arnica*, traces of it will pass through to your breastmilk and deal with any shock or bruising they have suffered. If the baby is more actively distressed, and this doesn't pass off, consider giving *Aconite* or *Staphysagria* depending on whether fright or anger is predominant.

Do
- ask your doctor or midwife to communicate with you as they are working through the above tests. You might ask them to give you a running commentary on their findings as they go along. You may have to keep asking, 'What are you doing now? What are you looking for now? Can you please tell me what you are listening for?' and so on. Doctors don't realise that their silence can be interpreted by some parents as a sign that some-

thing is wrong, when so much hangs on their pronouncement of health. Your doctor may be exhausted, busy and find it easier and quicker to work in silence, or may be used to working without communicating.

- step in if you feel your baby is being treated unnecessarily casually. Some midwives fling newborn babies around to demonstrate how resilient they are. This is unkind and unnecessary. You have every right to ask for your baby to be treated gently.
- hold your baby if vitamin K is administered and ask for reassurance about what is happening. Rub a little Rescue Remedy into the injection site and give *Aconite* if he or she is very upset.
- ask to hold the baby while the heel is pricked or an injection given so that you can cuddle, comfort and gently reassure, by talking calmly about what is happening and why.
- offer the breast once all the checks have been performed. Cuddle your baby close and let him or her suck for as long as they want. Some babies fall soundly asleep at this stage while others are curious about their new surroundings and take their time looking around.

NB You and your baby will be expected to attend a post-natal check with your doctor around six weeks after the birth (this is changing to a check-up after three weeks and one at eight weeks) at which your doctor will examine you to make sure you are recovering well. Your baby will not usually be examined unless there are any problems but will be weighed naked.

BIRTH PLAN

With all the information that's gone before you are probably ready to start preparing your birth plan. Before you do, though, read the birth chapter (pp. 105–15) to get more of a sense of what it is *you* are looking for, *you* are wanting for your birth.

Planning for birth requires careful thought. Fashions in childbirth change and contradictory information abounds on how to get it right. Your plan needs to reflect what you want and hope for as well as possible compromises.

If you are planning on a hospital birth ask your doctor or your hospital whether they have a birth policy. Check whether it is their policy to encourage women to be involved in their babies' births, to make a birth plan and for the staff to support it. If it isn't

and this is important to you, try to find a hospital or doctor who is sympathetic to your needs.

Discuss your plan with your partner and as many other people as you need. Use the following steps as a rough guide:

- Write down what you want the birth to be. If this is difficult, talk to women who already have children and use the Complaints section (pp. 107–15) to give you ideas of what you might want.
- Ask your partner to do the same.
- Read these out to each other so that you can start to work out what you want based on your shared ideas.
- Understand what really matters to each of you.
- Make a list of what you would particularly like to happen, and another of what you would particularly like to avoid.
- State these requests as 'preferences' to avoid being labelled as pushy.
- Write out your plan in the spirit of 'friendly co-operation', not as a series of demands, so as to gain the full support of the medical profession.
- Make sure you state that you are willing to make changes at any stage but would like to be consulted first.
- Discuss your plan with your midwives and/or consultant and be prepared to negotiate and compromise if they express concern over a particular request.
- Re-write your plan if necessary.
- Give a copy to the midwife, doctor or consultant and ask that it be attached to your notes.
- Don't forget to take a copy into hospital with you when you go into labour.

If you have given birth before, writing a birth plan will probably be easier: try to remember what worked and what didn't and just jot it down.

Specific issues to think about and include if relevant:
- Birth partners. Who will be attending the birth? Your partner, a friend or relative, homeopath, acupuncturist, active birth teacher? State their names and the roles they may have during the labour and birth. Stand your ground over having your partner plus one other supportive person (if you want one): some hospitals draw the line at one extra person only. If you have two, one can take a break without you feeling abandoned.
- How would you like to be treated? Be clear about the sort of birth you would like and therefore what sort of support you need from the medical staff. Make sure you can move around in labour and

give birth in a position that is comfortable for you. State your preference for a bed on the floor or a birthing-chair or birthing pool (if the hospital has these on offer). Ask that medical professionals communicate their findings in *all* their checks to you and/or your partner, that they do not, for example, remain silent after listening to the baby's heart and then leave the room. State your preference to be attended by a midwife or one of the midwives who has seen you through your pregnancy. Ask what your options are if you and a particular midwife don't get on.

- How would you like your birth partner(s) to be treated? Make sure that they won't be asked to leave the room for *any* reason, including a forceps delivery or a Caesarean, unless this is performed as an emergency measure.
- Are you willing to have medical students present if you are delivering in a teaching hospital? You have a right to refuse this. You may make your acceptance conditional on their attending the whole of your labour – relatively few medical students see a birth from beginning to end.
- State your attitude towards induction, routine procedures on admission such as breaking of the waters, shaving of pubic hair or enema (thankfully rare nowadays), and medical interventions in general (see pp. 58–64). State your preference, for example, not to be given an episiotomy, and be firm on issues that are important to you. 'If I tear I do not agree to being stitched by a student.'
- Make a list of what you will probably take in with you (see pp. 52–3).
- Which drugs do you hope to avoid? Which do you feel happy to use? Decide what you are willing to try, what you are willing to take and what you definitely don't want *unless all else fails* (see Pain Relief, p. 54). It doesn't matter *what* you have as long as you feel you need it, and you can always change your mind. Don't let yourself feel guilty or a failure if you eventually opt for something you had originally decided against.
- How do you want your baby treated at the birth? State your preference for soft lights and little noise. Ask that your baby be given to you without delay and for as long as possible: research has shown that breastfeeding is easier and post-natal depression less common in women who are able to bond with their babies immediately after birth. Ask that the cord be cut only when it has stopped pulsating, when the baby's own system is functioning fully, to minimise shock or trauma. Ask that the administration of syntometrine (to expel the placenta) be delayed for half an hour (see p. 115), unless there are complications, to allow the placenta to deliver naturally.
- How do you and your baby want to be treated after the birth? Think about the immediate post-natal period. Meeting your baby for the first time is a magical moment. Build what you want for the time just after the birth into your birth plan and try to anticipate any difficulties. Ask that you and your partner be left alone immediately after the birth, at least for a little while, and that your other child or children be able to visit as soon as possible after the birth. Ask not to be separated from your baby if all is well.

At the end of your birth plan make it clear that you are prepared to be flexible, to negotiate and compromise. Discuss your fears and build them into your birth plan: for example, 'In the unlikely event that I will need a Caesarean I'd prefer to be conscious and have it with an epidural anaesthesia. I'd like you to agree to both my birth partners being present. If I need a general anaesthetic I'd like the baby to be given straight to my partner and for my friend to take photos of my baby.' Think through possible difficulties – for example, what if your baby is premature and needs special care? What if you haemorrhage after the birth? – so that you can check out hospital policies and gain some idea of what you might want should you find yourself in this sort of situation.

If you are having your baby at home it is just as important to write up a birth plan, to try to establish what you would like and dislike, to negotiate the role your midwife will play and to have contingency plans for transferring to hospital if necessary.

Finally, this isn't going to be the perfect plan! It will act as a guide and help you to define what you want for your baby's birth. Women today have higher expectations. Hopefully your labour will be as you want but so often women have a very different experience from the one that they hoped for. Keep your expectations realistic, as almost anything can and may happen. Be flexible and go with the flow.

PREPARING FOR THE POST-NATAL YEAR

Becoming a parent changes everything: our lives are enriched in so many ways, *and* we are stretched and challenged, sometimes to our limits. The roller coaster of birth becomes the assault course of parenthood. Children bring us great joy and unconditional love – and their own demands and challenges. As they grow so do we alongside them. It is hard to prepare for parenthood because you don't know how you are going to feel and you can't predict how your new child will integrate into your and your family's lives, because of his or her unique character. Let your instincts guide you in how you respond – they are usually more reliable than theoretical advice. Do what *you* know is right no matter what others think. It doesn't make them wrong and you right, it makes you different – and that's fine.

Parenting ideas follow trends so question the style you choose. Do you want to do the opposite of your own parents or have you admired a friend's parenting style and want to emulate it? Don't be seduced into being an earth mother, full-time parent, or a Super mum, with a full-time job as well, just because you think you should. The stress of parenting in a style that doesn't suit you will cause tension and ultimately ill-health. Set yourself realistic standards that you know you can live up to.

Being a 'successful' parent is a question of balance – of finding your own way and of feeling confident in it. This book's aim is to offer advice to pick and choose from, so that you can begin to find out what works for you, and reject what doesn't. (See pp. 305–8 for a selection of support networks should you feel the need for 'hands on' help.) Listen to your children – they will teach you more than any child-care expert – and allow them to guide you.

THE JOB DESCRIPTION

Parenthood is a job *and* a way of life; although you can't prepare for it fully or train for it, there are ways in which you can become clear about the job you are taking on and *begin* to prepare for it so that it doesn't come as a complete surprise. The job description that follows is to give you food for thought, and provide a realistic framework for discussions – not to put you off!

Responsibility

You will be prepared to commit yourself for a minimum period of 16 years. The post necessitates a high level of executive ability and includes the following fundamental requirements:

- to feed and clothe the child or children adequately.

- to protect them from harm.
- to love them unconditionally.
- to teach basic survival skills, such as to communicate and to mix with others.
- to help them to form a belief system.
- to encourage them to achieve their full developmental potential, independence and high self-esteem.
- to look after yourself adequately to achieve the above and in so doing, create a healthy model of adulthood for them to aspire to.
- to protect yourself against burn-out.

The Hours

You will need to plan how a baby will fit into your existing life-style. Those who breastfeed may spend upwards of three to four hours a day doing just this. Time must also be allowed for bathing and nappy changing. Those whose babies like to suck or are slow to feed, or who feed little and often will find that feeding takes even longer. Previously successful job-holders have found that the new, often slower pace of life allows them time to sit and read, talk to other children, reflect or watch television, or simply enjoy the baby.

Caroline Flint (*Sensitive Midwifery*, Heinemann, 1986) suggests that midwives hand a note to new parents:

> Congratulations on your new baby. He or she will bring you great joy and pleasure and you will learn many new things from this experience. Having a new baby is like starting a new life or a new job which takes twenty-four hours a day. You will need someone to help you for at least two weeks after the birth and preferably longer. You will need to concentrate on the baby, feed her, change her nappies and talk to her. This will take about 12 hours a day. It will not be from 8 a.m. to 8 p.m., and then you are off duty. It is half an hour here, two hours there, an hour and a half next. This will take up nearly all of your time. You need someone to help by doing your washing, by cooking you nutritious meals, by shopping and keeping your home clean.

Life with a new baby may have little structure – some babies, for example, take a while to learn night from day – which can be a substantial challenge for the job-holder who has been used to working hard to a strict schedule and having large amounts of time off.

As your baby grows into a child the demands on your time decrease *but* they are rarely predictable, i.e. illness can 'strike' at any age and you'll be needed more or less around the clock for several days (and more) if your ten-year-old needs an emergency apprendicectomy. Be open (and prepared) for anything to happen and it generally doesn't. Plan for a quiet life and you may be surprised . . . !

Benefits

There are many, they include the following:

- the baby!
- being loved unconditionally.
- loving – the experience of loving a child, especially your own baby, is beyond description.
- increased emotional maturity. The challenges of parenthood help parents to grow up also.
- learning to do more than one thing at a time and to use small amounts of spare time to the fullest – whenever it comes.
- acquiring the arts of planning, strategy and diplomacy.
- responding to virtually any situation at any given time and resolving conflict without violence, either verbal or physical.
- developing organisational skills as well as those of negotiation and compromise.
- the ability to conduct at least two conversations at the same time.
- sheer, unadulterated enjoyment. The entertainment value of babies and small children (especially your own) is very high – they are infinitely more interesting than TV!

Tools of the Trade

The following will enable the job-holder to avoid burn-out and reduce stress:

- an open heart.
- a sense of humour.
- good health.
- common sense.
- patience and flexibility.
- constancy and a sense of perspective.
- respect and understanding.
- curiosity.
- the ability to listen and observe.
- a decent memory.

Age Restrictions

Women: approximately 16–45.
Men: no upper limit.

Job-share Opportunities

Job-share opportunities exist whether through necessity or choice with your partner, other parents of similar-age children, grandparents, friends or with paid help. Bear in mind, you should job-share only with someone who sympathises with your own goals in child-rearing.

It is recommended that those who decide to job-share negotiate carefully with their partner and older children so that household chores and responsibilities as well as childcare are equally shared, as the first year or two can be extremely exhausting.

The Equipment

You can prepare for the first year in this job by buying an enormous amount of equipment – a substantial carriage, a pushchair, crib, cot, baby carrier, car seat, swings, lambskin, reclining chair, bath, rattles and toys, clothes, toiletries and nappies.

Alternatively, you may buy very little. You will need a fair amount of equipment but as little of it wears out many parents willingly lend their baby gear to their friends in an endless merry-go-round where some eventually gets worn out and other bits get added. You can rent car seats, buy the bigger items, like carriages and strollers, secondhand through local newspapers, and buy slings and baby carriers.

It may be appropriate to ask family and friends to support in this new venture by buying specific items of equipment.

Experience Required

No previous experience is required. Some have had experience of caring for babies either within their own family or through friends or from having babysat as teenagers. Many, however, have never cared for a baby, may not even have held one until they had one of their own. This should not put you off, rather encourage you to seek appropriate support (see Back-up Support below).

Training

None needed, although you have an advantage if you had parents who were loving, caring and, by example, offered excellent preparation for this job. You should be willing to be at least partially trained by your children.

There is much reading material available on how to be successful in this job. You are encouraged to be selective regarding the theories put forward although you may find them useful for reference.

Back-up Support

See pages 305–8 for details of support organisations, but also available are women's groups, playgroups, mother and baby groups, toddler groups, nurseries and many others. Details of local ones can be found in newspapers, on doctors' surgery or clinic notice-boards, or at your library and from health visitors, GPs and homeopaths.

The lucky ones among us will have relatives or friends who love and respect them living close by, and are willing to help by being involved in the upbringing of the baby.

Salary and Conditions

Child benefit is currently fixed at £7.25 per child per week, rising at *ad hoc* intervals subject to government ministerial whim plus a small extra allowance if you are parenting alone. It is paid for all children under the age of 16. Those who decide to parent full-time should apply to their working partner for an allowance. A weekly maternity allowance (for a maximum of 18 weeks) can be claimed by women who have paid the necessary national insurance contributions. The following are free during pregnancy and for a year after the birth: dental treatment; all prescriptions; family planning services.

There are no statutory or agreed holidays, no paid overtime, no opportunities for profit-related pay. Promotion with greater responsibility does not attract any incremental increases. There is no super-annuation or pension scheme currently available!

PLANNING FOR PARENTHOOD

Partners can feel just as much at sea as new mothers while they get used to their new role in the family and much of the following suggestions are addressed to both parents. Check out the job before-hand by getting as much information as you can without getting overwhelmed. If you are a woman who has decided to parent single-handedly then make sure you have set up a solid support network of friends especially for the early weeks.

Do

- interrogate friends who are parents: ask them what worked and what didn't, what it was they wished they had known, how they would have liked to prepare for parenthood.
- dip into a book or two but stay with the ones that seem to mirror most clearly what you feel is right for you.
- find a friend with a baby, before you have yours, and ask to help out or babysit or be around when feeding, bathing and changing are going on.
- go with the flow: your life will change, a new baby is all-absorbing and you may wonder how you will ever manage to get dressed and wash your hair or cook a meal again. Your life *will* adjust, especially once your baby starts to sleep more at night so just hang on in there and enjoy the different pace of your life. The first year is a treasure chest of delight, which passes all too soon so make the most of it!
- use the post-natal support network that you set up when you were pregnant – friends to shop or clean, take your toddler out, etc.
- reassess your priorities. You'll find that they change as your family grows. Sleep and time with your family can become more important than almost anything else. The important people in your life may change as you seek out other parents to spend time with. Do make sure you look after yourself first, then your partner, and then your other children. Housework, three-course meals and entertaining can all go to the bottom of the list!
- avoid people whose advice makes you feel small, guilty, self-critical, bad or incompetent until you feel confident and your relationship with your baby is well established. It's normal to feel vulnerable after childbirth, especially to hurtful criticism from close relatives and friends – who should know better, anyway. Lack of sleep and the demands of a newborn baby are a special combination calculated to turn even the most stoic of women into emotional jellyfish. Protect yourself from unkind attacks by telling any critics, kindly but firmly, to leave you alone.
- build verbal encouragement into your life: parents can tell each other what a good job they are doing – frequently! Tell yourselves that day to day you are doing the very best you can.
- put your struggles in perspective by talking to trusted friends who share similar parenting

beliefs. Aim to be effective, good-enough parents, not perfect ones.

- accept your failings with goodwill and humour.
- start discussing what boundaries you are going to set for your children, and what consequences there will be if they break them. Decide how important it is that they don't eat sugar or don't swear, for example. If you don't want them to do it, you are going to have to stop yourselves.
- ask older children to help change and bathe the baby. Encourage them to express their feelings about the new one and listen to what they say, either positive or negative. It is normal for children to feel ambivalent about a new baby – and unusual for them not to.
- seek professional advice if you're not coping or finding it difficult to ask for help. Remember, it's a sign of strength, not failure, to ask for help.
- leave the baby with tried and trusted help from time to time so that you can go to the library, the hairdresser or have tea or go to the movies with a friend; spend time with your older child (or children) to give them the one-to-one attention they had before the baby came along, especially if you are a single parent.
- try to spend some time – an evening a week if possible – with your partner. Your primary relationship needs nourishing in order to survive and flourish.

Don't

- listen to theories expounded by professionals who haven't had children of their own, or read books that make you feel anxious or uneasy.
- listen to advice that overuses the words should, ought, must, or where they are implied or where you feel criticised or attacked.
- isolate yourself.
- fall into the trap of becoming a doormat, looking after everybody else's needs at the cost of your own.
- forget: *there is no such thing as the perfect parent.* Imagine what it would be like for a small child to have to live up to the impossible expectations of being a perfect adult. Your faults or flaws are like seams of gold and charcoal in the rock of your being and an important part of who you are. Let them strengthen you and adorn your personality by uncovering them and accepting them.

BONDING

Bonding is the process whereby you get to know another person very well and become very close to them and they to you. It is an essential ingredient in a successful relationship.

Some people have high expectations of falling in love with their new babies and are disappointed when that doesn't happen automatically. It can take days or even weeks, especially if you were separated shortly after the birth. You can encourage bonding to take place – both for yourself and for other members of the family.

Do

- be aware of the bonding process and nurture it consciously.
- ask that your baby be given to you immediately after the birth, if possible, so that you can 'connect' with each other – and with your partner.
- go home after the birth if you're in hospital, don't need to be and aren't enjoying it. It may not be appropriate for you to be surrounded by strangers at a time like this. You may have difficulty getting to know your baby if you are feeling tense.
- examine your baby: feel free to check out every inch of that little body, touch and smell him or her all over.
- make a calm nest at home. The first days and weeks after the birth are important for you and your baby to get to know each other. You need uninterrupted time together to nurture the bonds of intimacy. Encourage your other children to spend time with the new baby so that they can have an opportunity to become close.
- wallow in this time just after the birth if this is your first child. It's a very special time which won't come again; if you have another baby you'll have your older child to look after too.
- limit your visitors. Too many people at the wrong times will make you tired, tense and edgy, even if you enjoy them at the time.
- massage your baby. You can go to a baby-massage class or use one of the many books available as a guide.
- bath with your baby – the feel of your baby's skin next to yours is lovely for both of you. It's easiest if there's someone else on hand to take the baby out while you wash.
- exercise and play together: be creative and have fun doing it.
- hold your baby as much as you can. Remember, the familiar environment of the uterus consists of

constant contact, constant feeding and constant warmth. Carry the baby around in a sling, when you are shopping or when you make a meal if your back is up to it and your baby enjoys it.

- talk, sing, hum and whistle to your baby. Talk a combination of baby talk and ordinary everyday talk: if you talk only in baby talk they will take longer to speak proper language.
- look into your baby's eyes. They have difficulty in focusing during their early weeks and can see best at a distance of roughly 8 inches (20 cms).

A WORD ABOUT FEEDING

It is important that *you* are happy with how you feed your baby, whether that be by breast or bottle. Don't give in to someone else's dictates about what you *should* be doing. It is far more important that the relationship between you and your baby and between your baby and the rest of your family is close and loving than feeding in the 'right' way and feeling tense and anxious because it doesn't suit you.

You may choose to breastfeed fully or to mix bottle- and breastfeeding; to breastfeed for a short time and then transfer to bottle-feeding; you may decide to bottle-feed from the start, from necessity (because of, say, surgery) or choice. Be flexible: see how breastfeeding goes for you and continue if it works or mix it with bottles if it doesn't. If mixed feeding doesn't work, drop the breastfeeding. Bear in mind that if you introduce bottles early your baby may lose interest in the breast as getting milk out of a bottle is generally easier than out of a breast. Babies will thrive on either the breast or the bottle. The points which follow may help you to decide which is right for you.

Whether you opt for bottle or breast, feeding takes up so much time initially that it usually becomes the primary focus of attention. Those early weeks or months, where your life feels jam-packed with 'servicing' your new charge – feeding, rocking, changing and waiting for him or her to wake again – won't last – they are comparatively short-lived so try to enjoy them!

Bottle-feeding

Pros
- you don't have to do it all the time . . . your partner can do one or more of the night feeds.
- you have more freedom to leave the baby with

your partner, a friend or close family member while you have a break.
- you know exactly what your baby is getting. This may be a disadvantage for anxious mothers who become fixated on the quantity of milk their babies are taking, who panic if their baby doesn't finish a feed or still seems to be hungry when the bottle is finished.
- partners enjoy feeding babies too and can feel included in the feeding relationship.
- your exhaustion, emotional 'downs' or even illness can affect your breastmilk, sometimes reducing it. You won't have this worry to contend with if you are bottle-feeding.

Cons
- a lot of preparation, sterilising, measuring and warming bottles.
- an increased incidence of diarrhoea in bottle-fed babies.
- some babies are allergic to cow's milk and even one bottle is enough to set off a reaction (commonly causing colic and diarrhoea).

NB Don't automatically give soya milk. It is acidic which can make it difficult for some babies to digest. Only give it if you have a good reason and then select the brand carefully with the advice of your health visitor. Controversy recently erupted over the level of aluminium salts in one variety.

Breastfeeding

Pros
- the correct formula for baby humans (as opposed to baby cows) and has the right balance of nutrients.
- easily digested.
- the early pre-milk (colostrum) contains antibodies which boost your baby's immune system.
- always sterile.
- conveniently always there – anywhere, anytime – making travelling easy.
- always at the right temperature.
- an enjoyable intimate experience.
- it aids bonding, helping mother and baby to get to know each other.
- it is a good soother (dummy) and fulfils a baby's need to suck as well as the need for food.
- it helps the uterus to contract.
- it helps you lose the extra weight that you may have put on in your pregnancy. Breastfeeding uses 600–1000 calories a day, about an hour's worth of vigorous exercise.

- you can combine the best of both bottle and breastfeeding if you can express milk easily. Buy a manual breast pump, costing a few pounds, from your local chemist so that you can experiment once your milk comes in.

NB Research has shown over and over that breast-feeding (without supplements) even for the first two weeks of a baby's life, gives an extra boost to the immune system. So it's worth having a go – even if you know deep down that you won't continue for long.

Cons
- it's time-consuming.
- *you* have to do it – and that means every single feed, day and night. You are on duty 24 hours a day for an unlimited period of time unless you are able to express your milk.
- it can be painful. A minority of women find that breastfeeding can take a long time to establish and the pain of engorgement (when the breasts become overfull as the milk first 'comes in' after the birth) can be followed by cracked nipples and blocked ducts. These conditions are all treatable with homeopathic remedies so *don't* suffer in silence or give up if you find breastfeeding hurts.
- it can be confusingly sexual – especially for your partner.
- you don't know how much milk your baby has taken. This rarely matters because your baby will take what it wants and once breastfeeding is well established a system of supply and demand operates whereby you produce according to your baby's needs.

Breastfeeding Myths

Many myths surround breastfeeding.
Myth: successful breastfeeding is related to the size of the breast.

Women with very small breasts are able to breastfeed successfully even if their breasts do not change size markedly either during pregnancy or after the birth. There is, nearly always, an increase in breast size when the milk comes in but the breasts may revert to more or less their normal size when feeding is established.
Myth: either your breasts will become ugly as a result of breastfeeding or they won't change at all.

We learn from the media that breasts should be a certain size and shape and this changes accord-ing to fashion. In one decade breasts were out and

currently they are in. Women are frightened their breasts will sag and become unattractive to their partners. Their fears are often dismissed but it is true that breastfeeding may affect the shape and tone of your breasts. Some women have found that their breasts become more attractive not just during breastfeeding but afterwards too as they have retained some of their fuller shape. Others find that breastfeeding leaves them with smaller breasts. It is impossible to anticipate what will happen to yours. In any case, exercise will help to keep them – and you – in good shape.
Myth: your breasts will only produce the milk your baby needs, no more no less.

If you are anxious or under severe emotional stress your milk supply may reduce. Some women 'overflow' with milk which can be equally distressing. Homeopathic treatment will help in both cases.
Myth: your breast-fed baby can't get fat.

Yes they can! Some babies put on weight very quickly even with few feeds in a day. These babies have a slow metabolism (turn to *Calcarea carbonica* for a full picture of the constitutional type that puts on weight easily). As long as your baby is healthy and contented you do not need to worry whether they are taking too much milk.
Myth: the breast-fed baby will gain the correct amount of weight.

This is one to watch out for: the growth charts used to measure whether your baby is getting 'enough' milk do not take into account the indi-vidual variations of the breast-fed baby. Your baby's weight gain may not match your clinic's ideal but as long as your baby is healthy and contented *there is no need to worry*!
Myth: breastfeeding comes naturally – the 'perfect mother' doesn't need teaching – she can do it instinctively.

This isn't true. Successful breastfeeding *is* a learnt skill for mother *and* baby. Some women take to it like a duck to water, have relatively few difficulties and these are easily resolved. Some women struggle and need a lot of support. We all have different aptitudes in different subjects!

Physical problems such as cracked nipples or a breast abscess can make breastfeeding seem difficult so seek out the support and advice of a breastfeeding counsellor (see La Leche League or other childbirth associations, p. 305) to help you through.
Myth: breasts were made to feed babies with, there-fore breastfeeding is a natural function of the

body and it certainly isn't sexy.

The breast is associated with sex, reinforced through the media's frequent portrayal of women and their breasts as sexual objects, to sell anything from alcohol to cars. It is rare that we see images of women breastfeeding except in a Third World setting, with starving infants.

Some women are surprised and shocked to find that they become sexually aroused by breastfeeding. Few talk about this, especially if they also go off sex with their partners. They may even feel that there is something wrong or abnormal about them. There isn't.

Is Breast Best?

Breast is best *only* if you want to breastfeed. Some women breastfeed fully for a year and more. Others bottle-feed from the very beginning. Some mix breast with bottle in the knowledge that their baby may give up the breast sooner than if fully breastfed. Others breastfeed for a short time before changing over to the bottle.

The following dos are to help you to decide whether to breastfeed or not.

Do

- think through what messages, attitudes and beliefs you have about breastfeeding. Where did you get them? Are they true for you now? What do *you* want to do? What difficulties do you think or feel you might have? What are you afraid of?
- talk through any fears or anxieties to sympathetic ears. Get some help if you realise you are labouring under some prohibitive messages – like 'You'll never breastfeed because your breasts are too small,' or 'No one has ever breastfed successfully in your mother's family – you are just like her, I bet you'll find it difficult too' – and are not sure what you want to do.
- seek the help of a counsellor or psychotherapist if you feel revolted at the idea of breastfeeding but want to do it. They will help you to uncover the reasons for your feelings and help you to deal with them.
- breastfeed for two weeks if you can as that will give your baby the antibody-rich pre-milk (colostrum) specially designed to boost your baby's immunity to infection.
- know that you can switch to the bottle if you feel anxious, afraid, disgusted, angry, in pain or if any other difficult feelings surface while you are breastfeeding and you aren't prepared to see a

counsellor. You *can* stop if you feel that breastfeeding is not for you. If you know that you are going to be a better mother if you bottle-feed your baby then do that.

- seek counselling or psychotherapy help if you try to breastfeed and then decide not to breastfeed but continue to feel guilty that you didn't succeed or afraid that you've ruined your child's one chance at good health.
- decide to feed your baby with love and affection. It is this that counts more than anything.

Bottle-feeding

Bottle-feeding can be as enjoyable and soothing as breastfeeding, albeit in a different way: it is the sucking and the love bond between the mother and baby that is important. Feed your baby with love and let him or her suck as much as they need and you can't go wrong.

If you decide to bottle-feed, do try to breastfeed for the first two weeks because the antibodies your baby receives through the colostrum will help to build a healthy immune system.

Common complaints such as colic and diarrhoea may occur in babies who have difficulty in adapting to cow's milk formula. If the problem is mild and short-lived, you can treat it yourself but remember to take the whole picture into account.

Do

- be flexible.
- use bottles with disposable plastic liners if you are planning to carry on partially breastfeeding. Playtex teats are the closest in shape to your own nipples and the first size with the smallest hole allows milk through at about the same rate as breastmilk; your baby won't be encouraged to ditch the breast in favour of an easier option. The other advantages of these bottles are that your baby won't swallow air while feeding because the bag collapses as she sucks, and the bags are convenient for storing (or freezing) single feeds of expressed breastmilk or formula.
- give occasional bottles of *plain* water to encourage a thirsty baby to develop a taste for water. Sterilise the bottles and use cooled boiled water.
- be careful to sterilise all bottle-feeding equipment thoroughly to prevent the baby developing gastroenteritis – still a relatively common problem in bottle-fed babies. You can either use commercial sterilising solutions, or wash the equipment then

boil for 25 minutes with everything fully sub-merged.

- rinse bottles sterilised in commercial sterilising fluids with cooled boiled water before using them to wash off the chemicals.
- wash your hands before preparing your baby's feeds.
- use cooled boiled tap water from the mains cold tap, for making up his or her feeds.
- measure the formula accurately according to the manufacturer's instructions.
- make up each feed as you need it if you don't have a fridge.
- keep to the same formula, once you find one that suits your baby.
- keep extra formula milk in the fridge for up to 24 hours only, *no longer*.
- warm the milk by putting the bottle in a jug of hot water. Make sure it doesn't get too hot and only warm it just before it is needed.
- cuddle your baby while feeding – hold him or her nice and snug as you would if you were breast-feeding.
- stroke the baby's cheek or lips with your finger or the teat to stimulate the sucking reflex.
- hold the bottle firmly so that the baby can suck easily and tip it up so that the teat is full of milk. If it isn't he or she will suck in air with the milk, which may cause colic.
- turn the bottle round if the teat collapses during sucking to let air back into the bottle which will cause the teat to re-inflate.
- gently sit up and wind your baby if necessary during and after a feed.
- let your baby take what he or she wants at each feed: a bottle-fed baby, like a breastfed baby, will be hungry at some times and not at others. Let your baby regulate the amount of milk.
- let your baby take as long as he or she likes in the beginning to feed. Some babies stop and start or get distracted, by their mother or by strange noises.
- let your baby suck your finger or a dummy if the need to suck remains after the milk is finished.
- throw away *any* milk left in the bottle at the end of a feed: it can harbour harmful bacteria which will multiply rapidly in the warm milk.
- give formula until your baby is about nine months old. Consult your health visitor as to the right time at which to switch to cow's milk.
- consider taking advice about whether to give cow's milk formula if you or the baby's father is sensitive or allergic to dairy foods or if either of you has suffered from eczema, asthma, hayfever or digestive problems especially in childhood. 'Lactolite' formula, a lactose-reduced cow's milk for babies sensitive to cow's milk, is now available in many supermarkets and health-food shops, and the first goat's milk infant formula is being imported from New Zealand.
- let others feed your baby – your partner, older children, relatives or close friends. Be specific about how you want them to do it – don't assume they know. A child should be supervised.

Don't
- use the following waters to prepare your baby's formula: bottled mineral waters, as the minerals can be harmful; water from the hot tap (and preferably not from a cold-water tap that comes from the tank in the attic); water that has been 'softened' or 'filtered' with a plumbed-in water softener or plumbed-in filter because it will contain residues of the chemicals used; water that has been boiled more than once or has been left standing in the kettle.
- add extra formula to the bottle: you will make the mixture too strong, which can damage the baby's kidneys and make him or her more thirsty. If you give more milk than necessary your baby will put on excess weight and may cry a lot.
- add cereal, rusk, sugar or anything else to the formula.
- prop your baby (even an older baby) and the bottle in a high chair. The baby may choke.
- worry if the milk is a bit cool. Even cold milk won't hurt although the baby may refuse it if he or she prefers it warmed.
- give soya formula without taking advice from your doctor, health visitor or homeopath.
- encourage your baby to finish the bottle.
- encourage your baby to drink if he or she pushes it away, or turns away, or spits out the teat, or in some other way indicates the interest has gone!
- give fruit juice in any form (squash or diluted fresh fruit juices) in a bottle. This will encourage a 'juice addiction' that is very difficult to break and will contribute to your child's teeth rotting as they come through.
- keep bottles of formula for longer than 24 hours in the fridge.

Seek help if your baby
- isn't gaining much weight or is gaining too much weight.

- never finishes the bottles, doesn't seem particularly hungry.
- vomits the feeds.
- has consistently offensive-smelling stools.
- develops a rash.

Breastfeeding

Milk is manufactured in the breasts on a supply and demand basis – the more your baby sucks the more milk you'll make. Babies need to 'milk' the breasts by sucking in a particular way because milk isn't released if they suck on the nipples. They have to *draw* on the milk sacs lying behind the areola by taking as much of the nipple and areola into their mouths as possible. Small breasts have the same number of milk sacs as large ones. About a third of each feed is stored in these sacs; it is known as the foremilk and is thirst-quenching and low in fat. Sucking stimulates a hormone to be released (prolactin) which guarantees that milk will be stored after this feed is finished, ready for the next one.

As your baby feeds another hormone (oxytocin) is secreted which causes the fat-rich hindmilk to be released or 'let down' from the milk glands higher up into the milk sacs behind the areolas. This takes up to three minutes which is why limiting feeds to a few minutes each side can lead to 'failing' at breastfeeding because the hindmilk is essential for healthy growth. It is about three times richer than the foremilk and it will spurt out which is why a baby just has to swallow once this milk has let down. This let-down can be felt as a tingling sensation or a rush of warmth; some women feel nothing at all while others find it painful, especially at the beginning. Both breasts let down at the same time so if you are feeding on one breast, either catch the drips with a breast shell or in a breast pad or press the heel of your palm against the nipple to stop the milk leaking.

If your baby fusses and pulls on the breast after a minute or two it may be that the foremilk is all gone and the hindmilk has not yet been released. Once the milk has let down and after the initial rush of milk your baby will have to suck hard to get the rest of the feed.

Minor complaints in the early days of breastfeeding, especially with a first baby, are common. The points listed below are to help you to breastfeed successfully from the beginning. See pp. 117–23 for breastfeeding complaints.

Do

- let your baby have skin-to-skin contact with you immediately after birth. Offer the breast and let the baby suck for as long as he or she wants to. If you feed on demand from then on the chances are that your milk will come in quickly and your breasts will be less likely to become engorged (p. 118).
- decide to be relaxed about feeding. Remember that babies have been around a lot longer than clocks, that the timing of feeds was designed for bottle-feeding.
- use a breastfeeding counsellor for support and advice – many will visit your house after the birth especially if their telephone advice hasn't helped. La Leche League and other childbirth organizations have nationwide networks of counsellors. They are women with children of their own whose aim is to empower others to breastfeed successfully.

- rest, especially while your supply is building up. Breastfeeding is a lovely thing to do – enjoy it!
- drink plenty of fluids. You will need approximately 2 pints (1 litre) more every day than you have been used to while your milk supply increases and may feel thirsty for what feels like most of the time until it is well established.
- eat well (not necessarily a lot more) and regularly. Prepare a drink and a snack every time you feed your baby. Eat what you feel like as long as it includes some fibre and some fresh fruit and vegetables.
- wear a comfortable, supportive cotton bra. Many breastfeeding bras have zips which are easily done up and undone with one hand, although you have to be careful not to catch your skin in them. Some are made with Velcro fastenings and the more old-fashioned ones fasten with hooks. Make sure that your bra never cuts into your breast as this can cause a blocked duct (see p. 117). It is wise not to sleep in a bra for the same reason: they can pull around in the night and cut in. If your breasts are especially uncomfortable and need extra support both day and night, experiment until you find a bra that works for you – you may need a lighter one at night than in the day. It is worthwhile being measured and fitted properly by someone who knows what they are doing.
- position the baby's head by cradling it in your *left* hand when putting it to the *left* breast – holding

your breast from underneath with your right hand.

- bring your baby to the breast *not* your breast to the baby. Don't lean over to feed your baby as this will create tension.
- make sure the whole nipple and as much of the areola as possible (some women have particularly large ones), but especially the part below the nipple, is taken into the baby's mouth. Hold your breast from underneath to direct the nipple towards the back of the baby's mouth. Don't use your first two fingers as scissors to do this as the nipple will more easily point in the wrong direction.
- stroke your baby's cheek with your finger or nipple to make him or her 'root', turn the head towards your breast and open his or her mouth.
- make sure your baby's mouth is gaping wide when you offer the breast: this will encourage her to suck properly, with her mouth wide open. Rightly positioned you will see the muscles around the angle of the jaw, the temples and ears moving.
- take your baby off the breast (by breaking the suction gently with your little finger) if she is sucking with her mouth closed and therefore only chewing on your nipple and start again. Persevere until she has got the knack – some babies take days to get it. If the nipple is not far enough in, your baby will 'bite' you with its gums and your nipple will become sore.
- check that your newborn can breathe. If your breast obstructs breathing, reposition the baby's body or very gently press the area by their nose to give them some air (if you press too hard you can cause a duct to block).
- let your baby's head rest on your forearm, once latched on well, and *not* in the crook of your arm, which makes it difficult for all the ducts to be drained and may cause her to pull and fuss on the breast.
- position your baby so that its abdomen is facing yours otherwise it will have to twist its head to feed and may fuss and pull on your nipple.
- feed in different positions, sitting and lying, to find out which is most comfortable at different times.
- use the 'football' position, that is, with its legs tucked under your arm, especially if you have twins. This is especially good when you are trying to eat a meal and breastfeed at the same time!
- make sure you are comfortable when you breastfeed, whether you are sitting or lying down,

otherwise you will create pockets of tension in your own body that will drain you of much-needed energy. Organise yourself first and then latch your baby on. If you are sitting, have your feet flat on the floor (or on a small stool or a few telephone directories if you have short legs) and rest your baby on enough cushions to bring its head up to your nipple (newborns especially need plenty of support). Make sure your shoulders are relaxed and not supporting the baby's weight as this will give you backache. If you are lying down, bank cushions at your back and lay very small babies on a pillow.

- breathe when you breastfeed. It is amazing how many women hold their breath when they are trying to latch their babies on. This creates tension.
- respond to your baby if it is one of those who wants peace and quiet to feed. Some are distracted by noise and need you to be in a quiet place.
- invest in a rocking chair with comfortable arms – there are a number of reasonable kits around. It's very soothing to nurse and rock, sing or read, or watch the baby's face or the clouds . . .
- take your nipple gently out of your baby's mouth to prevent soreness developing, especially if your baby is still sucking. Put the tip of your little finger in the corner of her mouth: as you do so you will feel the suction breaking and you can take your nipple out without it being 'gummed'.
- let your baby suck for as long as he or she wants after at least some feeds to satisfy the need to suck. If your nipple is sore, you are in a public place or don't have the time, offer your little finger or try a dummy. You can use it after a feed (not before one) and remove it once the sucking has stopped or the baby is asleep.
- breastfeed in private if you feel inhibited or tense in front of others.
- take your emotional state seriously after the birth. Anxiety, resentment, shock and disappointment, for example, can all make it difficult for you to establish breastfeeding. See a homeopath or counsellor if you are struggling to understand what is happening to you.
- learn how to express milk (see below) as soon as possible as this will free you from being tied to breastfeeding and enable others to share the joy of feeding a small baby.
- use a Playtex bottle that has disposable bags (see also p. 73) for the milk. You can express your own milk and freeze it in the bags or put it in the fridge during the day ready for the night feeds.

- taste your own milk. It may look thin and bluish but it tastes good – incredibly sweet. No wonder children have a naturally sweet tooth.

Expressing Milk

Expressing milk is a learnt skill, which some women find easy to pick up while others struggle and never manage to do it. The following technique is worth persevering with if you are determined to express. Try a hand pump or an electric pump (from your hospital or the La Leche League) if you find it impossible to express by hand.

Apply hot flannels to your breasts for a few minutes and then massage the breast from the very edge towards the nipple all the way round. Repeat this ten times (or more) to encourage your milk to let down. If you find this difficult try doing it in the bath – the warmth will help you to relax. Stroke the breasts gently with your fingernails or 'comb' them (see p. 118) – again very gently and without applying pressure – all the way round just once or twice. Press gently with the thumbs and fingers of both hands on the area around the areola squeezing the thumbs and index fingers together and pressing backwards at the same time. Have ready a sterilised bowl to catch the milk! It should squirt out. Keep squeezing until you're only getting drops, making sure to squeeze at different places around the breast so that you empty the sacs as fully as possible. Repeat with the other breast.

· 3 ·
PREGNANCY

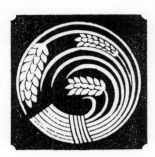

YOUR BODY AND PREGNANCY

These are some of the normal physical changes or 'symptoms' of pregnancy: you may experience some or all of them. Feet can spread a little, because of the extra weight and the loosening of the ligaments, becoming up to one shoe size larger; breasts may swell as the milk glands begin to develop and become more sensitive; nipples may exude a clear, yellow pre-milk fluid (colostrum); the area around the nipples (areola) becomes broader and darker and 'spots' will develop (Montgomery's tubercules); vaginal discharges may increase; an altered perception of taste or smell may develop; joints can become painful or stiff; sweat and saliva might increase; stretch marks can develop on the abdomen, breasts, thighs or buttocks; gums can become swollen and bleed more easily; a brown line may develop on the abdomen (from the navel to the pubis); brown patches may appear on the face typically in the shape of a butterfly; there may be an increase in moles or freckles; birthmarks may darken, although these usually fade after the birth; the external genitalia can become slightly swollen; there is usually an increased desire to pass urine (because of the additional load of fluid which the blood passes to the kidneys to cleanse); and towards the end of your pregnancy your belly button 'pops out'.

The human anatomy and physiology of pregnancy, childbirth and breastfeeding is complex, the product of millions of years of evolution. Most of the developments are hormone-related and include the following:

- All the connective tissue and smooth muscle of the body relax, including the ligaments. This enables the uterus and its supporting ligaments to soften, expand and stretch, and helps the spine and pelvis joints to become more flexible in preparation for birth. It also causes the walls of the blood vessels to widen and relax so that the blood circulates more freely and quickly, to carry oxygen and nutrients to your baby.
- The lungs automatically expand to adapt to the increased need for oxygen.
- The volume of body fluid increases dramatically. By the end of pregnancy your body carries about an extra 12 pints (7 litres) of water, half of which is taken up in the amniotic fluid, in which the baby floats in the uterus, and the rest is distributed throughout the body in the blood.
- The volume of blood increases by about 30 per cent to 9 pints (5 litres) by the end of pregnancy, so that both you and your baby have an adequate supply. The extra volume is made up largely of water but there is also an increase in the red blood cells, which carry iron (haemoglobin) and oxygen. The concentration of iron in the blood decreases by about 20 per cent because of the extra fluid.

Only about a quarter of the extra blood is lost during the birth, which allows for a safety margin in the event of more serious blood loss.

- Hormones are specifically responsible for the development of the placenta, which nourishes the baby in the uterus, and the baby; preparing the breasts for breastfeeding; preventing the uterus from contracting (it contracts continuously throughout a woman's life except when she is pregnant when the contractions slow right down).
- The increase of blood in your body means that the amount flowing to the surface increases about six times to help cool the body down – you may feel warmer and sweat more. This extra blood flow makes the skin glow and can cause red spots which disappear after the birth.
- The heart rate increases to deal with the extra volume of blood being pumped through the body.

COMPLAINTS

'Complaints' of pregnancy are always due to a combination of factors: the physical changes of pregnancy, hereditary factors and, of course, current stresses. They may include constipation, bleeding, cramps, frequent urination, involuntary urination (stress incontinence), swelling (oedema), piles (haemorrhoids), stretch marks, morning sickness (nausea and/or vomiting), emotional volatility and varicose veins, to name but a few! The extra weight can be tiring – imagine carrying a shopping bag strapped to your abdomen with 20 pounds (10–15 kg) of sugar or potatoes in it – and causes a shift in your centre of gravity.

Towards the end of pregnancy the baby's size pushes your internal organs out of position. Your lungs have less room, making breathlessness a common feature, and your stomach has less space to expand into if you eat a large meal – resulting in heartburn or indigestion. The complaints listed in this section are those most commonly experienced in pregnancy. I have not included those beyond the scope of the home prescriber (see p. 22). Homeopathic medicines are ideal for use in pregnancy because there is no danger of side effects: they offer a safe alternative to orthodox medicines, when used correctly, for a wide variety of minor complaints at a time when many women put up with the discomfort rather than risk harming themselves or, more importantly, their unborn child.

Most of the following complaints have more than one remedy listed in the Repertory. You will need to take the whole picture into account when prescribing

– including the general symptoms and the emotional state.

Read through Chapter 1 (pp. 19–20) for guidelines on potency and dosage before prescribing.

If you fall ill in pregnancy, deal with it appropriately and promptly: another person is now dependent on your well-being. Don't carry on regardless even if it is a relatively minor complaint like a cough or cold. If you have been under stress and your body needs a rest, that cold is a warning sign – ignore it at your peril! Rest when you need to even if you don't feel like it. On the following pages I discuss the common complaints of pregnancy and list practical advice for dealing with them. Only treat yourself for minor complaints that respond easily and quickly, and seek help if the complaint persists. *Always* seek medical advice for the following, more serious complaints.

Seek help if
- you have vaginal bleeding at any time during your pregnancy (because of the possibility of miscarriage or ectopic pregnancy early on in pregnancy or placenta praevia or abrupta (see p. 81) later on). You can self-prescribe *while* you seek medical advice.
- you suffer from abdominal pain, especially if it is continuous as it may indicate ectopic pregnancy or placental abruption.
- you suffer from persistent, severe back pain at about waist level (kidney infection).
- you suffer from severe headaches, blurred vision, chest pain or, your hands *and* face swell (which could signal pre-eclampsia (see p. 86) leading to toxaemia).
- you suffer from regular contractions before the 37th week, which may result in a premature labour.
- the baby stops moving or moves a lot less than usual; on average it should move about three times an hour.
- you leak amniotic fluid. The amniotic sac can tear but will usually mend itself and fill again with fluid, but if this happens it should be monitored.
- you have an unexplained and/or unusual symptom. Your doctor will be able either to put your mind at rest or to diagnose early the onset of anything that might need attention.
- you have a complaint that isn't listed in this section. I have only covered the common and mostly minor conditions of pregnancy that you can treat yourself, always bearing in mind that if they do not respond quickly, you should seek help.
- you feel anxious about the pregnancy.

NB I believe the routine administration of any medicines *at any time* to be inadvisable. Some people advocate the use of *Caulophyllum* (see p. 192) in the last few weeks of pregnancy or a homeopathic tissue-salt programme. Be aware of the dangers of 'proving' these remedies should you be tempted to try them and find another way of dealing with your condition.

ABDOMINAL PAIN

See Pain, pp. 96–9.

ACCIDENTS, AND INJURIES, MINOR

See Injuries, p. 286.

ANAEMIA, IRON-DEFICIENCY

Iron tablets are routinely prescribed for this common complaint. They are of questionable value as they commonly cause constipation (or occasionally diarrhoea) and can sometimes intensify the anaemia by blocking the absorption of iron.

During pregnancy the volume of blood circulating in your body increases gradually from about 7 pints (4 litres) to 9 pints (5 litres) by the end of the pregnancy. The haemoglobin (iron) content remains constant, however, which results in a normal drop in the level of iron per pint of blood of about 20 per cent. As long as you are fit and healthy, even if your haemoglobin level is low you need not worry. If you are suffering from symptoms of anaemia (exhaustion, palpitations, fainting, paleness and breathlessness) then you should take action, as a good supply of iron will help to promote a shorter labour with a decreased risk of haemorrhaging or infection after the birth.

The specific remedies for simple iron-deficiency anaemia during pregnancy are *Ferrum metallicum* (with exhaustion and pallor), or try alternating *Ferrum metallicum* with *Calcarea phosphoricum*, both in a low potency, to stimulate the body to absorb iron more effectively. These can be repeated whenever needed during pregnancy (see dosage chart on p. 20). However, there are other possible causes of anaemia like emotional stress or illness. In these cases you will need to take the whole picture into account and choose a remedy that covers all your symptoms – or seek professional help.

NB Thalassaemia and sickle-cell disease are both types of anaemia common in Asian, African, West Indian or Mediterranean women. They are inherited conditions and are not within the scope of the home prescriber.

Do
- eat a healthy, iron-rich diet. If you are a vegetarian eat plenty of greens and green vegetables (not spinach or watercress as the acid in them makes the iron difficult to absorb), cabbage, broccoli, eggs, molasses, wholewheat products (including wholewheat bread), whole grains, seaweeds, dried fruits (apricots/figs/prunes), almonds, sprouted grains and seeds.
- increase your intake of folic acid to help the absorption of iron. Folic acid is found in dark, leafy vegetables, root vegetables, whole grains, sprouted grains, whole milk, dates, mushrooms and orange juice, as well as salmon and liver.
- increase your intake of vitamin B_{12}, which is found in dairy foods and meat and is vital for the development of the brain and nervous system of your baby. If you are a vegetarian or vegan you might contemplate taking a supplement as about the only vegan sources of B_{12} are tempeh (a fermented soya product) or fortified nutritional yeast – consult a nutritionist for advice.
- rest as much as you need to.
- drink plenty of fluids but cut out tea: it contains tannic acid which prevents the absorption of iron.
- drink a fresh (citrus) fruit juice with your meals as vitamin C increases the absorption of iron. This is especially important for vegetarians.
- drink nettle tea as this is high in iron.
- take a herbal iron tonic such as Floradix if it suits you and you feel better for taking it. Stop if you become constipated.
- cook with iron pans. Your iron intake will increase because small quantities of the metal dissolve into the food.
- take your iron tablets with a meal if you decide to take those prescribed by your GP as they can irritate an empty stomach.

Don't
- take iron tablets routinely without trying the self-help measures outlined here and establishing the absolute necessity for them with your doctor/midwife. Ask your homeopath for an alternative, should self-prescribing have had no effect.

ANXIETY

See Emotions, p. 86–9.

APPETITE

See Food Cravings, p. 90.

BACK PAIN

See Pain, pp. 96–9.

BLEEDING

Spotting of blood is always a cause for concern although it is possible to spot – or even bleed quite heavily – in early pregnancy around the time when a period would have been due without losing the baby.

Other causes of bleeding are a burst varicose vein of the vagina, vaginal infections, a fall, cervical erosion or injury to the cervix, or a low-lying placenta (placenta praevia).

Light bleeding in the last three months of pregnancy can be caused by a vaginal infection or a burst blood vessel of the cervix caused by friction during sex. These are not serious. Heavier bleeding may be due to placenta abrupta, a rare condition where the placenta separates from the uterus prematurely before the birth. Repeated episodes of light bleeding or heavy spotting may indicate a placenta praevia, in which the low-lying placenta partially or totally covers the cervix. It can make itself known at about 24 weeks and will often migrate upwards later in the pregnancy. It will be spotted if you have an ultrasound scan (see p. 50).

Always take bleeding during pregnancy seriously as it *can* be a sign of miscarriage. Pain accompanying the bleeding (especially if the pains are like menstrual cramps) usually heralds a miscarriage, or more rarely, an ectopic pregnancy – a pregnancy developing in a fallopian tube – (the pains are felt more on one side if this is the case).

If you have a history of miscarriage caused hormonally then it is especially important that you seek the help of a professional homeopath for constitutional treatment. Homeopathic treatment, however, cannot prevent an inevitable miscarriage although careful prescribing afterwards may prevent another one. It is not within the scope of the home prescriber to treat a threatened miscarriage.

Advice and reassurance are essential if you bleed during your pregnancy – whatever the cause. Seek professional help, especially if the bleeding is heavy and accompanied by pain.

Do
- rest completely. Go to bed and stay there (leave only to go to the toilet) if you know instinctively that this is right for you. Young children are usually happy to play in and around a sick bed if there is a constant supply of interesting things to play with and eat. Get someone to move the television into the bedroom, stock up on videos, read or listen to tapes.

Don't
- rest if you are an anxious person. Staying in bed will cause more stress than carrying on being busy which may take your mind off your worries and keep you relatively relaxed. **But** don't
- ignore the symptom and carry on as usual hoping that it will go away.
- worry if the bleeding stops and you are still pregnant. No harm will come to your baby.

Seek help if
- bleeding is accompanied by fever.
- you have a history of miscarriage.
- there is heavy bleeding at any time, especially if it is accompanied by pain and/or the passing of clots.
- you are concerned for yourself – if you have a presentiment that things are not right. Women are generally more sensitive during pregnancy and often 'know' when something is wrong.

BRAXTON HICKS CONTRACTIONS

Sometimes known as false labour pains, these contractions occur painlessly and with varying frequency throughout pregnancy or not at all. They are attributed to the uterus practising for labour: your abdomen becomes hard and tight for a short time every now and then. Sometimes they can be bothersome, making sleep or resting difficult. They can come regularly, up to three minutes apart, for hours or even days at a time but the cervix doesn't dilate. It can be exhausting and dispiriting late in pregnancy to find out you are not in labour.

Do
- breathe gently and evenly with each contraction, just as you will need to do in labour – use them to practise on.

Seek help if
- there is bleeding or any unusual discharge from the vagina.
- the contractions become especially severe and/or prolonged.

BREAST PAIN

Sore breasts are common as hormonal changes are preparing them to feed the baby. They may or may not increase dramatically in size and become very sore – even painful. If the soreness is accompanied by fever then you may have a breast infection (mastitis) see p. 117.

Do
- wear a bra which fits well without cutting in anywhere. Buy new bras as your breasts increase in size.

Don't
- wear a bra at night as it can cut in inadvertently if you turn over.

Seek help if
- you develop mastitis and it doesn't respond to self-prescribing within 24 hours.

BREATHLESSNESS

Common in late pregnancy, especially after exertion (exercise or walking upstairs/uphill), it will also be worse if you were unfit at the beginning of your pregnancy and didn't take steps to improve your stamina. Breathlessness at any stage in pregnancy indicates simply that you are out of condition.

The extra load you are carrying makes the heart work harder and increases your need for oxygen. The pressure of the expanding uterus on the lungs also contributes. An extra large baby or twins can make this worse towards the end of pregnancy as your organs compete for the increasingly limited space in your abdominal cavity. Don't worry – this will pass after the birth.

There is no treatment for straightforward breathlessness, but if it is accompanied by exhaustion and pallor you may be suffering from anaemia (see p. 80). Self-prescribe on this condition taking breathlessness into account.

Do
- make sure you exercise regularly (walking, swimming, dancing, etc.) and gently to increase stamina. Remember that yoga builds suppleness and strength but not stamina.
- move more slowly towards the end of your pregnancy, using your breathlessness as a brake – walk at an easy pace. If you find yourself becoming breathless, pause and breathe slowly and deeply.

Seek help if
- you are breathless while resting or lying down.

BREECH BABY

Towards the end of pregnancy the baby settles into its favourite position. Ideally this will be with its head down and its back against its mother's abdomen, but it can adopt the 'breech' position with its head up, bottom down and its legs tucked up in front. A breech birth is more difficult and may result in the use of forceps or a Caesarean section. If your baby is still breech at 34 weeks it is worth encouraging it to turn round, although babies have been known to wait until labour to turn.

It isn't known why some babies settle in this position: one possible explanation is that the shape of the pelvic bones may make it more comfortable for the baby to be upright.

Pulsatilla 30, one dose every two hours for up to six doses (during the course of one day), has been highly effective at turning babies. Don't take it for more than a day.

Do
- exercise to encourage it to turn (postural tilting). Lie on the floor on your back with a pillow under your head and two or three pillows under your hips. Place your feet flat on the floor so that you feel comfortable. This will make a little extra space in your pelvis for your baby to turn – if it can. Encourage this to happen by massaging your abdomen gently, pushing your baby in the direction you want it to turn and *imagine* your baby turning. Rest in this position for 10–20 minutes several times a day. Use the time to practise your breathing and relaxation exercises.
- crawl around on hands and knees for 10 minutes every day, and carry on in labour if the baby is still badly positioned.
- talk to your baby – explain why you want it to turn and keep asking.
- ask your doctor or midwife to try to turn it. Some are skilled at this. If they succeed, some babies, irritatingly, will turn straight back again.

Seek help if
- the above measures haven't worked. Homeopathic treatment can sometimes help a breech baby to turn, even as late as the early stages of labour unless it is a footling breech (one leg born first), in which case you will have to be guided by your doctor as to what is best.

CARPAL TUNNEL SYNDROME

Numbness, pain and tingling in the fingers of the hand is common in pregnancy and is caused by a nerve being compressed as it passes through a space in the wrist called the carpal tunnel. A combination of swelling (oedema) and relaxed muscle tissue can easily press in on the nerve causing this discomfort which usually disappears after the birth. If the following suggestions don't help, ask your GP to refer you to a physiotherapist.

Do
- avoid movements that are painful.
- hang the affected arm out of bed at night.
- massage the hand and wrist gently.
- exercise the wrist and arms and stretch them up as often as you can.

COMMON COLD

A cold can be the body's way of letting you know you are run down, and that you need to recharge. You may catch more in pregnancy because the hormonal changes can cause the mucous membranes of the nose and sinuses to swell. Don't ignore them – neglected colds can turn into more serious chest infections, so treat them early.

Do
- take some time off, have early nights and deal constructively with some of the stress in your life (see pp. 44 and 88).
- get plenty of rest, especially if you have been overdoing it.
- drink lots of fluids.
- use steam inhalations to dislodge stubborn mucus. Sit over a bowl of just-boiled water with a towel over your head and the bowl and breathe in slowly and deeply.
- eat plenty of fruit and vegetables and avoid dairy products, sugar, junk foods and too much bread, all of which increase mucus production.
- avoid tobacco fumes.
- take some gentle exercise in the fresh air to see if this helps (and use the response as a symptom to repertorise).

Don't
- use decongestants. These only irritate the nasal membranes and make matters worse as soon as the effect wears off.

Seek help if
- you suffer from frequent colds ordinarily and start to get them in your pregnancy. You will benefit from constitutional treatment which will boost your immunity (see pp. 6–7).
- your cold seems unduly severe and isn't clearing with home prescribing and a large dose of tender loving care.

CONSTIPATION

The hormones which prepare and relax the pelvis for labour also cause the digestive processes to slow down. It is important to keep bowel movements regular to prevent a build-up of toxins and/or the development of piles and varicose veins.

Do
- drink plenty of water.
- make sure there is plenty of fibre in your diet from fruit, vegetables and whole grains except wheat.
- cut out bread and wheat products temporarily, as the gluten can have a clogging effect. If that helps, go easy on wheat products for the rest of your pregnancy.
- try eliminating dairy products or meat if you eat a lot of them, as they can also clog up the gut.
- avoid iron tablets: they are notorious for either causing constipation or making it much worse.
- eat stewed prunes in the morning or take a tablespoon of blackstrap molasses dissolved in hot water.
- use organically grown oat bran occasionally if you are desperate; it should only be taken regularly on the advice of a professional.
- make sure your feet are well supported when you are sitting on the loo so that the circulation to your legs isn't cut off, as this can cause varicose veins. You can put your feet on two low stools (or piles of telephone directories) either side of the toilet so that you are in more of a squatting position, which makes it easier for your bowels to work.
- try to make sure you are not interrupted.

Don't
- add wheat bran daily. It may interfere with the assimilation of vitamins and minerals, and your bowels may either be irritated by, or become dependent on, it. Oat bran is soluble and much gentler in its action.
- take laxatives, particularly if your diet is mainly of refined and junk foods. Make dietary adjustments first.

- strain when passing, or attempting to pass, stools as this can cause other problems such as piles (see p. 100). Be prepared to take your time – have a book handy to distract you!

Seek help if
- there has been no bowel movement for 24 hours and there is severe, unusual pain.
- there is difficulty in passing a stool and the stools are grey or white.
- your skin or eyes are yellow.
- there is a sudden and inexplicable change in bowel habit.
- there is alternating diarrhoea and constipation.
- your stools are extremely dark, almost black (unless you have been taking iron tablets in which case dark stools are not a cause for concern).

COUGHS AND CHEST INFECTIONS

Coughs are common especially during winter or a period of emotional stress. If the complaint recurs or stubbornly refuses to clear in spite of careful self-prescribing, seek professional homeopathic help.

Do
- follow the advice given for the common cold, p. 83.
- rest – it is even more important with coughs than colds.
- drink plenty of fluids as they will help to loosen the mucus.
- cough up the phlegm as often as possible.
- bend over or forward to cough so as not to strain the ligaments and muscles of the abdomen.
- use a humidifier or vaporiser in the bedroom to fill the room with steam, or use a simple steam inhalation; this will help the chest to expel sticky phlegm. You can put two drops of lavender or rosemary oil in the water or vaporiser, rather than coal tar or strong-smelling fumes, which will prevent a homeopathic remedy from working.

Don't
- suppress the cough with a cough medicine; this may prevent you coughing up phlegm which, if it is not expelled, may cause a more serious infection to develop. It is also important to avoid taking any medicines in your pregnancy that may cross over the placenta to your baby.

Seek help if
- you have difficulty in breathing, are wheezing, or have chest pain.

- the cough seems severe and doesn't respond to self-prescribing within 48 hours.
- your breathing is unduly rapid.

NB Pneumonia is a serious chest infection which is not always accompanied by a cough. Seek urgent medical help if you have a fever, are breathing rapidly and feel very unwell (limp and pale).

CRAMPS

Cramp is a sudden muscular contraction and is often caused by a change in body temperature or position, a loss of body fluids or when muscles are tired after exertion. It is a common complaint of pregnancy and more so in summer heat, because sweating can cause a drop in the level of body salts.

If your only symptom is cramp, take *Magnesia phosphorica* and *Calcarea phosphorica*, alternating them frequently, stopping and starting as needed.

Do
- straighten the affected part of the body, and gently massage the affected muscle.
- exercise gently and regularly, stretching your leg and calf muscles.
- increase your intake of calcium-rich foods.

Seek help if
- the cramps are increasingly severe, interrupt your sleep at night and do not respond to self-prescribing.

CYSTITIS

Urinary tract infections occur in pregnancy because the bladder and kidneys have to work harder to deal with the increased volume of body fluid and because of the pressure of the growing uterus.

Cystitis is an inflammation of the bladder and urethritis is an inflammation of the tube leading from the bladder to the urethra. The two can be easily confused but as they are closely related. First-aid advice and treatment is the same for both.

If left untreated, cystitis may develop into a serious kidney infection so great care should be taken with any urinary tract infection. I have included a few remedies for the treatment of simple cystitis (see p. 273), but symptoms should be carefully monitored and a professional homeopath or your GP consulted if there is no rapid improvement.

Do

- drink a large amount of water to flush out the kidneys and bladder, a glass every half-hour if you can, especially during the acute phase.
- keep your diet alkaline: eat lots of fruit, vegetables and whole grains, especially brown rice.
- cut out all acid foods and drinks, including tea, coffee, sugar, refined/junk food, alcohol.
- drink barley water. You can make your own by simmering a handful of organic whole barley in a pint (½ litre) water for an hour with a whole lemon cut into small pieces. Strain and drink a glass every half-hour during the acute phase.
- drink cranberry juice, either as it is or blended with fresh parsley, as it has been found to combat the bacteria that cause cystitis.
- take as much rest as you can. Go to bed and stay there!
- keep warm. Wear extra woollen clothing, especially around the bladder and/or kidney area; carry around a hot water bottle or use a heating pad.
- be sure *always* to wipe yourself from front to back after peeing so that bacteria from the anus cannot enter the urethra.
- 'bottle wash': fill a mineral-water bottle with warm water and pour over your genitals after you have peed and while you are still sitting on the toilet. Pat dry with soft white or unbleached toilet paper or a towel.
- pee frequently to keep the urethra free of bacteria.
- pee in the bath if peeing is painful – run enough warm water to sit in. Urine is sterile so don't worry about 'contamination'.

Don't

- use bubble baths or bath oils.
- wash the genitals with soap; just sponge down well with water.
- wear nylon tights or knickers or tight trousers or jeans.
- use vaginal deodorants.
- wash your underwear in biological washing powders.
- get chilled.
- use coloured toilet paper as the dyes in coloured loo paper have been known to aggravate.

Seek help if

- there are sharp pains in the area of the kidneys (in the back above the waist, on either side of the spine).
- the pains in the bladder (just above the pubic bone) or urethra (just behind the pubic bone) are extremely severe.

- there is blood in the urine – it looks pink, red or brown.
- the cystitis is accompanied by headache, vomiting, fever and chills.

DIARRHOEA

Because women are more generally sensitive during pregnancy, slightly 'off' food can cause more severe diarrhoea than normal. Make sure you give yourself adequate time to recover from it and take a remedy for exhaustion after diarrhoea if you still feel tired and listless within a day or two. The indicated homeopathic remedy will help your body recover much quicker – there are many for diarrhoea so you'll need to prescribe carefully, taking the whole picture into account.

Do

- limit the intake of food and drink.
- take water, freshly pressed apple juice, vegetable broth (simmer a selection of chopped vegetables in water for 15–20 minutes and strain), or rice water (white rice cooked in double the normal amount of water for slightly longer than usual and strained). Sip them initially and increase the quantity once the symptoms start to pass.
- introduce solid foods carefully, starting with white rice, toast or bananas. Eggs are also very 'binding' if the diarrhoea is persistent.

Don't

- let yourself become dehydrated.
- eat rich foods that are difficult to digest.
- eat if you are not hungry – a day or two without food will do no harm to you or your baby.

Seek help if

- the diarrhoea persists and fluids are not being tolerated (are being vomited or seem to pass straight through).
- you are exhausted and have lost your skin tone.
- there is acute pain in the abdomen which doesn't respond to first-aid prescribing within two to 12 hours, depending on the severity, or which is getting steadily worse.

DIZZINESS

Persistent dizziness should always be investigated by a professional. You can treat minor occasional vertigo yourself. In pregnancy it can accompany anaemia or exhaustion.

Do

- rest until the dizziness has passed.
- cup your hands over your nose and mouth for a few minutes as you breathe slowly and steadily if you suspect that the dizziness is a result of hyperventilating (see p. 40) as you may need to increase your carbon dioxide level.

Don't

- drive.

Seek help if

- there is severe vomiting with the dizziness.
- deafness or noises in the ear develop with the dizziness after an ear infection.

ECLAMPSIA AND PRE-ECLAMPSIA

Unique to pregnancy, it is not fully understood what causes this condition. However, in some studies it was noted that women with a diet high in protein were less susceptible to it.

Pre-eclampsia is fairly common – affecting up to one in ten pregnancies. The condition is fundamentally a disorder of the placenta and usually occurs at the end of pregnancy. It is a complex condition whose main signs and symptoms are oedema, *sudden* weight gain, headache, high blood pressure and protein in the urine (most likely to be diagnosed at an ante-natal visit); it is a combination of *three or more* of these symptoms developing quite suddenly which signals pre-eclampsia.

About a quarter of all pregnant women develop high blood pressure (who have previously not had it), and of these only about a quarter develop pre-eclampsia. If left untreated, about 1 in 20 of these women will develop eclampsia; adequate ante-natal care has made this condition relatively rare. The following characteristics can predispose some women to pre-eclampsia: height under 5 foot 2 inches (1.57m); first pregnancy; age under 20 or over 40; diabetes, kidney disease, migraine; a history of pre-eclampsia in a previous pregnancy; hypertension in the woman or in her family history; anxiety; under or malnourishment; sexual and emotional problems.

Eclampsia is life-threatening, with convulsions and coma consequently depriving the mother and baby of oxygen, which can lead to death. This is why it is cause for serious concern and must be spotted early. Women are most vulnerable to it just before, during and after childbirth. In some cases women are taken into hospital to monitor their condition carefully, as the only 'cure' for eclampsia is to induce labour early.

The traditional insistence on rest is now being questioned: because although rest can help bring down the high blood pressure of pre-eclampsia, it won't help much with placental deficiency.

The following self-help measures will help you to avoid pre-eclampsia. You can self-prescribe on simple oedema (see p. 96) if you can find a remedy in this book that fits, but generally it is beyond the scope of self-prescribing so consult your GP and your homeopath if you develop the symptoms.

Do

- pace yourself carefully in your working life and build substantial islands of fun and/or rest into your day.
- improve your diet – eat little and often and make sure you're getting plenty of protein.
- deal with the stress in your life – get some help with dealing with difficult in-laws, bosses, employees, teenage children, etc!
- seek counselling or psychotherapeutic help if you have strong ambivalent or negative feelings about your pregnancy, your body or your future role as a parent. This will reduce the pressure and will help you to adjust more easily in the post-natal period.

Seek help if

- you develop more than one symptom of pre-eclampsia. If you have been attending regular ante-natal hospital or GP appointments this will usually be spotted but it may be that you are the first person to suspect that it is developing. Make an urgent appointment to see your doctor if you think it is.

EMOTIONS

'Positive' Feelings

Pregnancy can be a magical, wonderful time, when you may experience a dramatic improvement in your general health, and feel unusually happy, harmonious and healthy, a pattern which may continue in subsequent pregnancies.

The positive feelings are many and glorious, and can be as overwhelmingly surprising as the negative ones. You may feel a heightened sense of awareness and perception, and respond more strongly or sharply than you would normally. You may feel powerful, full, rich, delighted, overjoyed, exhilarated, excited (and impatient!), elated, glowing, expectant and euphoric, but also peaceful, tender, vulnerable, calm and special.

Some women feel sensual and voluptuous, perhaps a primitive expression of fertility; others, who recognise an early strong connection or bond with their babies, feel a growing sense of falling in love, of walking on clouds – especially after the baby first moves. The magical feeling of the baby moving makes the pregnancy feel real, sometimes for the first time: it's hard not to feel special, harmonious, creative. When the baby starts to move is when feelings often surface more strongly: excitement may be tinged with fear, anxiety or resentment.

You may experience increased energy, especially after the third month, culminating in the 'nesting' instinct towards the end of pregnancy: you may find yourself tidying, cleaning and even redecorating your home, which can be a pleasure – or can be a real pain if it gets out of hand. Pregnancy is a time of preparation for the baby, for parenthood and for couples to grow closer.

I have included a few remedies for overexcitement, with consequent sleeplessness. If your good feelings get out of hand, if you become slightly manic and your health begins to suffer, get professional help from a psychotherapist, counsellor or homeopath.

Do

- acknowledge and express your positive feelings. Suppressed excitement can be as stressful as suppressed anger.
- include your partner in your inner life during your pregnancy, by sharing your feelings regularly.
- find a close friend to talk to if you are a single pregnant parent.
- keep a diary of your feelings and the changes that you go through – it will be a delightful reminder of this special time.
- use your energy creatively and don't squander it.
- tell the world how wonderful you feel and enjoy it. Sharing a good feeling doubles it and spreads it to others.

'Negative' Feelings

Pregnancy is a time of physical, emotional and even social change, which has different effects on every woman depending on her character and history, birth and childhood, unresolved and unvoiced traumas, and including ambivalence about motherhood. It may be a time of life-style change, from that of a relatively free single or married person to that of a parent. Finances may be tight, living quarters cramped, or friends thin on the ground because of a recent move to a new area.

Pregnancy brings so much into question.

Some women maintain that having a child won't change a thing, that life will carry on (or that they will carry on their lives) much as it always has and that the baby will fit in. But life *does* change – substantially for some.

Pregnancy can be awful if you feel unwell. Some women just feel fat and disgusting; athletic women may resent being slowed down and feel annoyed at the extra fat that develops – may dislike the 'softening' effect of pregnancy. Others look on the baby as a 'lump', which they take pride in not showing until the last month, and avoid looking at their bodies or talking about them: to them the baby may feel like a parasite. Being pregnant is confirmation of a woman's sexuality and her womanhood, which can be painful to some women who have not been able to accept or be open about this side of themselves.

Fears are a normal part of pregnancy: explore them with your partner or a good friend, being as honest as you can. Take your anxieties seriously and talk them through: they aren't irrational or neurotic, they always have a base in reality. The more that is questioned and dealt with in pregnancy the better: issues like money and childcare won't go away but at least the options can be explored when you have the time and energy to do so.

Don't forget that negative feelings can be viewed positively as an opportunity to grow and develop a deeper understanding of yourself – use them, don't ignore them.

While you are pregnant, you may be confronted by:

- anticipatory anxiety, accompanied or caused by low self-confidence about your ability to parent or to love. (Women who have written themselves a 'be perfect' script, with an I've-got-to-get-it-just-right message, suffer from this acutely.)
- denial, often associated with indifference or apathy. Some ignore the presence of the baby growing inside them – it is a relief not to think about the inevitability of what is to happen.
- confusion. Women who already have small children and are struggling to get by may be unable to imagine how an extra baby can possibly fit into their lives.
- depression, especially if fears or anxieties are not expressed.
- guilt – for any negative feelings!
- tales and beliefs passed down in families from generation to generation which may be hard to shift: 'All the women in this family have Caesareans.' Question everything your mother told you about pregnancy and childbirth unless it rings positive and true for you.
- resentment.
- shock. An 'Oh-my-God-what-have-I-done?' feeling.

You may fear:

- being trapped, losing your freedom, and the new and overwhelming responsibilities ahead – 'I won't be able to cope'.
- loss of control, events happening without being able to affect them.
- loss of libido (especially if it occurred in your last pregnancy and continued through breastfeeding).
- loss of identity or individuality as you realise your role is going to change whatever fixed ideas you might have had. Women whose own childhoods were spent trying to do the right thing for their parents often grow up insecure and not knowing deep down who they are. They may hide this by being successful and doing well but pregnancy may bring it out again.
- the baby being abnormal or deformed.
- death, either of the baby during or after birth or of yourself dying during childbirth. This can be strong in women who have had a previous miscarriage, abortion or stillbirth, partly through unresolved feelings of guilt or sadness.
- that the pregnancy will never end. The last month or two can feel endless, especially if it's summer and you've put on a lot of weight or are carrying twins. You may feel heavy, tired, awkward, hot, impatient and irritable.
- that the baby will be the wrong sex.
- that the baby will affect your relationships with your partner and/or your other children. It will: partners and children may have their own fears and anxieties so encourage them to speak out and prevent needless guilt or worry. The trick is learning to balance everyone's needs – the more people there are, the more difficult this is. Children, perhaps especially, may feel resentful and jealous – that they will lose their mummy – or scared that they won't like the new member of the family.
- your partner not wanting a child that wasn't planned. He may not. He may be negative for at least part of the pregnancy. Keep talking.
- physical changes, excess weight and stretch marks, etc.
- never having time to yourself, especially to rest if you are pregnant and have other small children to look after.
- becoming unlovable.
- childbirth.
- not being able to cope, especially if you are a single parent, when it is all the more important not to isolate yourself. Don't be tempted to work all the time.

Some women feel good in one pregnancy and terrible in another or fine in the early months and terrible as the birth draws near. There are no rules!

Your mental and emotional health has a very significant bearing on your physical health. Homeopathy is highly effective at helping with emotional stress but it is unwise to treat yourself as it is difficult to be objective about how you are behaving – for example, you may feel depressed but are actually being irritable. A trained homeopath will be able to differentiate and prescribe a remedy that fits the whole picture.

Emotional Stress

It is important to acknowledge and deal with stress in pregnancy especially if it is severe: anything that affects you will, to some extent, affect your baby. Now that you are no longer simply responsible for yourself, you cannot afford to ignore what is happening to you. Moving house, problems at work, conflict with your partner or the death (or illness) of a close friend or relative are stressful at any time but particularly in pregnancy. If you ignore or suppress your feelings, loss of energy or ill-health or both will very likely be the result.

Look in the Repertory under Complaints From (p. 269) where you will find many stress symptoms, including grief, anger, resentment, mental strain and bad news. Repertorise your symptoms carefully to find the remedy that best fits your whole picture. Seek the advice of a homeopath if you don't feel better quite quickly.

Do

- start by being honestly aware of your feelings. Be kind and compassionate towards yourself – and try not to be self-critical.
- explore your feelings regularly with your partner, a friend or a counsellor. Remember there is more than a little truth in the old saying that 'a problem shared is a problem halved'.
- find a close friend to talk to if you are a single pregnant parent.
- try to understand what lies behind your feelings. You may need professional help to discover unresolved emotional experiences from your past and childhood, difficulties you are having in your life now but not dealing with, anxieties and fears about the future that you are not expressing.
- assess and reassess your priorities regularly.
- reduce the stress in your life – right now, cross something off your list of things to do. It can be a heady experience: once you start you may find that other things can go too.
- reassess your beliefs and your life-style, what you want for your life ahead and for your family.
- listen to concerned friends or relatives if you are good at hiding your feelings when you feel

unhappy. Your emotional distress may not be evident to you. Depression can feel like tiredness – you don't want to get up in the mornings, or don't feel like eating, cooking or shopping because you're not very hungry, and you can't sleep. It's not a big deal but it is common and it is essential you deal with it *now*.

- write about what you are going through.
- understand what is happening rather than fight it.
- learn to laugh at yourself.
- slow down. Pregnancy helps in this automatically especially towards the end when you become heavier.
- read light-hearted books and avoid anything depressing or frightening.
- learn a relaxation or meditation technique and take time to do it at least once a day.
- seek the help of a counsellor or psychotherapist if your feelings are persistent and do not resolve through taking the above steps.
- seek alternative medical help to alleviate your symptoms.

Don't
- neglect your own needs. Now is the time, more than ever before, to put yourself first: you are *the mother* and you must be in reasonable shape to do your job properly. If there is something you really need and want, try to get it – it's easier than you think once you start talking. Even if you have to compromise, at least you were heard and that alone will help.
- talk to anyone who is critical and judgemental of how you are feeling or who adopts the 'count your blessings' approach. This person is trying to minimise and talk you out of your feelings. Don't listen.
- talk to people who give you constant, unwelcome advice. 'Your trouble is that you think too much. You need to dwell less on all these negative things. Remember there are a lot of people worse off than you.'
- cut yourself off from sympathetic friends and family. You need them even though your behaviour may be pushing them away. Tell them what you are going through, reach out and ask for their help. Start by making straightforward requests.
- hide, ignore or suppress any difficulties you are having.
- take anti-depressants, sleeping pills or other orthodox medication as these may not only affect your body but will suppress your feelings and make it more difficult for you to deal with them later.

Seek help if
- you are floundering and are finding that talking to partners/friends isn't helping. A counsellor or psychotherapist will be especially valuable.

EXHAUSTION

Tiredness can be completely obliterating in early pregnancy. Its major causes are hormonal and physical changes, unexpressed or unresolved emotional difficulties, and anaemia. I have included many remedies for exhaustion, some for tiredness after specific stresses like a period of hard work, an acute illness or after diarrhoea.

Look at the whole picture and repertorise carefully, bearing in mind that you may be anaemic or simply overworked. Be honest and realistic about why you are tired and take common-sense measures to look after yourself, as well as the appropriate homeopathic remedy to hasten your recovery. Many women have found that simply alternating the tissue salts *Kali phosphoricum* and *Calcarea phosphorica* (if suffering from nervous exhaustion) or *Ferrum metallicum* and *Calcarea phosphoricum* (if suffering from mild anaemia) is sufficient to make them feel better. Either may be repeated as often as needed throughout the pregnancy, stopping each time on improvement.

Do
- rest and sleep as much as you can and as you feel you need.
- eat especially well from a wide range of foods including plenty of protein. Eat little and often and drink plenty of fluids.
- delegate workloads for a realistic period of time while you recharge (at home or at work).
- vary your daily activities – boredom is tiring! Any activity that is stimulating (exciting) is energising *and* too much stimulation can be draining. It is the balance that counts – getting enough mental, emotional and/or physical stimulation to keep you from becoming bored without exhausting you.
- take gentle exercise, which will help to create energy.
- read undemanding books and magazines, the funnier the better.
- have a massage, facial or haircut, etc., at home, if you can arrange this.
- arrange to spend time with friends doing easy fun things unassociated with work or motherhood.

Seek help if
- the exhaustion persists in spite of following these guidelines.

EYESIGHT CHANGES

Contact lens wearers may develop problems with their lenses as during pregnancy the eye can change shape slightly due to fluid accumulation.

Do
- Consult your optician and keep in regular contact if you develop problems.
- bathe your eyes regularly with *Euphrasia* if they become sore (see p. 205).

FOOD CRAVINGS

Food cravings and aversions are mostly benign, aversions often being against foods contraindicated in pregnancy anyway, such as caffeine and junk food. Occasionally the reverse happens, which warrants attention. Morning sickness (either nausea or vomiting) can cause a change or total loss of appetite which should be dealt with. Cravings can be mild and amusing, like wanting shrimp and peanut-butter sandwiches at three in the morning, or positively self-destructive, when they are usually a symptom of emotional stress, exhaustion or dietary deficiency.

'Pica' is a craving for non-foodstuffs, such as earth or coal, and although I have included a few remedies for the treatment of this condition, I would strongly advise that if your appetite goes out of control during pregnancy you seek professional guidance.

Do
- eat regularly: five to six small meals a day rather than three large ones.
- make sure you have *plenty* of fresh fruit and vegetables.
- eat slowly and chew thoroughly as the saliva that is released will aid digestion.
- eat a varied diet from all food groups – fat, protein, carbohydrate, etc.

Don't
- indulge wild cravings unlimitedly.

Seek help if
- you cannot control a craving for a bizarre substance.

GROIN PAIN

See Pain, pp. 96–9.

HAIR AND NAIL PROBLEMS

Although many women find that their hair and nails are healthier during pregnancy than ever before, others find the reverse is true, perhaps because they neglect their diet, or because of emotional stress or hormonal changes. Hair can lose its shine and its curl and can fall out more heavily than usual. Nails can become brittle and break easily.

If the state of your hair is only a part of a larger picture of ill-health then you will need to prescribe on all the symptoms, seeking professional help if you are not successful. If you are generally healthy, both physically and emotionally but your hair is lank and your nails brittle, then a short course of *Silica* or *Calcarea phosphorica* may help.

Do
- make sure your diet is adequate. Fish, wheatgerm, yeast and liver are all said to provide the E and B vitamins essential for healthy hair and nails. Minerals like iron, iodine, zinc, silicon and sulphur are also important. A short course of multivitamins and minerals may help – apply the homeopathic principle of stopping on improvement.
- visit a qualified nutritionist if you are on a restricted diet – vegan, dairy-free, etc. – to ensure that you take the supplements you need.
- wash your hair frequently with a very mild shampoo – especially if you live in a polluted city, and massage your scalp thoroughly each time.

HEADACHES

Occasional minor headaches, resulting from such obvious stresses as overwork, loss of sleep or worry, can be treated with first-aid homeopathy. As well as finding the appropriate remedy, identify and remove or balance the cause of your headache – i.e. if you have been up all night with a sick child, have a nap.

Do
- rest and relax. Check your posture for tension if you feel a headache coming on and spend 10 minutes breathing deeply.
- have a nap – or at least lie down with your eyes closed – if you can take the time.
- get some fresh air if you've been in a stuffy atmosphere.
- have your eyes tested to make sure the cause is not a deterioration in eyesight – this is possible during pregnancy.
- seek counselling or psychotherapy help if you are under a lot of emotional stress.

- talk your worries, resentments or fears through with your partner or another sympathetic ear: tension building from unexpressed feelings commonly causes head and back pain.
- have a massage, if it helps. Ask an older child or your partner to rub your head, shoulders and back.
- rub your own shoulders, especially muscles at the base of the skull, or apply pressure around the temples – be guided by your instincts as to where to press.
- take a long bath.
- eat regular meals. During pregnancy the metabolism speeds up and you will need to stoke your 'energy fire' more often. Missing a meal can cause a headache: you can check this out by eating something like a spoonful of honey which will give your blood sugar an instant boost.
- ask people not to smoke around you if you know that tobacco is the culprit. During pregnancy many women are more sensitive to smoke and get instant headaches in a not very smoky room.
- exercise by rotating your head slowly and evenly, first one way and then the other, by lifting your shoulders as high as you can and then letting them slowly down. Exercise your head, neck and back in any other way that feels good; as you breathe out (see Breathing, p. 40) imagine the tension releasing.

Don't
- take pain-relieving drugs and carry on.

Seek help if
- the headache is severe.
- you are suffering from frequent or severe headaches, particularly if your eyesight is deteriorating.
- a headache is accompanied by a stiff neck.
- you have a high fever, visual disturbance, weakness or lack of co-ordination, or dizziness.
- a headache lasts more than three or four days.

HEARTBURN

Your stomach is under the breastbone, between and just under the breasts. Indigestion and heartburn are especially common in late pregnancy when the stomach has a smaller space in which to expand. Also, hormones relax the sphincter of the stomach making it easier for acid to escape into the oesophagus with consequent burning pain. Digestion slows down in pregnancy and the liver works less efficiently. Both are due to hormonal changes.

Do
- eat smaller more frequent meals, every three hours or so.
- eat slowly and chew thoroughly so that plenty of saliva is released and food partially digested before it reaches your stomach.
- cut down on fatty foods as the gall bladder works less efficiently, causing nausea and/or indigestion.
- avoid anything you know to cause more discomfort, such as spicy foods, onions and garlic, bread, dairy and other fatty foods, sugar or meat. Experiment to find out which foods you cannot tolerate.
- relax before meals and eat sitting down at the table.
- avoid bending over – to wash the bath or pick up toys from the floor – as this will cause acid to escape from the stomach. Squat down instead, keeping the trunk of your body upright.
- lie down on a wedge of pillows so that you are not sleeping completely flat, which can also encourage acid to leak into the oesophagus.

Don't
- take antacids without professional advice as they can upset the balance of the acidity in the stomach even further and contribute to anaemia by affecting your iron absorption.
- drink a lot of fluids with meals as this can bloat the stomach and make the heartburn worse.

Seek help if
- symptoms are accompanied by a cough, loss of appetite or loss of weight.
- there is severe abdominal pain.
- the heartburn is severe and doesn't pass off (with or without first-aid prescribing) within two or three hours.

HERPES, GENITAL

Genital herpes is caused by the same virus that causes herpes (cold sores) on the lips. It is spread by sexual contact and can lodge in the nervous system breaking out at times of stress. The first attack can occur months or even years after infection. It may be a one-off or recur cyclically. The symptoms are mild (a small blister that itches and doesn't even come to a head) to severe (extremely painful blisters preceded by pains in the buttock and leg and accompanied by exhaustion and flu-like feelings). There is no cure although constitutional homeopathic treatment can help decrease the severity and frequency of attacks. If you have a blister at the time of giving birth your baby will be delivered by Caesarean because of the risk to its life if it contracts the disease.

Do

- tell your GP if you have ever had an attack of genital herpes.
- advise your GP immediately if you have your first outbreak in the first three months of your pregnancy as it may cause damage to the baby.
- the following if you have an outbreak (a blister): anything you can to boost your immunity – eat well, rest and sleep well, take some extra vitamin C, garlic or *anything* that you know makes you feel better – this will help reduce the severity of the attack; keep the affected area dry and cool; avoid nylon underwear and tight trousers and try to spend as much time as possible without underwear to expose the blister(s) to the air; avoid hot baths; add a handful of sea salt to a tepid bath to aid healing; avoid intercourse until the sores have healed; be vigilant with hygiene if you have an open blister.

HIGH BLOOD PRESSURE
(Hypertension)

This is beyond the scope of the home prescriber and should always be treated seriously. On its own a small rise in blood pressure isn't a cause for concern, but it can precede the development of more serious conditions, which is why your doctor or midwife will want to monitor your blood pressure carefully throughout your pregnancy.

The doctor will write down two numbers when taking your blood pressure. The high one (systolic) reflects the heart at work (how well the body deals with exertion) and the low one (diastolic) reflects the heart at rest (a sort of baseline of physical tension). The numbers should read around 120/80 (with individual variations). High blood pressure is diagnosed if your blood pressure rises to 130/90 or more, or if the systolic reading rises 30 points above its norm and the dyostolic 15 points or more, based on your blood-pressure readings from early pregnancy. Your blood pressure may take a natural dip in the second trimester of your pregnancy.

Do

- ask if your midwife will come and take your blood pressure at home. The curious phenomenon known as 'white coat hypertension' refers to the stress of a lengthy wait in a hospital or doctor's surgery, which can cause a temporary rise in blood pressure. (The diagnosis of 'high blood pressure' can in itself be stressful, causing anxiety in a nervous woman, which forces the readings higher still.) If your blood pressure is higher than usual at an ante-natal check-up, ask yourself if you felt anxious or pressured beforehand.

- rest. If your blood pressure is high go to your sofa or bed and stay there until it starts to come down.
- cut down the stress in your life. Working women juggling home and office may need to stop work temporarily. Get clear about your priorities – and the consequences of ignoring your body's early warning signals. If you are very stressed, and you have high blood pressure, your body needs rest and you *must* take the pressure off yourself. Or is your work more important than you and your growing baby? Remember – when everything becomes so pressured that you can't possibly take time off, *that's* the time to take time off.
- relaxation exercises and/or meditate regularly.
- cut out *all* stimulants (tea, coffee, chocolate, tobacco) if you haven't already done that.
- cut down on your salt intake if it is high. Cook without it, adding a *little* sea salt, if you really need it, at the table.
- make sure your diet has plenty of protein each day, enough calcium and lots of fruit and vegetables. Talk to a dietician or nutritionist, if in doubt.
- drink relaxing herbal teas in moderation – chamomile and hops are good.
- increase your fluid intake.
- exercise as well as rest. Brisk walking or swimming are both good but build up slowly.
- ask friends and family to help out with your other children and/or household chores until your blood pressure comes down.
- seek counselling help if you are under a lot of emotional stress.
- seek alternative medical help with bringing it down as quickly as possible.

Seek help if

- you also have a sudden weight gain and puffy wrists or ankles which don't disappear after a night's sleep. This could herald the onset of preeclampsia (see p. 86).

INCONTINENCE

'Urinary or stress incontinence', that is, leaking when you cough, sneeze, laugh or exert yourself, is common in pregnancy partly due to the pressure of the growing uterus on the bladder, and partly because the pregnancy hormones relax the muscles and sphincters. See also pp. 78–9.

Do

- Your pelvic-floor exercises (see p. 43) religiously –

even if you don't exercise a single other muscle in the body.

- urinate frequently so that your bladder doesn't become stressed.

INDIGESTION

See Heartburn, p. 91.

INSOMNIA

We all have different sleep requirements. In the early months of pregnancy most women need more sleep than previously – up to 10 hours a night with a day-time nap. If this sleep (and nap) refreshes then no treatment is necessary. If you are getting plenty of sleep but are still exhausted and dragging yourself around during the day, prescribe on your low energy (see Exhaustion, p. 89). Your sleep pattern may have been disturbed by illness or small children so that you find it difficult to get to sleep, and/or wake early. Emotional stress can also affect sleep patterns. If you are a long-term insomniac, you need to consult a professional homeopath if you continue to suffer during your pregnancy. If, however, you are coping well on four or five hours' sleep a night, don't worry. Your moods and your energy level will let you know if lack of sleep is taking its toll.

Do

- develop a regular bedtime relaxation routine, including deep breathing, gentle exercise such as a walk round the block or some yoga positions, a warm bath and a hot caffeine-free drink such as hot milk with honey or a cup of chamomile tea. *Don't* drink chamomile every night unless it really helps: you may find yourself becoming unusually irritable – the reverse of the effect it is meant to have – and are, therefore, 'proving' it (see p. 10). If this happens, stop at once.
- read boring books or magazines in bed.
- wear earplugs and an eye mask to cut out noise and light if necessary.
- make sure your mattress is right for you, neither too hard nor too soft.
- make sure you are warm enough, but not too hot, and that your room is well ventilated.
- do some basic relaxation exercises. Tense your whole body and then relax your muscles one by one, starting at your head and moving down your body. Then imagine you are very heavy and are falling through the bed – tense people can 'hold' themselves just above the bed.
- count backwards in threes from 600!

- put the light on and read or listen to the radio if you can't sleep, and try again when you feel ready.
- clear any 'niggles' with your partner well before you go to bed so that you aren't keeping yourself awake by chewing over resentments.
- sit up and make a list of all worries and frustrations if you can't sleep because of them and make an action plan for dealing with them.
- seek counselling or psychotherapy if your sleeplessness is due to emotional distress such as anxiety, depression or bereavement.

Don't

- worry or panic! This always makes sleeplessness worse.
- read thrillers, ghost stories or stories that upset you in bed.
- have a large meal close to bedtime.
- drink tea, hot chocolate, coffee or Coca-Cola during the evening (or at any other time) as all contain caffeine.
- watch too much television.
- work in the evening or take material connected with your work to bed.
- get into taking long afternoon naps or sleeping very late in the morning as this can make it more difficult to get back to a normal sleeping pattern, especially if this is your first pregnancy.
- take sleeping pills. Apart from the effect they may have on your unborn child they can affect your dream life so that you wake feeling unrefreshed. Many have side effects, causing drowsiness and dependence.
- drink any alcohol.

INVERTED NIPPLES

See Breastfeeding problems, pp. 117–23.

ITCHING

Itchy skin without a rash is common in pregnancy especially towards the end. The skin can itch all over, or just on the abdomen where it is being stretched, and can be made worse by heat. Take a short course of *Sulphur* and, if it helps, repeat if the itching returns.

Do

- keep cool.
- try a tepid bath with half a cup of cider vinegar.
- keep your skin well oiled if it is getting dry and

itchy – you can put some oil in the bath or massage it in afterwards.

Don't

- use coal tar or hydrocortisone creams on your skin.

Seek help if

- a rash accompanies the itching.
- home prescribing doesn't help and the itching is preventing you from sleeping.

JOINT PAIN

See Pain, pp. 96–9.

LOSS OF LIBIDO

Sex can be entirely spontaneous – and especially with a first baby (there aren't other small persons liable to wake in the middle of the night and interrupt you).

It can be health-promoting, energising, as you renew physical and emotional bonds with your partner, and active sex counts as physical exercise: it is very good for the pelvic-floor muscles (see p. 43) – *and* it's relaxing and sleep-promoting!

You cannot harm the baby while making love: the uterus thoughtfully moves up and out of the way when you are sexually aroused. Also the hormones in semen that help the cervix to soften and dilate in early labour will *only* have that effect when you are in labour. If penetration is painful, experiment with different positions; take your time with foreplay and adopt a slower, gentler pace of lovemaking than perhaps you were used to before your pregnancy.

Loss of libido can be due to unexpressed feelings which cause you to withdraw sexually *and* emotionally, or you may be having difficulty getting used to your constantly expanding body: talk to your partner or to a psychotherapist or counsellor. It is important to try to identify the cause: maybe you feel fat and unattractive, tired or nauseous or have been influenced by ancient unfounded taboos against sex during pregnancy.

Causticum, *Natrum muriaticum* and *Sepia* can all help with loss of libido, but only if they fit your picture in other ways as well. If you have, say, cramps, depression *and* loss of libido, *Causticum* will help both you and your sex drive.

Do

- familiarise yourself with your changing body. Look at yourself in the mirror without your clothes on. Massage yourself after your bath or shower.

Talk about these changes with your partner: be honest about how you feel about them. Ask your partner to massage your body; talk about which parts are sensitive and be specific about how you would like to be touched.

- find ways of being close to your partner without necessarily leading to sex (learn to separate affection from sex and sex from penetration).
- tell your partner how you feel, if you have gone off sex, when and why you think it happened, and what you need. Express any resentments and ask for your partner's support and understanding.
- encourage your partner to share their feelings also – some find their pregnant women incredibly sexy and others quite the opposite.
- find some time each day to be by yourself, to have a bath, read a book or go for a walk, even if only for fifteen minutes.
- deal with any tiredness.
- get seriously into pleasure and sensuality – there's nothing sexier! Shared baths (if it's big enough), massage, breakfast in bed, hugs and strokes, etc.
- let yourself go!
- choose a time to make love when you know that you will not be interrupted by your other child or children.
- seek the help of a counsellor or psychotherapist who is trained to work with sexual difficulties if you go off sex in your pregnancy.

Don't

- make love (with penetration) if you experience pain no matter what position you try; if you are bleeding, even if it's only spotting; in your early pregnancy if you have a history of miscarriage and feel you want to play safe; if your waters have broken in late pregnancy/early labour as there is a risk of infection.
- feel guilty if you don't want penetrative sex. There are other ways to give each other pleasure: masturbation won't make you blind and neither will oral sex.
- abandon your partner. Continue to show affection. If you don't want to, you are holding in feelings that need to be expressed.

Seek help if

- you experience feelings of disgust towards your body and sex.
- your partner associates affection with sex and you feel you can't be affectionate because of what it will lead to.

LOW BLOOD PRESSURE (fainting)

The symptoms of low blood pressure are feelings of faintness and dizziness on standing up quickly from sitting, stooping or lying down. It can be a nuisance in pregnancy but is rarely a cause for concern. Blood pressure always drops between the third and the sixth month of pregnancy due to hormonal changes.

Faintness and dizziness may be associated with anaemia (see p. 80). If you have this condition, repertorise carefully to find a remedy that matches all of your symptoms.

Do
- use your pregnancy to become more graceful and to take life at a slower pace.
- sit down immediately if you feel faint – even if it means sitting or lying on your side on a supermarket floor (preferable to passing out and hurting yourself by falling clumsily). If you can find a chair, sit down with your legs apart (to accommodate your abdomen), breathing deeply and evenly, and bend forward, placing your elbows on your knees. Get up *only* when you feel ready.
- stand up slowly from sitting, stooping or lying down, at any time, including the morning when you get out of bed. Take your time.

Seek help if
- you often feel faint and dizzy and not just when you stand up quickly.

MORNING SICKNESS

Usually associated with the first three or four months of pregnancy it can, for some poor unfortunates, last most of the nine months. In some women it occurs only in the morning but in others lasts all day while still others suffer at different times of the day and even night. In the first three months it feels unfair because it comes at a time when you don't look pregnant and therefore don't automatically collect sympathy from, say, people sitting down in rush-hour trains or buses while you die on your feet.

The causes were commonly thought to be related to hormonal changes but it is now known that the emotional state also has a significant bearing on morning sickness: doubt, ambivalence, fear, resentment, disgust and denial can all contribute to or aggravate it.

The nausea is often accompanied by one or more of the following symptoms: an increased sensitivity to smells – particular smells, strong smells, or even any smell – and to noise – loud noises or the slightest, softest sound; a foul, metallic taste in the mouth which is only relieved while eating; a funny smell *in* the nose which taints all other smells; and alteration in appetite (see Food Cravings, p. 90). Many things can worsen nausea like eating, drinking, motion, sleeping, emotional upsets, etc.

When you self-prescribe on this unpleasant condition, do search into your soul and record honestly your secret thoughts and feelings about the baby and take them into account. If you don't succeed quite quickly and the nausea is severe, don't hesitate to get professional advice.

Do
- talk through ambivalent, difficult feelings with your partner or a close friend – they are quite normal, even if they are intense.
- eat plenty of fresh fruit and vegetables for a day or two and introduce unrefined carbohydrates (wholewheat bread and pasta, and unpeeled potatoes) for a couple of days. If that doesn't help introduce a high-protein diet (fish, cheese, eggs and meat, if you eat it). Tune into the inner voice that tells you what you can and can't eat.
- try eliminating fats and rich, fatty foods, dairy foods, sugar and even fruit.
- make sure you are getting enough calcium elsewhere if you cut out dairy foods, and iron if you cut out meat and wholewheat.
- have a drink with a dry biscuit or piece of dry toast on waking. Eat the biscuit lying down, before you lift your head off the pillow, very slowly and thoroughly and have your drink sitting up but before you get up. Some women have found this trick to work wonders. Instead of tea or coffee, try a glass of hot or cold lemon and honey, a cup of herbal tea or a teaspoon of cider vinegar in warm water – with or without honey. Ginger tea is a good alternative to lemon and honey, made with powdered or freshly grated ginger and a little honey to taste. Don't make it too strong and avoid it altogether if you are a warm-blooded person as it can make you feel even hotter. Honey tea – hot water, milk and honey – is also good.
- eat little and often, slowly, and chew thoroughly. Sit down and enjoy what you eat.

Don't
- fast unless eating aggravates your symptoms, in which case you must get professional help.
- let yourself get hungry, which means that your blood sugar levels have dropped and it will be harder for your body to bring them up again.
- worry if you lose some weight in the first three months of your pregnancy. Your baby will get what it needs from your fat supplies and you will put on weight once the nausea has passed and you can eat normally again.

Seek help if
- the nausea is accompanied by vomiting, especially if you are vomiting everything you eat and are keeping very little fluid down. A professional homeopath can usually help with this condition, with no harmful side effects to your baby.
- you are unable to talk to those closest to you or have feelings that you can't put into words. A counsellor will help you to understand and resolve them.

NOSEBLEEDS

These can be troublesome in pregnancy due to hormonal changes and the increased blood volume. As a preventive measure, blow your nose more gently.

It is important to prescribe on the loss of blood if you have bled copiously (see Complaints from loss of body fluids in the Repertory, or *Ferrum metallicum* if you have a tendency to anaemia).

Do
- sit with your head tilted forward and breathe through your mouth (spit out blood that drips into your throat).
- pinch together the soft part of the nose for about 15 minutes, or less if the bleeding stops sooner.
- hold a cloth wrung out in very cold water or an ice-pack over your nose for a few minutes and then pinch your nostrils again.
- sit quietly and repeat the above if the bleeding starts again.

Don't
- blow your nose if you start a nosebleed, or for a few hours after it stops bleeding.
- sniff or swallow the blood if you can avoid it.

Seek help if
- the bleeding doesn't stop.
- a lot of blood is lost and you become pale and dizzy.

OEDEMA

A common pregnancy complaint, the cause of which is not fully understood. It is thought to be due to the pull of gravity combined with the increased volume of body fluids and fluid retention. A slight puffiness or swelling develops in the feet, ankles and/or hands which disappears after a rest or a night's sleep. Women who are overweight or carrying twins or large babies are more susceptible. Hot weather and standing for long periods usually make it worse.

Many homeopathic remedies are appropriate to this condition so the whole picture counts. What *else* have you got? If a bit of swelling is all – and I mean all – take a short course of *Natrum muriaticum* and stop if it helps (repeating as needed). Other remedies like *Apis mellifica* or *Phosphorus* may be useful depending on the whole picture.

Do
- exercise.
- wear comfortable, flat shoes.
- wear support tights. Before you get out of bed in the morning, raise your legs to empty the veins before you put them on.
- take off your rings to avoid them getting stuck if your fingers swell badly.

Don't
- stand if you can sit.
- sit if you can lie down (or sit with your feet up).
- cross your legs when sitting down.
- wear high-heeled shoes.
- wear socks or stockings with tight tops, or any tight clothes, especially tight trousers.
- restrict your intake of fluids in the belief that it will help the swelling as reduced liquids may even aggravate the condition.

Seek help if
- swelling is as bad in the morning in spite of a good night's sleep. Excessive swelling can be a warning sign of a more serious condition developing, such as pre-eclampsia.
- your fingers leave an indentation mark when you press a puffy area (like your ankle). This is called 'pitting oedema' and may also indicate pre-eclampsia (see p. 86).

PAIN

The main areas in which you may experience either transitory or prolonged aches and pains are the abdomen, back, groin and joints. The bones of the pelvis form a cradle shape, which is lined with a complex criss-crossing of muscles and ligaments which holds the contents of the pelvis securely in it. The uterus floats fairly freely in the abdomen attached by ligaments to various of the organs, including the bladder and rectum, and the pelvis. Ligaments are fibrous tissue with very little elasticity whose job is to hold firm. The uterus is held mainly by two pairs of ligaments: the round ligaments which run from the front of the uterus down into the groin and the broad/flat ligaments that run from the sides of the uterus to the lower back (sacrum). They work in pregnancy like sail ropes – holding the uterus firm once it's full! As it expands the ligaments are stretched, which may cause pain. It is important to exercise the muscles of pelvis and spine throughout your pregnancy so that they are strong and supple enough to cope with the added weight. One of the functions of the hormones produced in pregnancy is to soften bones, joints and ligaments in preparation for the birth of the baby, which adds to the likelihood of minor discomfort developing.

The following general suggestions are to help you cope with the annoyingly debilitating pains which may accompany pregnancy. Try them as a first resort and if they don't help, consult the sections which follow dealing with specific pains which offer further self-help measures and suggestions for homeopathic treatment. Or self-prescribe, taking the whole picture into account.

Do

• rest as much as you need to. Make sure your mattress supports you without being too hard.
• exercise gently and regularly to build healthy, strong, supple muscles, joints and ligaments.
• breathe deeply, slowly and evenly through the pain. Pain can make you tense so that you breathe too shallowly, which will increase tension. Breathing deeply will bring oxygen to tense muscles and help you relax.
• relax: tension increases pain. Try lying down, stretching or having a hot bath. Imagine your muscles relaxing as you breathe out and let go of each breath.
• find sitting, standing and lying positions that ease the pains and use them.
• lift using your legs to avoid unnecessary strain on your back and abdomen.
• think before you bend, twist, turn or lift and take it more slowly than you would normally.
• know your body's limits, be 'careful' with it in pregnancy and 'listen' to it.
• try massage to help relieve pain and soreness. Your partner or a close friend can give your back and shoulders a comforting rub.
• maintain good posture when sitting or standing and seek the help of an Alexander-technique teacher if you slump when sitting or walking or find yourself being dragged forward by the weight of your uterus as it gets bigger. He or she will help by giving you advice and exercises to help you correct your bad habits (see Posture, p. 43).
• carry two bags when shopping rather than one heavy one.
• consider wearing a girdle or 'maternity belt' for the relief of abdominal and/or back pain if: you are carrying a big baby (or several); you were over-

weight and out of condition before you became pregnant; if you have put on a lot of weight; if your muscle tone is poor; if you are having to be active or on your feet a lot; if your tummy is uncomfortable towards the end of the day – especially towards the middle of your pregnancy; if you *feel* instinctively that having some light-weight abdominal support would be very comforting. It can be. Unfortunately it is a fashion that has fallen out of favour in this age of 'flat tummies'. If you do decide to wear one then put it on at the beginning of the day so that your muscles don't get a chance to become tired and achy. Mothercare stock a pantie-girdle for pregnant women; specialist corsetry stores sell various products, including lightweight maternity briefs or girdles with soft, elasticated front panels and maternity belts (a strip of adjustable webbing with Velcro fasteners).

Don't

• lift heavy weights – especially towards the end of your pregnancy and if lifting has caused problems in the past. Ask for help in carrying and make more journeys rather than doing it all at once.
• continue a movement that feels even slightly uncomfortable, as this is how ligaments are strained. A strained ligament takes a surprisingly long time to heal and is vulnerable to further strain.
• grit your teeth and carry on (working/washing/running around after small children) if your body 'complains'.

Abdominal Pain

Common but unwelcome, especially towards the end when you seem to be stretched to your limit! It is often caused by the stretching and straining that occurs as your body accommodates the growing uterus: muscles, ligaments and nerves have continually to adapt. Sometimes they complain!

The pressure of the baby or parts of its body (especially its head) can cause discomfort in the abdomen if it presses down on the bladder, kidneys, ovaries, rectum or up on the ribs. This is normally transient and the 'pain' can be relieved by changing position. Some babies love to kick and depending on the position in which the baby is lying muscles or even organs like the bladder can become quite sore and bruised. Take *Arnica* (6, 12 or 30) if you simply feel sore and bruised but if you feel really 'abused' by, say, a sharp kick in the bladder, take *Staphysagria*. If, however, the baby becomes very active after you have had a shock, you should repertorise carefully, taking the whole picture into account.

The weight of the expanding uterus stretches and can strain the ligaments, resulting in stiffness and soreness. (Even turning in bed at night needs to be done carefully, especially towards the end of your pregnancy.) If you let the weight drag you forward the broad bands of ligaments attached to the spine are pulled, causing discomfort and pain.

Look up sprains and strains in the Repertory and choose between the remedies listed using your general symptoms.

Unusual and distressing, although not dangerous, are sharp abdominal pains which dart about, too fast to be pinned down or properly described. They come and go and you can do nothing about them except take a homeopathic remedy and perhaps, if they persist, see a masseur. The specific remedy for this complaint is *Cimicifuga*: take it in a low potency (6 or 12) for up to a week, stopping on improvement and repeating if it has worked well and the symptoms return.

Do
- ask your doctor or midwife for an examination if the pain persists, even if it is not severe, because a mild infection of the bladder or urethra (urinary tract infection) can cause abdominal pain.

Seek help if
- pain is severe and continuous.
- pain starts suddenly, is sharp and felt more on one side of the abdomen (indicating a possible ectopic pregnancy).
- pain is accompanied by vaginal bleeding.

Back Pain

Common in pregnancy, especially towards the end when the weight of the growing baby pulls on the lower spine and the muscles and ligaments of the pelvis and spine are weak. Exercise these muscles (ask at your ante-natal class) so that the extra weight is carried rather than dragging on the ligaments, which can cause backache. Don't forget to check your posture (see p. 43). Backache is common after childbirth along with the other aches and pains. Be gentle with your back until you have built up your strength and take extra care when lifting or carrying your baby, especially when getting the carrycot in and out of cars, buses or trains. Make sure you always change your baby at a good height where your back is straight and not bent forward. Small babies can be changed on your lap – this takes a little practice but is an easy option especially when away from home.

Back pain can be isolated in the lower back, can radiate to the hips or the abdomen or down into the legs, and can be accompanied, or caused, by 'complementary' pain in the upper spine/neck. Sciatic pain is caused by pressure on nerves that pass through the lower spine into the legs and is usually one-sided. Pains in the ribs are also a possibility towards the end of the pregnancy when the uterus expands, pushing the ribs up and out. There are many remedies for back pain – choose carefully to find one that fits your whole picture.

Do
- consult an osteopath (or cranial osteopath, chiropractor or physiotherapist) if the pains are severe and you have a recurring problem that you know responds well to osteopathy, or if you know you have lifted too heavy an object or done something else that may have 'put your back out'.
- use heat (baths, compresses or hot-water bottles) or cold (showers, compresses or ice-packs) to relieve pain.
- make sure your mattress is supportive and right for you – for some people with backache lying on a hard surface (the floor or a futon) is best, for others a mattress with some give in it (so that lying on one's side doesn't distort the spine) is better. Experiment to find the right sort of mattress for your needs.
- have a massage if the pains are due to emotional tension.
- go swimming, an especially beneficial form of exercise as the spine is relieved of the pull of gravity. Make sure you don't keep your head out of the water all the time when you breaststroke as this can strain your upper back. Swim occasional lengths of backstroke if you can.
- build into your 'exercise' routine some exercises specifically designed to strengthen the lower spine.

Don't
- further stress a strained back by lifting or pulling, etc.
- maintain positions that are painful as this will make your condition worse.

Seek help if
- back pain is accompanied by fever.
- the urine smells strong or is bloody (it looks pink or is flecked with red or brown).
- you are having difficulty with either the bowels or bladder.
- it is difficult to move your legs or they feel numb.

NB Never attempt to treat a serious back injury yourself.

Groin Pains

Towards the end of pregnancy, especially after the baby's head has engaged, the round ligaments that run into the groin can be stretched and strained and the uterus may press down on the pelvic nerves causing excruciatingly sharp but short-lived and harmless pains which sometimes radiate down into the legs. They usually occur while walking and are often severe enough to stop you in your tracks until they are over. They sometimes occur earlier in the pregnancy when they resemble a 'stitch'. Homeopathic treatment can be extremely effective. *Bellis perennis* is the one remedy indicated for this. If it doesn't help you will need to seek professional advice.

Do
- sit down if you experience a groin pain – wherever you are – until it is over. If you are in a shop, ask for a chair or stool.
- exercise to strengthen the pelvic-floor muscles (see p. 43) during pregnancy – this will not only help to prevent groin pains, but will make labour easier and enable a faster healing after the birth.
- bend your knees or bend over to cough, sneeze and laugh – as a preventive measure to avoid straining these ligaments. Roll on to your side and use your hands and knees to stand up from lying down.
- see an osteopath to check that your spine is in good order.

Don't
- carry on walking if you are in pain.

Seek help if
- the pains don't respond to homeopathic treatment within five days.

Joint Pain

Joint pain is relatively common due not only to the relaxing properties of the hormones (see pp. 78–9) but also the extra weight; unfitness; change in balance which can mean you will fall over more frequently, leading to joint injury; a sprain or strain. Women who have a tendency to joint problems may find they worsen during pregnancy. The joints of the hips, knees and back can all be affected as well as those of the hand and wrist and foot and ankle, with soreness and stiffness accompanying a sensation of looseness.

Numbness and tingling of the hands can accompany pains in the wrist, known as carpal tunnel syndrome (see p. 83). It is usually worse in the morning because of the build-up of fluid in the tissues overnight.

Do
- use heat or cold to relieve pain. Try heating pads, hot baths, ice-packs, etc.
- keep your diet healthy and reduce your intake of 'acidic' foods such as sugar, refined or junk foods, red meat and citrus fruit. Eat plenty of fresh (non-citrus) fruit and vegetables, or put yourself on a short fruit fast if you feel like it, preferably under the guidance of a naturopath.

Don't
- use a painful joint more than is absolutely necessary.

PALPITATIONS

A not uncommon feature of pregnancy related to the extra strain on the heart from the increased blood volume. You can treat occasional minor palpitations yourself, especially if they have been brought on by excitement, fear, shock, or the suppression of these feelings.

You will need to use differentiating symptoms to choose between the remedies listed in the Repertory. Identify what brings on the palpitations and what eases them.

Do
- rest and recharge.
- sit quietly and breathe deeply, slowly and evenly.
- practise relaxation exercises or meditation.

Seek help if
- the palpitations persist over several hours.
- they are accompanied by chest pain.

PILES

Piles (or haemorrhoids) are varicose veins of the rectum/anus. You may have had piles before your pregnancy or for the first time in pregnancy or labour. They are caused partly by the increased pressure of the growing uterus on all the veins of the pelvis, partly by the hormonal changes which cause your muscles (and the walls of the veins) to relax and also by a poor diet lacking in fibre. They can manifest as small round lumps, bluish or reddish or purply, around or protruding from the anus, or can remain internal – you may suspect they are there if you have pain and/or itching and/or bleeding on passing a stool. Piles can be painless or may itch, burn, hurt intensely, bleed copiously or scantily. They can give a feeling of fullness in the rectum.

Do

- increase the fibre/roughage in your diet dramatically to keep your bowels moving and your stools soft. Decrease your intake of refined foods and fats.
- take a natural laxative, such as oat bran or prunes, at the first sign of constipation.
- use a homeopathic or herbal piles cream or ointment (see pp. 162–3) to relieve pain and encourage them to shrink if they are external or to ease external itching.
- apply piles cream to the anus before passing a stool to ease its passage.
- clean your anus after a stool but not with hard dry paper which can break the piles open. Use soft, damp toilet paper (wet it a little with water) and then pat dry.
- pop them back in if they protrude, especially after passing a stool. Smear them with cream or soapy water and push back using a wet sponge.
- apply witch hazel or *Hamamelis* (see p. 208) compresses if they are inflamed and swollen. Cut some lint, a sanitary pad or a piece of cotton wool into a small square. Saturate with witch hazel and leave in place for half an hour at a time. If it helps repeat frequently – it should ease the pain and help to shrink the piles.
- sit in a bidet, bath or bucket of cold, cool, tepid or hot water to find out which temperature soothes them.
- avoid standing for long periods of time.
- exercise the pelvic-floor muscles and especially those around the anus (see p. 43).
- see also Constipation, p. 83.

Don't

- take iron pills as they have been known to cause piles or worsen them.
- strain when passing a stool – take a book or magazine to the loo with you and let your bowels do their best (or worst).
- squat, as this will encourage piles because of the additional pressure. Semi-squat trying a low stool or pile of books for support.
- sit on hard surfaces – use a cushion or fold a coat or sweater into one.

Seek help if

- you can't push the piles back or if they'll go back but won't stay up.
- the pain is not relieved by self-help measures.
- you bleed copiously and regularly.

RESTLESS LEGS

This unpleasant (but not serious) syndrome is commonly associated with old age . . . and pregnancy. The legs feel as if they *have* to move – it is an awful, uncomfortable feeling inside the muscles of the legs which can get so bad they ache. When it's bad they have to be constantly on the go. The cause is not fully understood but thought to be a combination of factors including tension and dietary deficiencies.

Homeopathically there are several remedies for this distressing complaint. Differentiate carefully to find one that fits.

SINUSITIS

See also Common Cold, p. 83.

Sinus congestion can occur more readily in pregnancy due to hormonal influences, especially towards the end and in those who are already prone to sinus problems. When you have a cold, you will know if your sinuses are infected because your head will feel heavy and you may be aware of pressure above the eyes and in the cheeks by the bridge of the nose, which may also be tender to the touch.

Do

- use a humidifier or steam inhalations to relieve congestion.
- drink plenty of fluids.
- avoid tobacco smoke and builders' dust.

Don't

- use decongestants.
- blow your nose too hard.

Seek help if

- the sinuses are tender, you have a fever and there is a smelly discharge from the nose which does not respond to self-prescribing within 48 hours, or less if you are in severe pain.

SKIN COMPLAINTS

Women who suffer from chronic skin complaints may find that they miraculously clear up during pregnancy, but occasionally they become worse. Always consult a professional homeopath in such cases.

Minor skin complaints are commonly experienced in pregnancy by women who have not previously suffered from them.

Pigmentation

During pregnancy the skin produces more pigment which may help you tan more easily. It can also cause dark patches to develop on the face: a mask or 'saddle' over the nose and across the cheeks and a 'moustache' on the upper lip. Birthmarks, freckles and moles may all become darker as may the area around the nipples. There is nothing you can do to prevent this from happening and the skin will mostly revert to its normal colouring after the birth.

Take a short course of *Sepia 6* if the dark patches on your face bother you and you have another symptom or two which fits the *Sepia* picture. If it helps, repeat it as needed.

Rashes, Itching, Flaking, Roughness

Increased skin sensitivity can lead to the development of mild allergies to soaps, soap powders, perfumes, cosmetics, the metal on watches or jewellery, etc. Women with a tendency to dry skin may be worse affected. (See also Itching, p. 93.)

Take a short course of *Sulphur 6* if your skin is dry, itchy and worse for heat and bathing. However, look at the whole picture to see if another remedy fits you and other complaints you may have better, even though skin complaints are not mentioned. Take a short course of your indicated constitutional remedy. If it helps *you* but your rashes are getting worse, consult a professional homeopath.

Do
- wear cotton next to your skin and avoid nylon.
- use a simple, refined oil, such as almond oil, on dry skin, or aqueous cream, available from chemists, if your skin is also itchy.
- wash your clothes and bedding in non-biological powders (Ecover, Dreft, Lux, Fairy Snow, etc.), or experiment to find out which powder is the culprit if you are sure that that is what is causing your skin problems.
- experiment with your diet: have you had a craving for orange candies, frozen peas, cream? Are you suddenly eating something in particular? If so, cut it out for a few days. If your skin improves, you can double-check by reintroducing the rogue food item as you habitually ate it before. A mild sensitivity won't usually show itself immediately on reintroducing the food you eliminated – it will take a few days to build up again.

Don't
- use hydrocortisone creams or coal-tar preparations on your skin.
- use bath oil, bubble bath or perfumed soap.

Seek help if
- itching is preventing you from sleeping.
- a rash is spreading all over your body.

Spider Veins

These are caused by hormonal changes and there is little that can be done about them. They will disappear after the birth.

Broken Veins

Also caused by hormonal changes, they will not disappear after the birth.

Take a short course of *Arnica* at the first sign of broken veins as this will help 'mend' damage already done and prevent them developing further. You can also rub some *Arnica* cream into the skin.

Spots

A short course of *Calcarea sulphurica* or *Silica* may help to clear them up. If the spots are especially bad don't attempt to treat yourself but consult a professional homeopath.

Do
- cut out all sugar, including chocolate and biscuits, and cut down on fat for a week or so.
- drink the juice of half a freshly squeezed lemon in water first thing in the morning and last thing at night.
- wash your hair regularly if your spots are on your face.
- let the sun get to your skin regularly for short periods of time.
- use a good skin-care routine, cleansing thoroughly at least once a day.
- make sure your diet is rich in fruit and vegetables.

Don't
- squeeze or pick at spots as this can cause scarring unless they are absolutely 'ripe', in which case very gentle pressure will encourage the pus to discharge. Apply *Calendula* cream immediately.
- use antibiotic ointments.

STRETCH MARKS

Almost nothing can be done to prevent stretch marks. Some women have more elastic skin which stretches without marking. Others are less lucky. Stretch marks usually appear on the abdomen, buttocks, thighs, breasts and upper arms. They are reddish or purplish when they first appear and may itch. After the birth they will shrink and fade to white.

Calcarea fluorica will help prevent stretch marks. Don't take it continuously, but if you have dry skin and are prone to stretch marks anyway, take it for regular short courses throughout your pregnancy.

Do
• use an oil or oily cream on a dry skin to help keep it reasonably supple. Any cream or oil containing vitamin E is helpful, both as a preventive and once the marks have appeared.

Don't
• put on too much weight as this can exacerbate stretch marks.

TEETH AND GUM PROBLEMS

Your gums may swell and bleed more easily in pregnancy, due to hormonal changes. See your dentist and hygienist regularly to maintain a healthy mouth during your pregnancy. Dental treatment is free throughout pregnancy and the post-natal year.

Do
• ask your dentist to use a rubber 'dam' if you need an amalgam filling or a filling replacement. This is a rubber sheet that protects your mouth and prevents amalgam dust from being swallowed accidentally.
• have your teeth overhauled when you are *planning* to get pregnant.
• avoid X-rays. Discuss with your dentist the possible alternatives to amalgam fillings as their toxic effects are being increasingly noted.
• brush your teeth regularly and floss at least once a day. Some dentists recommend a brush and a floss after each meal to keep teeth and gums in really good condition. Massage your gums with your finger after you brush your teeth.
• use a mouthwash of salt water or *Calendula* tincture if your gums are sensitive or bleeding.
• watch your diet and limit your intake of sweets and sugary products such as biscuits, soft drinks and ketchup.
• eat plenty of fresh fruit and vegetables.

Don't
• forget that emotional stress affects teeth and gums. If your toothache is not related to a cavity, try to identify what is really causing your pain.

THRUSH, Vaginal/Yeast Infection

Because the acid/alkaline balance of the vagina changes in pregnancy, thrush is another common complaint. Vaginal discharges can become heavier, smell different and be mildly irritating.

Several remedies are indicated for the treatment of acute thrush. Differentiate between them carefully, using the symptoms of the thrush as well as any general and stress symptoms and your emotional state. Remember that the onset of thrush can occur without a discharge, and don't ignore soreness, redness and itching.

Do
• put half a cup of cider vinegar or a tablespoon of bicarbonate of soda in your bathwater.
• cut out sugars and refined breads, cakes and biscuits until it has cleared up. The yeast in wheat products can exacerbate thrush.
• wash the genitals after urinating and after making love: the acid/alkaline balance of semen can aggravate thrush. 'Bottle wash', see p. 85.
• use condoms (without integral spermicide) with plenty of lubricating jelly (such as KY-Jelly) until the thrush has cleared so that you don't pass it on to your partner, unless penetration (and/or the condoms themselves) aggravate the thrush, in which case have non-penetrative sex until the condition has cleared up.
• wash cotton underwear with unscented soap or soap flakes, not detergents, and rinse well.
• apply live yoghurt to ease itching and discomfort. You can smear some in and around the vagina with your fingers or insert a mini tampon or a small natural sponge (which has been boiled to sterilise it) dipped in yoghurt. Remove tampons or sponges after an hour or so.
• eat lots of dark green vegetables and whole grains.
• try adding acidophilus – powdered, live dried yeast cultures, available from health-food shops – or live yoghurt to your diet.

Don't
• make love without a condom until the thrush has cleared up as you can pass it to your partner.
• wear knickers if it is practicable and the weather hot as sweating can make it worse.
• use vaginal deodorants or soap.

Seek help if
• mild thrush hasn't cleared up within a week.
• the discharge begins to itch, smell unpleasant or changes colour to yellow or green and becomes thick and lumpy.

TOXAEMIA

See Eclampsia, p. 86.

URETHRITIS

See Cystitis, p. 84.

URINARY TRACT INFECTIONS

See Cystitis, p. 84.

VARICOSE VEINS, of legs and vulva

The softening of tissues in pregnancy can affect the walls and valves in the veins. The extra weight you are carrying added to increased blood volume plus, perhaps, constipation may stress the leg and pelvic veins. If the veins are weak, blood may 'pool' (instead of being returned to the heart) in the leg and pelvic area, and stretch the veins into the unsightly knots and lumps.

Varicose veins may be sore or acutely painful, can itch or cause the whole leg to ache especially if you stand for long. Those of the vulva are usually even more painful because it is harder to take the pressure off the area without lying down. You may feel as if there is a fullness and heaviness in and around the vagina, as if 'everything will fall out'. Varicose veins of the legs may become less 'knotty' after the birth but they are usually 'here to stay' whereas those of the vulva disappear quite soon after childbirth. They won't cause any trouble during labour because the perineum stretches so much that they disappear at that point and never return! See also Piles, p. 99.

Do

- exercise regularly to keep muscle tone healthy, especially the pelvic-floor muscles (see p. 43), and walk briskly to keep the blood circulating.
- wear support tights. Put them on *before* you get out of bed in the morning.
- splash or shower with cold water (if you can bear it) from the waist down, which will temporarily alleviate the soreness of inflamed veins in the pelvis and/or legs.
- elevate your legs as often as possible.
- raise the end of your bed with bricks or a block of wood (6–8 ins/15–20 cms high) so that you sleep at a slight angle with the blood draining more easily back to the heart (without having to be pumped).
- apply witch hazel compresses to painful veins to reduce inflammation. Soak lint, cotton wool,

hankies or soft thin teatowels in witch hazel and tie loosely around the veins. Remove when dry. Repeat as often as needed.

- avoid becoming constipated as this will aggravate them.
- try to control your weight.
- flex your feet and leg muscles if you are having to sit or stand for long periods of time. You can rotate feet, walk around, flex on to your toes, shake your legs, etc.

Don't

- sit with your legs crossed.
- stand for long periods.
- constrict the flow of blood to the legs in any way – through wearing tight clothes, or by sitting on chairs that press into the backs of your thighs. Make sure your feet can be flat on the floor with your thighs comfortably free while sitting (on chairs or the toilet). Use fat books or telephone directories if you've got short legs, especially if you have a desk job.

VOMITING

See Morning Sickness, p. 95.

WEIGHT GAIN

The increased weight in pregnancy is *not* all baby! It is also composed of increased body fluids including blood, fat deposits (on the belly, buttocks and thighs), enlarged breasts, amniotic fluid and placenta. (Amniotic fluid is 98 per cent water with the other 1–2 per cent composed of fetal hair and skin cells, enzymes, urea, glucose, hormones and lipids. It is completely replaced about every three hours.)

A 20–30-pound (10–15-kg) gain is normal, although some women put on a lot more and others considerably less. Extra fat is laid down for breast-feeding, and, during the initial post-natal period, will help you avoid becoming run down and exhausted.

If you are putting on a lot of weight check your diet, but if it is balanced and healthy don't worry. You can begin to lose any excess weight straight away if you decide to breastfeed, which uses at least 600 calories per day.

Do

- eat a balanced diet (see p. 41).
- eat little and often.
- keep physically fit however much weight you put on. If you turn into a couch potato, the labour itself may be more arduous. If you are not keeping

fit because emotional stress is draining you, consult a psychotherapist, counsellor or professional homeopath to help you deal with it.

Don't
- gain too much weight *and* become sedentary.

- diet. If you put on too much weight cut out sugar and refined/junk foods, cut down on fats and increase your intake of fruit, vegetables, fish and whole grains.
- worry if you do gain a lot of weight – concentrate on getting fit.

· 4 ·
BIRTH

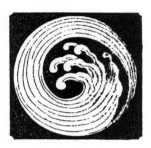

YOUR BODY AND BIRTH

This chapter is not about how to have a perfect birth: there is no single 'right' way to give birth. Each woman has different strengths, weaknesses and beliefs and therefore different needs. What works for one person won't necessarily work for another. Also, what works in one birth won't necessarily work in the next.

Birth can be a wonderful, extraordinary and powerful event, a truly mysterious rite of passage. On the other hand, it can be miserable, painful and lonely. Either way, it is unforgettable. The presence of a healthy baby can transform or, at least, soften the memory of a long, arduous labour.

I am going to look at some of the possible difficulties surrounding birth and share ideas and tips I have gathered over the years during which I have been working with women in labour. My aim is to encourage you to find your own way to give birth – with confidence and conviction. I hope that from reading this chapter, and the sections on birth in Chapter 2, you will gain a balanced sense of what you *might* need in labour and therefore how best to prepare for it. Take time to reflect on what *you* really want, and remember to keep an open mind. Labour is a process in which you can be fully involved, not an acute illness that you have to lie back and endure!

It is important to be aware of what is happening to you and your body during childbirth so that you can picture in your mind's eye what is happening and not feel frightened or powerless through ignorance. First births can be made unnecessarily difficult if you don't understand the physical processes.

PRE-LABOUR

Labour takes place approximately 280 days (40 weeks) after the first day of your last period. It is usually preceded by one or more of the following:

- practice contractions (Braxton Hicks), which are felt as a tightening or hardening of the abdomen and may be uncomfortable but are rarely painful. Use them to practise on: breathe (see p. 40) into them and relax with them.
- a 'lightening' as the baby's head drops down into the pelvis (engages) towards the end of pregnancy (if it is head down). It feels as if a little more space is suddenly available in the abdomen. It is!
- fewer movements from your baby who usually becomes less active.
- a 'nesting' compulsion – an unexpected pre-labour surge of energy. Women have been known to redecorate or springclean their houses during this period, which usually lasts a few days. Don't overdo it – you need to express your elation while

conserving your energy. Be careful with your body – don't paint ceilings, for example, as you don't want to fall off a ladder!

- loose stools or diarrhoea.
- a 'show': the plug of mucus that stops up the neck of the uterus may come away.
- the waters breaking or leaking of amniotic fluid, as the baby's head engages.

All the above symptoms of impending labour can come and go and nothing happens – carry on as normal. Pack your case if you are going into hospital. If you are having a home birth, organise your house and make sure you have all the bits and pieces that you need, including those that your midwife has instructed you to have ready.

NB Complications such as a breech baby or a small pelvis require expert attention throughout.

LABOUR

First Stage: Labour

True labour is precipitated by:

1 A mechanical process: when the baby reaches a certain size the pressure of its head and body against the walls of and entrance to the uterus are thought to stimulate reflexes which set off contractions. The contractions push the baby down, which stimulates more contractions.
2 Hormonal changes cause the uterus to contract.

Both processes work together to expel the baby.

During the first stage, the cervix – the neck of the uterus – softens, opens (dilates) and pulls up so that the baby is able to emerge. It is the longest stage of labour. Generally this stage takes longer with first babies and is quicker in subsequent labours.

The contractions are felt initially as low abdominal or low back pain, not unlike period pains. They increase, usually gradually, in frequency and strength as the cervix dilates. The waters (amniotic fluid) may leak or break.

Transition

Transition occurs between the first and second stages once the cervix is fully dilated and can last for one contraction or continue for several hours. The contractions are irregular and usually close together and may be accompanied by an overwhelmingly strong urge to push. They mark a change from first stage contractions which open the cervix to second stage contractions where the longitudinal muscles of the cervix actually shorten with each contraction thereby automatically pushing the baby out.

The altered rhythm as the contractions change over can go unnoticed or it can be hard to deal with. Everything may feel out of control as the body takes over to complete the most physically arduous task it ever accomplishes. Many women become irritable or even abusive to those around at that time.

If the cervix isn't fully dilated at this stage your midwife will ask you to pant to prevent you from trying to push your baby out when your body isn't quite ready.

Second Stage: Birth

The baby moves out of the uterus and travels the 4 curved inches (10 cms) of the birth canal (vagina) into the world. Each contraction automatically pushes the baby a little further down. The contractions are regular and usually come several minutes apart. The baby moving down the vagina can feel as if you are about to pass a large grapefruit or melon – even a football. You will usually feel a strong urge to push, accompanied by any number of sensations – stretching, bulging and burning are all common. Your midwife will ask you to pant if she doesn't want you to push, so that the baby is born nice and slowly without tearing your perineum or vagina. A burning sensation may indicate that your baby is emerging too fast and not giving your muscles a chance to stretch.

It is tiring and therefore important to drink something, to take some honey or sugar for energy and to rest completely between contractions. Because of the shape and position of the vagina, lying down to give birth is not necessarily the best position – taking gravity into account by squatting or semi-squatting can help enormously. But do lie down if you want to. Squatting or standing are good positions if this stage is slow. Get on to all fours if it is very fast. Many women instinctively find the position that suits them during this stage: a semi-squat is good as you can see what's going on and reach down to touch and lift up your baby and also helps your midwife. Your partner can sit behind you and support you from behind. Go with the flow, follow what your body and your midwife tell you to do. The emotions that accompany this last physical hurdle are many and glorious. This is a most wonderfully empowering moment in a woman's life. Some women love this second stage while others find it a painful last straw and are glad when it's over at last. Whatever – you are shortly to greet your baby for the first time.

Third Stage: Afterbirth

The placenta comes away from the wall of the uterus and is delivered. Contractions may cease temporarily after the birth itself; they can be re-stimulated by putting the newborn baby to the breast which will cause the uterus to begin contracting again and, as the uterus decreases in size, the placenta to detach from the wall of the uterus. Sensations at this stage of labour are coloured by the excitement of the birth; the contractions are considerably less demanding but may not be regular. The vagina may feel numb.

How long this stage lasts very much depends on your medical attendants. If you have negotiated for syntometrine not to be administered immediately after delivery of the baby (see p. 66) then your body may take its time. If syntometrine is given, your midwife will 'encourage' your placenta to deliver by pulling very gently on the cord while you are having a contraction: syntometrine causes the uterus to contract very efficiently and the placenta must be out promptly before it contracts. If you wish to breastfeed after the birth *and* for the cord not to be cut, you must ask that syntometrine be administered *after* the cord is cut to prevent the drug passing through the placenta to your baby.

Do not try to prescribe on yourself when you are in labour: leave it up to others. Once labour starts you need to put all of your energy into what you are doing. Your partner or homeopath should take responsibility for prescribing homeopathic remedies. Many midwives are now becoming interested in how homeopathy can help during labour and some have a basic kit, which they use according to their knowledge and skills.

Birth partners should read through the following section to get an idea of what might happen and what might be needed in labour, to become familiar with the labour sections in the Repertory (p. 288) and the Materia Medica (read up each remedy that may be needed for the birth). See also p. 302 on how to put together a homeopathic kit for labour and make a list of the remedies you want to have to hand. You may ask a professional homeopath to help you with this if you find yourself confused.

COMPLAINTS

The complaints section deals with the events of labour and makes suggestions for dealing with them, both practical and homeopathic. Play the 'What if' game: read through each complaint asking yourself and your partner, 'If "this" happens, what will we want?' You are not allowed to answer 'Give up'! This will stimulate you to think through some of the problems you may encounter so that they won't take you by surprise, which will help you feel more in control.

BACKACHE LABOUR

See Labour, p. 111.

CAESAREAN

See Medical Interventions, p. 58.

CONTRACTIONS

See Labour, p. 109.

EMOTIONAL DISTRESS

Emotions can run deep, strong and unexpected. Some or all of the following feelings can and do surface: anger, rage, fear, panic, despair, excitement, apathy, shame, embarrassment and so on. You may find it easier to express yourself at home but don't let a hospital environment inhibit you.

During labour so much is going on that it is almost impossible for a lay person to stop and work out a first-aid remedy to help. I have listed below some commonly needed remedies for emotional distress in labour to choose from. They should be taken fairly frequently – and either will or won't work. If the emotional distress accompanies physical symptoms it is best if you build those symptoms into your prescription for it to be truly effective: if *Pulsatilla* seems right for the emotional distress look it up in the Materia Medica (p. 239) to check whether it also has the physical symptoms.

Aconite Anxiety, fear and panic. Fear of dying, of the baby dying.
Arnica Suppresses feelings (esp. shock). Says she is OK when she plainly isn't.
Arsenicum Anxious, fussy, bossy and irritable.
Belladonna Angry and abusive. May throw a tantrum (rant and rage).
Chamomilla Abusive, angry. Impossible to please, asks for things then rejects them.
Coffea Over-excitable. Excitement alternating with fear. Talkative and jokey.
Gelsemium Lifeless, apathetic, despairing and dazed.
Kali carbonicum Irritable, anxious and bossy.

Lycopodium Pre-birth nerves. Lacks self-confidence. Feels exposed.

Natrum muriaticum Closed up emotionally. Feels shy and exposed. Wants to be alone.

Pulsatilla Weepy, clingy and pathetic. Despair. Changeable moods.

Sepia Irritable, anxious and despairing. Sluggish. Worn out.

Do

- go with the flow.
- be true to yourself. Find a way to express what is happening to you wherever you are.
- keep talking, keep communicating about what is happening to you – emotionally as well as physically.
- be assured that you won't feel like this for the rest of your life!
- use your feelings to empower you. Don't suppress them to make others feel better. This is one of the few times in your life when you'll be forgiven for behaving badly!

EPIDURAL

See Pain Relief, p. 54.

EPISIOTOMY

See Medical Interventions, p. 58.

EXHAUSTION

A common problem in labour, simply because of the arduous physical job that has to be accomplished, so it is vital to keep the blood sugar level high enough to provide plenty of energy, especially in the early stages, and if the cervix is dilating slowly – even if contractions are coming thick and fast. If you don't eat, you may need an intravenous drip if the blood sugar level drops, which is worth avoiding if at all possible.

Put 4 drops of Rescue Remedy in all drinks if tiredness sets in; physical tiredness may be alleviated by *Kali phosphoricum 6X* between every contraction for up to 6 doses, repeated fairly often, if it works. *Arnica 30*, taken from time to time, may also help, or can be alternated with *Kali phosphoricum 6X*.

If other symptoms accompany the exhaustion, like despair and weepiness, or terrible backache with a badly positioned baby, work out a remedy for the whole picture and take practical measures to deal with the situation. (See also pp. 53–4.)

Do

- eat, little and often, light, easily digestible foods. Some women only want liquids, others like proper meals at regular intervals. If you're at home and you want food, try soup, puréed vegetables or fruit. Ask your birth attendants to make themselves useful in the kitchen cooking exactly what you want. If you are in a hospital, you may not be allowed to eat much, if at all, because of the possibility of your needing an anaesthetic but have on hand a selection of small pieces of fruit to dip in honey in case your midwife has no objection. Dried fruit and nuts or biscuits are another easy alternative, although their chewiness can be irritating.
- drink often to prevent dehydration. Lemon or orange juice, freshly squeezed if possible, diluted with a little hot water (if you want a warm drink), with honey or sugar makes an ideal source of energy. Diluted stocks or soups, herb teas, ordinary tea or even coffee are all fine if that is what *you* really want. A word about honey: you can buy honey from wholefood shops which has not been 'heat-treated', but pressed out of the combs and has retained more of its goodness. You won't give birth often – get a pot for your labour if you can find it.

  NB Many women don't want to eat or drink in labour: it is important that your partner, friend or midwife regularly feeds you tasty morsels to keep you going.
- rest between contractions if you feel tired.
- sleep between contractions.
- have a long, warm bath or shower.
- take some gentle exercise – a walk in the fresh air, around the garden, up and down your street – or even in the hospital corridor!
- express any feelings that surface, like anger, to release tension, which is tiring.
- laugh – ask to be told corny jokes, if you really want!
- have a change of scene – if possible.
- ask your partner to touch, massage, hold, kiss you.
- breathe deeply and evenly.
- do *anything* that you know energises without draining you.
- consider medication.

Don't

- fast during labour or deprive your body of food and/or drink.

FALSE LABOUR

See Labour, p. 111.

FAST LABOUR

See Labour, p. 112.

FORCEPS

See Medical Interventions, p. 58.

HAEMORRHAGE

It is unlikely that you'll be able to treat this condition because your medical attendants will administer an injection of syntometrine at the first sign of serious bleeding (see p. 115). However, homeopathic treatment works extremely fast: the right remedy will work within 30 seconds. You might ask for a minute's grace before syntometrine is administered. I have also included the following remedies just in case you do not have immediate access to medical treatment:

Phosphorus 200, one dose, is indicated if the blood is bright red, there is a lot of it and it gushes out; have *Phosphorus* to hand during labour if it has worked well in the past, and you have a history of bleeding easily (nosebleeds, profuse menstrual periods, etc.); if *Phosphorus* hasn't worked, follow it with *Ipecacuanha 200*, one dose, after 30 seconds. If there is a lot of dark red blood with clots that gushes out, try *Belladonna 200*, one dose, instead.

LABOUR

Contractions

The sensations accompanying contractions are different for every woman and in every labour. It is not possible to know ahead of time what your baby's birth will be like and it is best therefore to be aware that it might hurt. Although painless labours are not unknown, I have found, from my own professional experience, that childbirth without pain is rare.

It is useful to have a reality base to measure yourself against. If you know that it is likely that you will experience pain, you can plan accordingly and confront your fears and/or anxieties *before* the event. Start by building a picture of your own response to pain: ask yourself what you know about your pain responses. Are you good with pain? Do you have a high pain threshold or do you suffer easily? How do you

cope at the dentist? Can you have a filling without an injection or do you need a lot of local anaesthetic to cope with the pain?

Pain in childbirth can be managed so that it is not overwhelming and one of the best aids is to understand the process of childbirth fully so that you can work with the contractions. Overwhelming, unexpected pain causes tension and muscle-tightening, resistance, which increases pain. Learning techniques for coping with pain whether you are at home or in hospital is an important part of preparing for an active birth. Our bodies' automatic response to pain is to secrete hormones (endorphins) which relax *and* ease it – their action is similar to that of morphine. The more serious an injury the more hormones are released: after an accident, victims report afterwards that they felt nothing, numb, and as if they weren't all there.

In labour we hope to draw on this natural mechanism, which is easier for some women than others. All the techniques for helping with pain in childbirth are designed to relax, distract (so that relaxing is easier) and make a woman feel more at ease so that she *can* relax. We all have different ways of alleviating pain: think back to what has worked for you before as it may help when you are in labour.

The following guidelines for dealing with pain may help you to think ahead to what might help you: file them in a reasonably accessible part of your brain so that your body can tell you what it needs when the time comes (see also pp. 53–4). Once labour is established some of the following suggestions will become neither possible nor appropriate, but by then you will have found a rhythm and discovered the things that help most. Forget the things that don't work and keep trying new ideas until you discover the right ones. Then keep doing them!

There often comes a moment in labour when the intensity of the pains and the loss of control become overwhelming and a woman says she can't go on, which *may* come close to delivery. *Pulsatilla* (if she is pathetic and weepy) or *Arnica* (if she is more irritable) taken then can give her the emotional strength to carry on. If another strong emotional picture surfaces then prescribe the appropriate remedy.

I have included several remedies for labour pains where a pattern is emerging: where the contractions stop, come at irregular intervals, are ineffective in dilating the cervix or are exceptionally painful. You will find these in the Repertory under Labour pains. Observe carefully the pattern of the pains as well as the general and emotional symptoms to make a good prescription.

Do
- see pp. 37–77.

- use distraction. You can learn a mantra, poem or line of a poem which you speak, either aloud or in your mind, with all your attention during the contractions to take your mind off the pain. Say it with your full concentration on the words alone. Pre-natal classes often teach this method.
- use breathing techniques. A variety of techniques are taught so learn one and try it out. If it works use it, if it doesn't try something else.
- take one step at a time, one contraction at a time.
- bath or shower. Once labour is well established many women spend much of the painful part of the first stage in a bath. It's a wonderful way of relaxing and relieving pain especially in a long labour. For some women though, lying down isn't a good position, especially if the baby is posterior presentation. In this case you can kneel on all fours in the bath (rest your knees on some soft padding like folded hand-towels) and get your partner or midwife to direct the shower on to your back, especially the parts that hurt. Try warm, hot and even cool water: pain is sometimes relieved by cool or even cold bathing – this could guide you to a helpful remedy as well as easing the soreness. The bathwater should be warm (not too hot) and deep so that you can change position easily. Block the overflow with Blutack to get a deeper bath. Wait until the contractions are really well established before getting in the bath as this has been known to slow labour in the early stages. You can rent good-sized pools specially designed for labour: they are compact enough to fit into a small-ish space in your home (6 feet/2 metres in diameter) but large enough to contain three people comfortably! It is possible to be on all fours with the water covering you in a pool like this, which gives considerable pain relief; some women give birth to their babies under water. A few hospitals have installed birthing pools while others have jacuzzis available for women in labour. Many hospitals will ask you to get out of the pool for the actual birth.
- bite on a twisted towel or a leather belt, making sure that you don't stop breathing at the same time. This helps release tension, especially if you grunt or make growling noises at the same time.
- make a noise – find your own sound. Pain is greatly relieved by releasing tension through making a sound. Go with the flow and see what sounds come out. You may be surprised. Don't scream or constrict your throat: let sounds bubble up from deep inside you – let them out and then let them out louder. This can be a brave new thing to do – you may need encouragement, may feel self-conscious about being noisy. At the end of the first stage you may not be able to suppress noise,

anyway – women grunt, groan, moan, shout and make the most wonderful sounds when they are in labour. They 'cancel out' the pain.
- sing. Connect with a favourite song and just sing it over and over again.
- move. Experiment with finding different movements at different stages and go with the contractions.
- dance. Let your body move to music, or to the rhythms of your labour: follow those movements with and through each contraction. Many women find themselves circling their hips or their whole bodies. Belly dancing was designed for women in labour because it was observed that those natural movements actually helped with the process of labour itself.
- let your body hang, by holding on to door handles or the bars of a ladder or bed. This allows your spine to stretch and is very relaxing. In some countries a rope or sheet is slung over a high beam and women spend much of their labours hanging in a relaxed but upright position.
- relax. Release your pelvis and hips during a 'contraction', let them loosen, soften and widen.
- eat calcium-rich foods as calcium helps to raise your pain threshold. Yoghurt is ideal because it is also easily digestible. Eat carbohydrates for energy.
- walk. Especially in early labour, you can take a walk outside if you feel like it – especially if you have a garden. Or you can simply potter about inside.
- exercise gently – to relieve stress and keep supple. Do your yoga positions, any stretching and contracting of muscles that feels good. If it hurts stop immediately. There will be times in labour when you feel like moving and others when you want to rest.
- experiment with different positions to relieve pain. Try kneeling; kneeling with a midwife or your partner fully supporting you or holding you from behind, kneeling on all fours, kneeling or squatting with your partner or midwife supporting you from behind or in front, lying – every which way – leaning against a person, bed or wall; sitting on a birthing stool; sitting forward over a bean bag or a heap of cushions or pillows; sitting on the toilet!
- use touch and massage. Ask your partner to touch you in different ways and places, at different times. Try tender-light touch – very gentle feather-light stroking – especially on your abdomen, face and back. Try firm massage in places where there is pain – experiment with the pressure till you get it right. Massage another part of the body completely, like the feet. Pressing or pushing can be

wonderful, especially for a backache labour where the palms of the hands pushed hard against the small of the back can ease the pain of each contraction. Remember, you may not want to be touched at all at times – perhaps during your entire labour.

- massage the perineum with lots of oil (almond or olive) to help avoid tears and also to focus some energy on that area, to encourage you to relax it. Visualise the muscles of your vagina loosening as you massage the area.
- canoodle: kissing, hugging and holding are wonderful for encouraging a person to relax. If you feel like it and have a willing partner handy, go ahead!
- get some pain relief if you are not coping, if the pain is much worse than you had imagined, if you are finding it too much or if it has gone on for too long, you are beginning to lose hope and your vitality.

Don't

- feel bad if you have to 'resort' to drugs. Remember, you have done your best – you prepared yourself for this labour, not knowing how it would go or what would happen and you have done as much as you can to go it alone. It is OK to accept help: if you were running a marathon and began to flag as well as get cramp in your legs you would stop and get help. You cannot choose to stop in labour but you can get help and *whatever help you need is OK*.
- hang on to unrealistic expectations of a pain-free labour, a painful labour or any particular type of labour. Disappointment can increase tension and intensify pain.

Backache Labour

This is caused by the baby being in the posterior position, its back against your back. The pains are doubled, felt in the uterus, the abdomen *and* in the back.

Several remedies are indicated for back pain in labour, including *Causticum, Gelsemium, Kali carbonicum, Nux vomica, Petroleum* and *Pulsatilla*. It is the individual symptoms of the contractions as well as any general and emotional symptoms that will guide you to one of the above remedies. If another remedy is indicated on the general symptoms and the emotional state then consider it instead.

Do

- follow the guidelines for pain in labour (p. 110).
- find a position that eases the pain without taking the pressure of the baby's head off your cervix. Kneeling on all fours, with pillows under your

knees, or draping yourself over a bean bag are two of the most comfortable positions.

Don't

- lie down on your back as this will increase the pressure on your spine and take it away from your cervix.

False Labour

Established labour is diagnosed if the cervix is 3 centimetres or more dilated. If after four hours at 3 centimetres there is no further dilation then it is assumed that true labour has not yet begun.

Braxton Hicks contractions (see p. 81) can develop into what feels like labour and continue for several days or even weeks, coming every 10–20 minutes and feeling as if they might be the real thing. They are frustrating because nothing – or next to nothing – actually happens.

Remedies for getting labour going include *Belladonna, Calcarea carbonica, Caulophyllum, Chamomilla, Cimicifuga, Gelsemium, Kali carbonicum, Natrum muriaticum, Nux vomica, Opium, Pulsatilla* or *Sepia*. Take into account the individual symptoms of the contractions, any general symptoms and, of course, the emotional state to guide you to one of the above remedies. If another remedy is indicated on the general and emotional state then try it instead. During labour emotions run deep and strong and helping a woman 'feel' good in herself is as least half the battle.

Do

- carry on life as usual.
- go for long, brisk walks, round several blocks, or take longer walks of at least a mile, or do something special for yourself like painting your toenails, going to the hairdresser or on an impromptu outing with any other children (not too far away).
- dance or engage in vigorous exercise.
- encourage labour to 'get going' by kissing, stimulating the nipples, masturbating or having sexual intercourse. Kissing on the lips is very relaxing, nipple stimulation and masturbation can both encourage the onset of labour. Privacy is an issue in a hospital labour ward but kissing, nipple stimulation and masturbation can be successfully done in the bath or under a sheet, by the labouring woman or her partner.
- make love if you are still at home and your waters haven't broken. Semen contains a significant quantity of the hormone that helps stimulate labour (prostaglandin).
- encourage it to 'go away' if it is night-time or if

true labour is plainly not going to start. Have a warm bath, go to bed and try to sleep. This is the one time when you can either take a couple of paracetamol with a hot drink or drink a tot of whisky or glass of wine. It is better to have a small quantity of alcohol now, sleep and have a manageable labour, than to end up with a lot of medication in labour because you are exhausted.

- consider going into hospital rather than carrying on alone if you are at home, you can't sleep or rest, and are finding that you are becoming increasingly exhausted. You may benefit from having help in establishing your labour.
- talk about your fears for the labour with your partner or your midwife.

Don't
- panic.
- give up!

Fast Labour

A very fast labour can be frightening. It can feel like a roller coaster out of control with contractions coming one after another without a break in between. After a fast, violent labour some women report feeling shell-shocked: there's no time to assimilate or integrate anything. Typically, a second or third birth will be fast if the first or second was fairly quick – but, as always, there are no rules here . . .

Aconite is nearly always indicated during a fast labour. Even though everyone else knows it's not true women *know* they are going to die and say so. It should be taken frequently, every 5–10 minutes, until some sort of shelter is reached from the storm: it will slow down the contractions and make them manageable. Rescue Remedy in the drinking water or massaged into any part of the body will also help.

Do
- get on all fours as that will help to slow things down a little and help with the contractions, or try the 'frog' position: kneel down with knees apart to accommodate your belly and lean forward until your head rests on the ground, arms outstretched or folded under your head. This will take the pressure off your cervix.
- breathe as slowly and deeply as you can.
- go with the flow: imagine you are on a boat on a stormy sea and try and ride the waves – or create a different visualisation that works for you.
- remember to urinate. You don't have to pee on the toilet if there's no time; squat over a bucket, a washing-up bowl, potty or bedpan.

Don't
- panic and hyperventilate. If you find yourself getting dizzy, with tingling in your fingers, then breathe into your cupped hands (to take in more carbon dioxide – see also p. 40).

Late Labour

A high percentage of first babies are late, according to dates, so it is not worth worrying about. Only a tiny percentage of babies arrive on time – a normal pregnancy can range from 240 to 300 days. You can negotiate with your doctor or midwife to go up to two weeks over before they begin to suggest induction. Some women seem to have longer pregnancies than others.

A close relationship develops between mother and baby from the outset of pregnancy and if one or other is frightened or anxious then this can delay the onset of labour. If your baby is overdue by dates, and you are *absolutely sure* your dates are correct, ask yourself whether you are hanging on to your baby because of one of the following: this is your last planned pregnancy; you are scared – it's either the first one or the previous one was a bad experience; you're anxious about the responsibility of parenting, of your changing role; you don't want to stop being pregnant because you've enjoyed it so much; you don't want to lose your pregnant 'status' and stop receiving the special attention that pregnancy has conferred upon you; you had to work right up until the end of your pregnancy and you need some time to rest and relax.

See Inductions/Breaking the Waters, p. 63. Prescribe on fear or anxiety – some women need *Argentum nitricum*, *Gelsemium* or *Lycopodium* before their due date (or after it if they are still pregnant) because they approach it rather like an important exam and get the all-too-familiar exam nerves. Homeopathic help at this stage relaxes, enabling the body to go into labour if the baby is also ready. Take up to six doses of *Caulophyllum 30* over the course of a day if you are late and not frightened. If the baby is ready to be born it will help to establish labour. You can repeat it 2 days later.

Do
- deal with any of the above that apply to you. Talk about your feelings with your partner and your midwife; spend some time saying goodbye to your pregnancy and inviting your baby to come out; take time to do something nice and relaxing.
- ask for two weeks' grace after your due date – unless, of course, there are symptoms indicating that an induction is advisable.

- follow the Dos for False Labour (see pp. 111–12).
- contemplate a castor oil induction if you are desperate, bearing in mind that you will almost certainly have an unpleasant attack of diarrhoea that may or may not precipitate labour. Take two tablespoons of castor oil in orange juice. Half an hour later take one tablespoon of oil with juice and repeat this again, half an hour later. Relax in a bath (as long as your waters haven't broken). Do check, with your doctor and/or your midwife, that it is OK for you to try this.
- remember – you *and* your baby are going into labour together and you both need to be ready.

Don't
- be panicked into a hospital induction without taking a second opinion if you feel instinctively that it isn't necessary.

Premature Labour

The main danger with going into labour early is that your baby's lungs will be under-developed and it may have trouble breathing after the birth. Babies of 34 weeks' gestation or over are usually OK.

There are many causes for premature labour, the most commonly known of which is multiple births of two or more babies. Your doctor will be on the lookout for other complications later in your pregnancy that may lead to a premature labour so you don't need to worry about it. There's not a lot you can do homeopathically, as far as self-prescribing is concerned. Take *Nux vomica* if there is no apparent reason for labour starting, or *Opium* if labour started after a shock, and follow the advice of your midwife and/or doctor.

Do
- go to bed if you are in premature labour – and stay there.
- take a couple of stiff drinks (vodka or whisky). It's better to have a drink now and stop this process than end up with an early labour and a premature baby that needs intensive care. Alcohol relaxes the muscles of the uterus and stops the action of oxytocin, the hormone responsible for getting labour going.
- spend 20 minutes several times daily doing the postural tilting exercise (see p. 82).

Slow Labour

The early part of labour, where the cervix dilates, can seem endless, especially with first babies. If labour slows down or goes on for ever and you are 3 centimetres or less dilated, then:

Do
- remind yourself of the anatomy and physiology of what is happening. You, your body and your baby are working together for this birth and your body has been designed to give birth with little assistance. The contractions, plus the pressure of your baby's head on the cervix, will cause your cervix to open and the muscles of your uterus to thicken and shorten, which pulls them up and automatically pushes the baby out. You have to do very little apart from surrendering yourself to what is happening.
- rest to build up your energy reserves and sleep if you can between contractions.
- have a glass of wine to help you sleep and recharge the batteries.
- talk through any unresolved conflicts with your partner. Express any unexpected emotions.
- take a *long* walk outside.
- organise a change of scenery: settle yourself in a different room for a while, open the curtains if they are closed, or close them if they are open.
- ask new people to leave if your labour slowed down after their arrival.

If labour slows down when your cervix is 4–5 centimetres dilated:

Do
- try a different position: sit cross-legged for a while, letting your shoulders and hands loosen. Your partner can sit behind you supporting your back with their back; or squat for a short time; or walk about for a bit.
- be still. Slow down if you have been very active so far and retreat inside yourself.
- focus on the rhythm of your breathing rather than actively 'doing' the breathing method you have learnt. Allow your body to go with the flow of your breath.
- urinate every hour.
- talk through your fears with your midwife or partner. Some women can keep 'hard' labour at bay because of a fear of losing control. Fear can cause the muscles to tighten against the body's efforts to expand.
- allow yourself to melt and soften all over your body – your uterus, your back, your legs, your vagina and your mouth.
- ask for help – any help will do – some women need to reach out in labour to be able to let go and allow their bodies to work effectively.
- make sure you are eating and drinking.

If labour slows down after the cervix has dilated 6 centimetres, your uterus may be exhausted. You should follow your midwife's recommendations and your own instincts about what you need to proceed. Take *Arnica* alternating with *Kali phosphoricum* frequently (every 5–10 minutes) to help restore your exhausted muscles and nerves; or *Sepia* if indicated.

Do

- rest between contractions: give your body permission to slow down and recuperate.
- ask your partner to massage or hold you.
- drink and/or eat something nutritious.

Don't

- worry if labour slows down from time to time if it is generally progressing well. It can even stop for short periods of time while you and your body integrate what is happening and gather your forces to move on. It can commonly slow down when the cervix has reached 4, 6, 7 or 9 centimetres in dilation.

MEDICAL INTERVENTIONS

See pp. 58–64.

NAUSEA

Nausea and vomiting, relatively common in labour, especially towards the end of the first stage, can be caused by tiredness, stress leading up to the onset of labour, hormonal changes, fear, low blood sugar and the side effects of pain-relieving drugs.

Retching or vomiting can help by relaxing some of the muscles of the stomach and abdomen and vomiting can also be nature's way of emptying the stomach before the second stage (the birth).

If the nausea is constant and distressing, or the retching painful, or if the vomiting is preventing you from keeping any food or drink down, it is important to try to deal with it.

Put Rescue Remedy into drinks to combat panicky feelings and rub a few drops of it (neat) into the forehead, the back of the neck and the abdomen.

Ipecacuanha is indicated if the nausea is constant and unremitting; *Arsenicum* if it is accompanied by fear and anxiety; *Phosphorus* if the vomiting occurs a short while, but not immediately, after eating or drinking anything; *Pulsatilla* if it is accompanied by whingeing and thirstlessness. If none of these remedies is indicated, or if the indicated one doesn't work, look up the symptoms in the Repertory to find a remedy that fits the whole picture, perhaps *Cocculus* or *Tabacum* if faintness or dizziness is a problem.

Do

- drink frequent small quantities of anything you fancy.

- take small spoonfuls of honey or sugar water if you can't take anything else.
- breathe into the nausea (see Breathing, p. 40).
- relax between contractions.

PAIN RELIEF

See pp. 54–8 for a synopsis of drugs and techniques.

PREMATURE LABOUR

See Labour, p. 113.

RETAINED PLACENTA

After the baby has been delivered, the placenta can take up to three hours to separate from the wall of the uterus. During that time the last of the amniotic fluid drains away and there is some blood loss as the placenta separates, leaving a raw 'wound' which takes up to six weeks to heal (see Lochia, p. 128). The uterus will carry on contracting (although it may 'rest' for a while) after the baby has been born to encourage the placenta to separate, which you can promote by putting your baby to the breast. The sucking will stimulate contractions to start up again, or help make them stronger. In the process of separation, however, the placenta can tear the wall of the uterus more seriously and cause a haemorrhage (see p. 109), a serious cause for concern: in the past women regularly bled to death after childbirth if this happened.

The drug syntometrine is often administered routinely to deliver the placenta as fast as possible. It is a life-saver as it causes the uterus to contract very fast and prevents the possibility of haemorrhage but this third stage of labour becomes a more rushed affair which can spoil the beautiful atmosphere of a calm delivery. Most placentas deliver themselves within half an hour of the birth, with others taking up to two hours. Some midwives and doctors are happy to wait for up to two hours if all is going well and there is no bleeding. The side effects of syntometrine are not well recorded, but include nausea, after pains, headaches, jaundice in the baby, three-month colic and emotional disorders. It can apparently pass through to the breastmilk and cause colic in babies whose digestive tracts are sensitive or immature.

Many remedies are indicated for this condition. It is important that you take the whole picture into account: give *Cimicifuga* if there is shaking, trembling, soreness and a retained placenta; *Nux vomica* if there is great irritability; or *Sepia* if there is a great sagging as if all the energy went down the 'plughole'.

Do

- be patient after the birth – it's not all over yet!

- relax and enjoy the post-natal period to the full if all has gone well and you are able to. It's a birthday!
- ask for a delay in the administration of syntometrine of up to one hour (at least half an hour) with the proviso that if you start to haemorrhage, you will accept it immediately (see opposite).
- remain in an upright position to encourage the placenta to separate, to make expulsion easier and to reduce the risk of haemorrhaging.
- put your baby to the breast immediately after the birth as the sucking will stimulate your uterus to contract. If your baby doesn't want to suck, stimulate your nipples yourself and relax.
- have it written in your notes that you are not to be given syntometrine for the time that you have negotiated and remind each midwife of this. Write it in your birth plan.
- watch closely after the birth that it isn't 'accidentally' given to you anyway. You'll feel numb for a while after the baby has been born and are unlikely to notice the injection, which is given in the thigh.

Don't
- give up now!

RETCHING/VOMITING

See Nausea, p. 114.

RETENTION OF URINE

Immediately after the birth it is common to experience difficulty in urinating, at least for a short time, because of the combined soreness and numbness in the whole pelvic area, possibly accompanied by a feeling that those muscles will never work again! If you go for too long without peeing then your doctor or midwife will insert a catheter into your urethra and draw off any urine to prevent your bladder from becoming over-stretched. This is an uncomfortable and occasionally painful procedure and is worth trying to avoid.

Take *Arsenicum 30* every 10 minutes if you can't pee and you're feeling scared, *Arnica 30* if you are sore and bruised but feeling OK, *Staphysagria 30* if you feel disappointed or resentful, if you have had a forceps delivery and/or your body feels all 'beaten up', or *Pulsatilla 30* if you feel very sorry for yourself, weepy, clingy and thoroughly miserable.

Do
- ask for a tap to be run as you try to pee, whether on a bedpan or on the toilet.
- 'bottle wash' on the toilet if you are mobile (see p. 85).
- pee in a warm bath if you are mobile enough to have a bath.

SLOW LABOUR

See Labour, p. 113.

SYNTOMETRINE

See Retained Placenta, p. 114.

TREMBLING

It is not uncommon for women to have an attack of 'the shakes' before, during or after labour. It may be uncontrollable and you won't necessarily feel cold. It is generally your body's way of releasing tension and doesn't usually last long. It can accompany other symptoms, a slow, fast or backache labour, where a lot of tension is building up, or fear.

Take *Cimicifuga 30*, one dose every 10–20 minutes for up to 6 doses if the trembling comes on its own with no other symptoms and hasn't passed of its own accord after a few minutes. Take *Gelsemium 30* if the trembling accompanies a backache labour or a terrible exhaustion. If the shaking is accompanied by strong feelings that point to another remedy then take that instead.

Do
- rest and allow your body to express itself with the trembling.
- breathe slowly and deeply.
- ask someone to massage your back.
- find a comfortable position in which to sit or lie where your limbs are well supported.
- drink or eat something with sugar or honey in it.
- follow the dos and don'ts on p. 108 if you are also exhausted.
- put on some warmer clothes, a cardigan, some woolly socks, a heated towel or blanket, if you feel at all cold.

Don't
- tense up against the movements your body is making. Go with them, let them develop if you can as they may be part of a process whereby your body is letting go of deeper tensions and may therefore be helpful to you.

· 5 ·
THE POST-NATAL PERIOD

YOUR BODY IN THE POST-NATAL PERIOD

After birth your body goes through a series of physical, emotional and hormonal changes, some of which relate directly to the birth and some of which are part of the post-natal adjustment to not being pregnant. They include:

- complaints from the birth itself, which take variable lengths of time to heal, for example, piles (see p. 131), episiotomy (see p. 61), general bruising, pain as the body heals (see p. 127), numbness in the genital region with difficulty in urinating (see p. 132), exhaustion (see p. 125), involuntary urination (see p. 132) and prolapse (see p. 131).
- afterpains, as your uterus contracts back to its pre-pregnant size (see p. 117).
- the production of colostrum, which began in pregnancy and continues for 2–3 days after the birth to provide the antibody-rich fluid which boosts your baby's immunity, followed by the swelling of your breasts as your milk comes in on the third to fifth day after the birth (see Engorged Breasts, p. 118). Your baby's sucking stimulates the hormones which

cause the milk glands to produce milk. If you don't breastfeed then your breasts will return to their pre-pregnant size.

- an increase in urination as your body gets rid of the extra fluid accumulated during the pregnancy.
- a rounded abdomen which can feel flabby for a while after the birth until the muscles regain their former tightness.
- your vulva and vagina may have changed their shape through the process of birth with the stretching and especially if you have torn or had an episiotomy. If you have had a Caesarean then your genitals will be intact but you'll have an abdominal scar to get used to.
- a feeling of tightness in the joints as the hormones that helped them soften during pregnancy (in preparation for birth) adjust back to normal.
- hair loss, again because of hormone changes (see p. 127).
- skin changes that were caused by the extra hormones during the pregnancy (discolouration on the face, nipples and abdomen) will gradually fade.
- stretch marks will fade but not disappear.
- varicose veins in the vulva will have disappeared during the birth.
- varicose veins in the legs will take a few months to

settle down as the hormones and the fluid levels adjust and as your weight drops. They may improve and ache less but they won't disappear.

- ankles and feet will take a few days to return to normal if they swelled during your pregnancy.
- you'll bleed after the birth as your uterus contracts, sheds its lining and heals (see Lochia, p. 128) and this will turn to a brownish discharge before stopping.
- complaints of pregnancy, such as heartburn and breathlessness, due to the extra weight and the size of the baby in the abdomen, will disappear.
- emotions can be extreme partly because of the nature of the experience itself but also because of the hormonal changes. Euphoria often gives way to a day or two of the 'blues' on about the third to fifth day after the birth (see pp. 123–5).

COMPLAINTS – MOTHER

After birth, so much is happening and so fast that it can be difficult even to think of what remedy to take and when. You may find that you have after pains, piles and are sore around any stitches. Where do you start?

You may find that one remedy fits your whole picture in which case take it until you feel better. More often, however, different pictures emerge on a daily (and sometimes hourly!) basis. The guiding rule is to deal first with whatever is most distressing. If two remedies are strongly indicated, you can alternate them. If you find that you are taking one remedy after another and they aren't helping, consult a professional homeopath who will be able to prescribe on the whole picture.

AFTERPAINS

The uterus continues to contract after the birth until it has regained its pre-pregnant size. This process, involution, can take up to two months. Your GP will want to see you when the baby is about six weeks old to check, among other things, that the uterus is contracting as it should.

Afterpains may resemble mild period pains or be surprisingly painful. With a first baby they often pass unnoticed; with subsequent births, however, the afterpains are worse each time as the uterus has to work harder to contract back to normal. If you have had a large baby or twins, it will have stretched more and will take longer to contract. The pain is usually worse during breastfeeding as the baby's sucking

stimulates the contractions, but they can come on at other times and may be noticeable for up to a week after the birth. They can be the last straw after a difficult birth and a serious block to successful breastfeeding.

You may be taking *Arnica* for bruising which will also help with afterpains but if it doesn't, take *Magnesia phosphorica* just before and during breastfeeding. If neither helps, you will need to work out a remedy specifically for you and the pains. You may be feeling weepy, in which case consider *Pulsatilla*. Other remedies indicated are *Chamomilla, Cimicifuga, Cuprum, Rhus toxicodendron, Sabina, Silica,* or *Secale.* Make time to differentiate between these remedies to find the one that fits your picture and take it instead of *Arnica* every two hours for one day, stopping on improvement and going back to *Arnica,* if necessary, once the afterpains have eased.

Do

- breathe through them or move your body as you did in labour to help ease the pain.
- make sure you are comfortable when you breastfeed (see p. 75).

Don't

- tense up against them as this can increase the pain.

BREASTFEEDING PROBLEMS

Blocked Duct (mastitis/breast abscess)

Prompt treatment can clear up a blocked duct and prevent a more serious breast infection (mastitis) or abscess from developing. The first signs are soreness and a lump in the breast, with or without redness on the skin above the lump. Fever is a sign that you have developed mastitis and need to take it seriously. Homeopathic treatment is highly effective at dealing with breast infections and abscesses and is a safer option than antibiotics but if self-prescribing doesn't help quickly seek the advice of a professional homeopath if you don't want to take orthodox medicines.

Do

- see Breastfeeding, pp. 71–7.
- check that your bra isn't cutting in and causing the blocked duct.
- rest more if you suspect a duct may be blocked. They can be a sign that you are overdoing it.
- apply hot and cold compresses alternately to the sore breast every 2–4 hours for 5–10 minutes each time. Dip a flannel in a basin of very hot water, wring it out and lay it over the breast until the flannel cools. Replace with a flannel that has been dipped in ice-cold water and wrung out.

- increase your fluid intake.
- breastfeed more often and in a variety of positions to drain the milk from all the ducts.
- massage your breasts as the baby feeds (especially if and when you feel the milk let down, a prickling sensation). Massage gently from the highest or lowest point to the nipple to encourage the duct to clear: if the blocked duct is in the side of your breast massage from your armpit, if it is in the top massage from your collarbone, etc.
- use a breast pump if your baby isn't feeding much and your breasts are engorged.
- express or breastfeed in the bath to encourage your milk to flow strongly.
- pull a plastic fine-tooth comb through a bar of soap and 'comb' your breasts very gently from the highest or lowest point to the nipple – some women find this more effective than massaging. You can 'comb' or massage your breasts in between feeds as well as during feeds.
- position your baby on the breast so that her chin points across from the blocked duct.
- try some vigorous arm-swinging exercises to encourage blood to pump into the area.
- breastfeed from the affected breast first at each feed until it starts to clear and then alternate. Make sure that the affected side is fully emptied at each feed.
- go to bed and stay there if the duct doesn't clear up with the above self-help measures *and* you develop a fever. Call around and get help with your chores. A day or two in bed now will prevent a more serious abscess developing.

Don't
- stop breastfeeding.
- automatically take antibiotics.

Seek help if
- self-prescribing hasn't helped within 24–48 hours.
- you develop a fever that doesn't respond to self-prescribing within 12–24 hours.
- the glands in your armpits are swollen: you may have developed a more serious infection.

Engorged Breasts

This common condition often occurs within a few days of the birth when the milk first comes in. Homeopathic treatment can alleviate the pain and discomfort and help to stabilise the milk supply. The two main remedies for this condition are *Belladonna* and *Bryonia*. *Belladonna* is more restless, and the breasts may have red streaks on them. *Bryonia* pains are much worse for movement; the breasts are usually pale. You'll need to stop taking *Arnica* or any

other post-natal remedies while you self-prescribe on the engorgement.

Do
- reassure yourself that this is a temporary condition. It won't last.
- encourage your breasts to soften so that your baby can latch on easily by: expressing some milk either by hand or with a pump (often easier if done in a warm bath); applying hot flannels to your breasts just before a feed; stroking the breast *away* from the nipple, lightly with your fingertips, to make the nipple more accessible.
- breastfeed frequently – wake the baby to feed her or feed her while she is asleep – until the engorgement has passed.
- apply ice-cold flannels to the breasts after a feed to reduce the blood supply.

Don't
- give up!

Seek help if
- you are engorged and have a fever. You may have mastitis (see Blocked Duct, p. 117).

Inverted Nipples

Some women's nipples remain flat or even inverted after the birth. Breastfeeding may be more difficult in the beginning but not impossible. *Sarsaparilla* or *Silica* may help the nipples to come out.

Do
- get support from a breastfeeding counsellor if you are determined to continue.
- remind yourself that you are breastfeeding – not nipple feeding!
- bring the nipple out before a feed by: using a hand or electric breast pump immediately before a feed; placing a pad soaked in cold or ice-cold water over the nipple; rubbing an ice cube gently around the nipple.
- try using a nipple shield when feeding. Ask a breastfeeding counsellor or your health visitor or midwife to help you with this.

Mastitis

See Blocked Duct, p. 117.

Pain on Feeding

Some women suffer from pain in the breasts unassociated with a blocked duct, breast abscess, sore nipples, or the let-down reflex. This distressing condition can make it difficult to establish breastfeeding. Seek professional help if self-prescribing doesn't help within a few days.

Do

- be aware of your breathing (p. 40) while you are breastfeeding and use any breathing techniques you learnt for labour.

Sore/Cracked Nipples

The cracking of nipples has nothing to do with their colour but reflects their sensitivity. Relatively insensitive nipples – those that do not become particularly aroused during love-making and are not sore from brushing against rough clothing – are less likely to become sore and cracked with breastfeeding. If your nipples are sensitive study the general breastfeeding guidelines especially carefully.

Sore nipples can crack so look after them. Some of the points below will help prevent soreness developing and also help heal if it does.

Phytolacca, Borax, Silica, Castor equi and *Sulphur* are all indicated for this condition and the right one for you should help quickly. If not, consult your homeopath, especially if you are in great pain.

Do

- see Breastfeeding, pp. 71–7.
- let your baby suck for as long as she wants at a feed and feed her when she first cries rather than wait until she is screaming. This will avoid her latching on desperately and with great force which can injure the nipples.
- settle yourself and then bring your baby to the breast.
- offer the breast that is least sore first, as the baby sucks hardest at the beginning of a feed.
- distract yourself as you did to deal with pain in labour if your nipples feel sore.
- listen to music, breathe easily, use your relaxation exercises as you begin to feed, imagine the milk flowing easily into and out of your breasts.
- feed your baby in the bath if you are sore, engorged and desperate and a hot bath is soothing for you. If no one is available to help you get out, put a few pillows beside the bath to lay the baby on before you try to get out yourself. *Take great care when getting in and out of the bath.*
- limit the amount of time your baby sucks if your nipples are sore as long as she is taking milk (gulping or swallowing), usually about 10 minutes on each side, and after that encourage her to find her thumb, or let her suck a pacifier or your little finger.
- try feeding your baby when she is sleepy or even asleep as her suck may be gentler then.

- switch sides frequently to encourage your milk to let down several times, especially if you suspect that the baby is sucking voraciously because she is hungry and you are not producing enough (see also p. 120).
- try a nipple shield to protect the skin from direct sucking. Feeds take longer if you use one.
- spray ice-cold water on your nipple before a feed to numb it enough to allow your baby to latch on, or rub your nipple and areola with an ice cube. Don't do this if you are super-sensitive to cold!
- feed in different positions to distribute the sucking pressure to all areas of the areola.
- express a little milk first if your breasts are very full so that your baby can latch on more easily.
- keep the nipples dry by: exposing them to the air after a feed; drying them with a hair-drier; using disposable breastpads without plastic backing between feeds (change them frequently if your nipples 'leak', or put a one-way diaper liner between nipple and pad, or try a piece of toilet paper or a cotton handkerchief instead of pads); wearing a loose shirt without a bra at home unless your breasts are large and heavy; wearing plastic tea strainers with the handles cut off inside your bra to let the air circulate without anything touching the nipples (only do this for short periods during the day).
- moisten a bra or pad which has stuck to the nipple with water before removing.
- expose your nipples to sunlight or sit with your breasts uncovered a foot (30 cms) away from a 40-watt light bulb for a few minutes four or five times a day.
- stop using all your usual creams and sprays as you may be allergic to one of the ingredients.
- try using a cream if you have not been using one (see External Materia Medica and Repertory). Experiment until you find one that works and stick to it. *Calendula* or Rescue Remedy creams are the most helpful. Rub in after a feed. Otherwise rub a little expressed milk into your nipples.
- stop wearing a bra at night to allow your nipples to heal in the air.
- stop feeding for 48 hours to rest your breast if all else fails. Express the milk by hand or pump and give it to your baby in a bottle. Resume breastfeeding once your nipples have healed.

Don't

- pull your nipple out of the baby's mouth (see p. 76).
- use creams other than those suggested in the External Materia Medica.

- use a nipple cream with chamomile as it can give some babies colic.
- wash your nipples more often than once a day: too much washing will dry the skin and make it sore.
- use *any* soap on your breasts.
- wash your bras in biological soap powders.
- wear nylon bras.
- press the top of your breast away from the baby's nose. This will direct your nipple towards the top of its mouth where it will get sore and bruised. Reposition or place another pillow under the baby or hold your breast from underneath with your whole hand.
- give up!

Seek help if
- there is bleeding or severe pain.

Too Little Milk

Getting the hang of doing breastfeeding can take a little time and patience initially but if your baby isn't gaining weight satisfactorily or you know that your milk supply is down, try some of the following self-help ideas. If your only symptom is not having enough milk, take a short course of *Urtica urens*. Otherwise repertorise carefully before self-prescribing.

Do
- see Breastfeeding, pp. 71–7.
- have a nutritious snack with every feed – you will need about 600 extra calories a day to breastfeed.
- feed your baby often to build up your supply.
- drink plenty of fluids. You will need about 2 pints more per day than you normally drink.
- cut out caffeine (tea, coffee, Coca-Cola and chocolate) and tobacco as it can reduce your milk supply by overstimulating your nervous system. See p. 42 for alternative ideas for drinks.
- see if your baby is producing roughly the same number of wet diapers per day as before your milk supply dropped and try to build up your supply, or give extra fluids, if there are fewer than usual. There should be roughly 8–10 wet diapers in a 24-hour period with breastmilk alone.
- try a complete rest in case you have been over-doing it. Go to bed with the baby and eat and sleep for a day or two (both of you!).
- use your relaxation exercises before and during a feed – and at other times if you are feeling tense and anxious. The more you worry, the less easy it will be to build up your supply.
- remember that babies have growth spurts – at around three weeks, five to six weeks, three months and six months – when they will want to feed more. Increase your food and fluid intake and resting time for 24–48 hours.
- switch your baby from one breast to the other often during a feed. This will encourage your milk to let down several times, which will in turn increase your supply and stimulate a baby with a weak suck to suck more strongly.
- use a pump to increase your supply after a feed if your baby sucks infrequently or has a weak suck.
- encourage the milk to let down before a feed by using warm compresses on your breasts before-hand, having a warm bath, thinking 'baby' or 'milk', or imagining milk flowing into your breasts. Breathe!
- listen to music or the radio, watch TV or read a favourite book, and take your time.
- start each feed on alternate sides.
- feed in a quiet room if the baby fusses or doesn't seem interested, or if you are shy feeding in front of others. Your feelings will inhibit the let-down.
- make sure you are not interrupted. Unplug the phone or switch on the answering-machine, pin a note on the front door that says something like 'Please do not disturb, baby resting – call back later. Thank you'.
- trick your baby into feeding from a breast that he or she goes off: move the baby in the same pos-ition across your lap to your breast, or use the football hold (see p. 76) with the baby under the arm on the side he or she is feeding on.
- give a bottle of formula at night if you know that your busy day has caused a drop in your supply which you are not going to make up. Use a teat with a very small hole that takes as much energy to suck from as the breast and position it carefully, as you would your own breast, so that the baby sucks on the bottle, mouth wide open and the teat at the back of the mouth. (See also p. 73.)
- leave the baby with your partner, a tried and trusted relative, friend or childminder *and* a bottle (of expressed milk or formula), and go and do something completely different. If your life is nothing but breastfeeding and baby, plus your other children, you can quickly become burnt out – a break really is as good as a rest.
- deal with any emotional trauma as a shock or distress can affect your let-down reflex (see p. 75). Talk to your partner, friends and your baby about what is happening – don't keep it to yourself.
- ask yourself if you really want to breastfeed, or carry on breastfeeding.
- check that your baby hasn't got thrush in her mouth.
- wean your baby off a nipple shield if you have been using one as the nipple may not be receiving

enough direct stimulation. Do this by smearing a little sterilising fluid on your nipple or starting to feed with the shield and removing it quickly once your baby has latched on, or cutting away the tip of the nipple shield very gradually over a number of feeds.

- ignore unhelpful remarks from relatives or professionals who are obsessed with your baby's weight and whether he or she is getting enough milk. Your baby's weight gain is always going to vary and the charts in your clinic are only a guide. You will *know* if things aren't right.

Don't

- worry if you have small breasts. The amount of milk they produce is not related to their size.
- worry if your milk looks thin or bluish. This is normal and healthy.
- worry if your breasts become smaller a few weeks (or months) after the birth. This is a sign that your milk supply is well established, the milk letting down when the baby feeds; even though your breasts may feel empty at the end of a feed there is always some milk in them.
- time feeds. Let your baby decide when the feed is over, even if it seems to take for ever, especially with the first breast.
- use soaps, perfumes or sterilising fluids on your breasts as it may make them smell or taste unpleasant to your baby.
- worry if your baby seems to go off your breast when you are menstruating or ovulating – some babies do temporarily.

Seek help if

- you know something is wrong and can't sort it out on your own.
- you suspect that your baby is ill.
- you are getting into a cycle of anxiety about breastfeeding and need a reassuring counsellor to help you break it.
- you are on medication such as diuretics, the pill, antihistamines, laxatives or antibiotics as these may affect your milk supply. Your doctor may suggest an alternative or you may decide to take a break from the medication while you are breastfeeding.
- your milk isn't letting down. You will be able to tell if this is so because your baby won't be swallowing or gulping during a feed. If you have taken steroids before your pregnancy this may have affected your let-down reflex: consult a professional homeopath or see your GP for a syntocinon spray to use until it gets going.
- your baby is producing fewer wet nappies than usual.

- your baby isn't gaining weight and stools are consistently green.
- your baby is sleepy from drugs you had in labour and doesn't respond to the treatment outlined in this book (see p. 123).
- your milk smells or tastes different from usual.

Too Much Milk

When your milk comes in, it might spurt everywhere at the slightest opportunity and cause the baby to choke at the beginning of every feed, or you may be producing so much so quickly that the baby takes too much, becomes too full, feels uncomfortable and cries. He or she may gulp desperately, take in air and then get colic. This usually settles down within a few days but some women consistently produce more milk than their babies' need. You may suffer from a temporary overabundance of milk if you miss a feed. Try the suggestions given below and choose a remedy to help decrease your supply or, if it worries you, get in touch with your homeopath, breastfeeding counsellor or midwife.

Do

- be reassured that your milk supply will probably even out by the time your baby is around eight weeks old.
- use the heel of your hand to press on the nipple of the opposite breast to the one your baby is feeding from so that when your milk lets down it doesn't spurt out; or hold a sterilised container under it to catch the 'overflow', which you can freeze, store in the fridge for use later, or donate to a milk bank.
- express a little milk before a feed if it flows too fast and makes the baby choke and splutter.
- position your baby to suck 'uphill': lie in bed with the baby on your tummy, supporting his or her forehead with your hand – gravity will help to slow down the gush of milk.
- sit your baby upright to feed so that swallowing is easier.
- let your baby feed on one breast at one feed and offer the other at the next. This will encourage your milk supply to diminish. Be careful, though, not to let your breasts become lumpy – express a little milk off the unused breast, if need be, at each feed.
- encourage your baby to suck a pacifier or your finger if she wants to suck but isn't hungry. Continued sucking after she has fed will stimulate your supply.
- use a nipple shield to restrict the flow of milk and decrease the supply.
- talk reassuringly to your baby about what is happening. Your anxiety or panic is contagious and

you may find that your calm voice will help you as well!

- use cold compresses after a feed to slow down your milk production.

Don't

- cut down your fluid intake.
- worry if your breasts become temporarily lop-sided if you are only feeding from one breast at a time. They will even up once you are feeding from both breasts again.

Weaning

Whether you have decided to breastfeed or bottle-feed, when to wean is a matter for you and/or your baby to decide. Some babies love to suck and hang on to the breast or the bottle for years, given the chance! Others can take it or leave it, losing interest from eight or nine months onwards making it perfectly clear that they wish to drink out of a cup like every-body else! Eating is a social activity and some babies cotton on to this early.

Weaning follows fashions so it's useful to remem-ber that around the world babies are weaned onto the local fare, be it raw fish or curry. However, it is worth giving a little thought and care to your baby's early solid diet to avoid illness such as gastro-enteritis or allergies. Packaged or tinned foods are usually high in carbohydrates (some are also high in sugar and salt) and low in vitamins and minerals, so use them as occasional convenience foods rather than for everyday eating. Your baby will want to eat what you eat so it is best to start as you mean to continue and introduce foods that, roughly speaking, you eat as well. Fresh foods are good for adults and babies alike: start your baby on fruit and vegetables (organic if possible – most supermarkets stock them now) and delay introducing wheat, eggs, meat, sugar and refined foods for as long as possible. You can give your baby a good start and the rest is up to him or her!

To help your milk dry up quickly, you can take *Lac caninum* once you have stopped feeding. You can help your baby adjust by giving a constitutional remedy to deal with any upset after weaning. Some children promptly go down with a cold or become clingy or angry or develop diarrhoea: take the whole picture into account when prescribing. Seek pro-fessional advice if your baby is having difficulty digesting 'real' food or if a food intolerance or allergy develops.

Do

- what is best for you, your baby and the rest of the family.

- stop breastfeeding if you have had enough, what-ever the reason.
- breastfeed for as long as you are *both* happy to do so. It is unusual for both mother and baby to want to give up at the same time: sometimes it is the mother who is ready to give up first and some-times the baby. Perhaps you have decided to go back to work and find expressing difficult – or you may simply have had enough.
- wean your baby from the breast gradually if you can. Try cutting out: daytime feeds first and replacing them with something nice – a special drink, a cuddle, a new toy, or a distraction such as an outing; or the bedtime feed first by letting someone else put the baby to bed for a week or so; or night-time feeds first, in the knowledge that nights could be noisy until your baby is used to the new regime; or the last feed of the day first, as that is when your supply will be at its lowest, and give a bottle of expressed milk or formula. Substitute a bottle for another feed after a few days and carry on until your baby is only getting one breastfeed a day. This will help your milk supply to diminish gradually.
- let your bottle-fed baby decide when to give it up. For some children it is their major comforter and they will drop it when they feel independent enough to do so.
- be careful how you introduce solids once your baby is old enough to avoid allergic reactions and digestive problems. Start with small amounts of one food at a time. Go as slowly or quickly as your baby wants – some are cautious while others are instantly wildly enthusiastic. Try fruit or veg-etables first and introduce the following foods carefully, one at a time and one a week, because of the allergy risk: yoghurt; milk; cheese; egg; wheat; fish; tomatoes; strawberries; tofu; meat; nuts (but not peanuts, and any others should be finely chopped or ground). Make sure your baby's food doesn't contain salt, sugar or spices and introduce cereals or fatty foods gradually: young babies don't need them before they are four to five months old if they are still on milk and these foods will encourage unnecessary weight gain. Don't forget to offer extra water to a baby who is having solid food, but you should avoid giving sweet drinks altogether, either juice or squash, however much they are diluted in the interests of prevent-ing sugar addiction and early tooth problems. Give instead the fruit to eat and water to drink. Make mealtimes as relaxed as possible – times to chat and laugh and share news as well as eat. And never make your baby's eating dependent on *your* approval as this will have repercussions when the child grows up.

Don't

- feel guilty because you haven't let your baby decide when to stop breastfeeding.

CONSTIPATION

Constipation after childbirth is an occupational hazard. The vagina and perineum may be sore and swollen for several days, in spite of taking *Arnica*. You cannot imagine that you will ever go to the loo again because everything feels numb, or painful or both. And to top it all you may have piles and/or stitches as well.

You will probably have emptied the contents of your bowels during the course of your labour and also if you have eaten little since it is unlikely that you will either want or need to do so again for several days. If you want to but can't, see also Constipation in Pregnancy, p. 83 for suggestions which may help.

If constipation does not clear quickly with self-prescribing, consult your GP or homeopath.

Do

- take heart if you become constipated – it will pass. As all your muscles and organs snap back to their usual places and the bruising heals, your bowels will regain their former health and strength.
- support any stitched episiotomy or tear by holding a pad (sanitary or piece of felt) against it when you go to the loo to pass a stool, which will make it less painful and less likely that stitches will give way under the pressure.

DETOXIFICATION FROM DRUGS TAKEN DURING OR POST-LABOUR

Pethidine or a general anaesthetic can make you and/or your baby feel nauseous, 'high', intoxicated, or sleepy, or conversely tense, irritable and unable to sleep. Pethidine remains in the system of an adult for up to about five hours but it can affect an infant for as long as 24 hours.

Opium, Chamomilla, Nux vomica or *Phosphorus* are all remedies that may be needed after labour to counteract the effect of anaesthetics or pain-relieving drugs. Choose between them noting your general and emotional symptoms. *Secale* will counteract the ill-effects of syntometrine (see p. 115). Seek the help of a professional homeopath if you feel 'toxic' after the birth or if you have had medication which *you* think is still hanging around.

Don't

- automatically take laxatives, sleeping pills or pain-killers without questioning carefully whether you need them and also whether they will affect your baby if you are breastfeeding.

EMOTIONAL DISTRESS
(Post-natal blues)

The feelings you experience after the birth may be the most intense you have ever encountered: overwhelming extremes and upsurges of emotion. A great unadulterated joy, a love beyond your wildest expectations, contentment, fulfilment, waves of happiness that wash over you whenever your baby smiles or whimpers . . . And babies are hugely entertaining – their antics make you laugh for hours on end. The funny expressions their faces make when they yawn and sneeze and wrinkle up against a bright light. The infectiousness of a baby's laugh is heartwarmingly delightful. Your own baby is delicious – the best thing since freshly baked brown bread!

It is common, too, normal even, to feel depressed after childbirth. It can pass by fleetingly as post-natal blues on about the third day after the birth when your milk comes in, or span a longer period while your hormones sort themselves out and you are beginning to make the emotional adjustments to having a new person in your life.

A satisfying birth will leave you feeling strong and empowered, and strengthen your relationship; a difficult one followed by post-natal stress and a demanding baby may leave you feeling shipwrecked and drive a wedge between you and your partner that is difficult to deal with. There is a sensation of emptiness after the birth that can come as a relief and a shock. Women need to transform that shock by holding their babies and connecting with them. If they are not able to after a difficult birth depression may set in and last for weeks or even months.

Babies come in all shapes and sizes: some are supremely needy and demanding, emotionally and physically. They can make you feel frustrated and angry, fearful, anxious, guilty, confused and depressed over how to cope with them – all entirely normal and part of the package deal that is parenthood. Women with demanding babies need lots of support, more than those whose babies are accommodating and easy to please. Even so-called 'good' babies make what seem like unreasonable demands at times when you are exhausted and need to rest.

It is vital that you remind yourself continually that all healthy relationships involve compromise so that everyone is satisfied, and one person isn't having all their needs met at the expense of another. Your own needs are terribly important: when they are met you can feel good about yourself and cope easily with the baby. It is not appropriate to meet all your baby's needs all the time. Sometimes you will come first, sometimes the baby, and at others your partner's or other children's needs will take priority.

> My two children have instructed me in the arts of motherhood. They have taught me more than a million textbooks could . . . They continually take me on a guided tour of my limits, physical, emotional and intellectual, and having demonstrated these, revealing my inadequacy, they then proceed to love me despite everything.
> (Jane Price,
> *Motherhood – What it does to your mind*,
> Pandora, 1988)

Some women are particularly vulnerable to post-natal depression, especially those with poor self-esteem; those who had a difficult childhood themselves; single mothers; women whose partners are not supportive; very young women; those lacking a strong support network of family or friends; some older women who have concentrated on their career; any who suffered a lot of stress, such as moving house, a bereavement, an unexpected change in circumstances, during pregnancy and/or shortly after the birth; women who have had an unexpected Caesarean or a disappointing or downright awful labour; those whose own feelings of distress during the pregnancy or around the birth were denied by being encouraged to suppress their emotions or to 'snap out of it'; and women who feel confused about feeling sad at the loss either of the pregnancy itself, or freedom and the carefree independent life they used to live, or their former pre-pregnant, tight-muscled body, or attention, especially if visitors focus only on the baby.

Post-natal blues is often misdiagnosed as exhaustion or anaemia. If you are dragging yourself around and not sleeping well, or lacking in energy however much rest you get, you may be depressed. Common symptoms of post-natal depression are:

- a creeping sense of hopelessness.
- low self-confidence.
- anxiety about the baby.
- exhaustion accompanied by an inability to sleep; waking in the early morning, not necessarily to feed the baby, and being unable to sleep again.
- mood swings.
- gloom – a lack of joy or a sort of flatness.
- feeling numb and dazed.

- a feeling of being unable to cope with anything, especially any extra demands.
- everything seems to take a long time, even small tasks.

We all have different resources for dealing with parenthood: it's a mistake to assume that because you have undergone a lot of stress, you will feel depressed – just as it's a mistake to assume you shouldn't be depressed because things haven't been that bad.

Homeopaths take emotional injury as seriously as physical injury. If you break a leg (a serious physical injury) then the care and attention you receive is necessarily considerable. Emotional injury is not visible in the same way but it needs as much if not more time and support to heal. The following suggestions are to help you process the emotional impact of childbirth and to take any distress seriously so that healing can take place.

The range of emotions that follows childbirth is extensive. Here are some common to depression in the post-natal period that you may experience: anger; anxiety; apathy, indifference (cut off/numb); aversion to family members, to visitors (company); confusion: thinking and concentrating are difficult; absent-mindedness; depression; despair, especially of recovering; exultation – over-excitement or euphoria; irritability; lack of confidence; loneliness and feelings of abandonment; resentment: dwelling on past events; regret; shock; weepy or sad; sentimental. All these are included in the Repertory (see pp. 264–99). It may be that one emotion predominates or that you feel a complex mixture of different ones. In taking the whole picture into account, if the remedy that is strongly indicated sounds just right when you read it through in the Materia Medica (pp. 169–263) take it according to your needs – *but please seek professional advice if your self-prescribing doesn't help you within a week or two.*

Do

- see Emotional Stress, pp. 88–9.
- be open to the feelings that come your way on a day-to-day basis. Acknowledge and accept them. Talk about how you are feeling with people you trust, who care about you.
- debrief: you need to talk and talk, as much as you want, to tell the story of your baby's birth over and over again. This will help you integrate the experience into your life and understand how it has affected and shaped you.
- reach out to the support network you set up during your pregnancy.
- use your telephone support system if you don't have close friends or family living nearby.

- keep in contact with at least one other mother and baby so that you can talk 'babies' and not feel isolated with your small charge.
- seek the help of a counsellor or psychotherapist to help heal and integrate a particularly difficult birth experience if you are in distress and finding it difficult to bond with your new baby and/or reconnect with your partner.
- see a masseur or cranial osteopath if you feel that your distress is linked to physical tension or injury from your labour.
- listen to those you love and trust if they tell you that you are looking rough.
- write (or type) an account of the birth, putting in as much detail as you can remember. As you write, notice your feelings and write about them too. If you feel sad, allow yourself to cry. If you feel angry, kick a cushion around or have a good shout. If you feel inhibited about expressing your feelings and they are very strong, seek the help of a counsellor or psychotherapist.

Don't

- get orthodox medical treatment if you are depressed or in distress after the birth of your child and the measures outlined here do not help. In the long term orthodox medicines can make it difficult for this raw wound to heal. Seek alternative help as a first measure.
- wait until you are desperate to ask for help. If you get help early it will be easier for you to heal.
- ignore your distress by saying things like 'Many women have to cope with far worse than this' or 'I'll get over it'.
- listen to people who say things like 'It wasn't that bad, you are both alive and you have a healthy baby with all its bits and pieces in the right places', or 'It will heal, time will heal – you will soon forget about it – stop thinking about it and it will go away'.

Seek help if

- you feel you've lost touch with reality, that there is an unpleasant feeling of distance and unreality that permeates your waking life and keeps you feeling separate from everybody and everything.
- you find it difficult to feel the floor or pavement solidly under your feet, or the bed solidly holding your body when you lie down.
- you are also suffering from inexplicable fears and worries.
- you feel repeatedly angry with the baby.
- you feel cut off and unable to respond to your partner or the baby.

NB Severe post-natal depression – that is, severe emotional/mental problems surfacing after childbirth – always needs the help of competent professionals.

EXHAUSTION

With a first baby you may wonder how you will wash your hair or cook a meal or do anything else ever again! Second or subsequent babies are usually easier to integrate, although the demands of a toddler who is still in diapers alongside a newborn who is being fully breastfed are as impressive as the demands of a first baby who feeds every two hours around the clock.

Exhaustion is an occupational hazard at any stage of parenthood. Less sleep and more demands make it difficult to get the rest you need when you have babies and small children in the house. They are either breastfeeding or teething, suffering from a cough, cold, nightmare, inexplicable loneliness at 3 a.m. or a childhood illness, involving round-the-clock nursing care and attention. You may be lucky enough to have a baby who sleeps through the night from early on or a partner who wants to share the childcare and is not bothered by broken nights. It is easy to become run down when you are breastfeeding, especially if you are feeding on demand: irritatingly, babies have growth spurts, one at six weeks and one at three months and will want to feed more often just when you are beginning to feel like a human being again and wanting to get out and about. Extra activity may decrease your milk supply when you need to build it up to meet your baby's increased demands.

Use common-sense measures to look after yourself and take the appropriate homeopathic remedy to hasten your recovery. You may need to repeat it relatively frequently while you are breastfeeding, especially if you find it difficult having your sleep disturbed at night.

Several remedies are indicated for the treatment of exhaustion after childbirth, which may stem from loss of blood, breastfeeding or broken sleep, including *Cocculus, China, Kali phosphoricum, Nitric acid, Nux vomica, Staphysagria* and *Phosphoric acid*. Seek professional advice if self-prescribing doesn't help as exhaustion is often the first symptom of stress and can lead to depression. You must deal with your tiredness to avoid the development of physical complaints such as mastitis.

Do

- go with the flow. Again!
- get your priorities right. Look after yourself, eat, drink, rest and sleep so that you have enough energy to care for your new baby.

- rest and sleep when your baby rests and sleeps.
- remember your partner and other children. Have a bit of fun.
- ditch the housework. It will still be there tomorrow and *you* are much more important right now than a clean kitchen floor.
- get a close relative or good friend to live in for the first two weeks after the birth so that you and your partner don't have to do *anything* except recover from the birth and get to know the baby.
- be strict with visitors. Either get them all over and done with in a 'visit-the-new-baby' day or restrict yourself to one set of visitors a day: ask them to stay an hour at the most and to bring a small present for an older child or children. You could also ask for a contribution to your kitchen – a cake or casserole. Yet another option is to make a 'provisional' time for a visit and either confirm it on the day, or put if off if you are too tired. Visitors have a neat habit of turning up when you and your baby are settling down for your first peaceful nap in what seems like 24 hours. Your partner can always ask them to come back later, or entertain them with stories of the birth while you sleep.
- eat well – little and often is better while you are breastfeeding. Have a snack every 2–4 hours. Listen to your body: hunger pangs are a symptom that *you* need feeding – don't ignore them when you are breastfeeding.
- drink plenty while you are breastfeeding – you will feel more thirsty anyway, so make sure you have a snack and a drink on hand whenever you sit down with the baby.
- negotiate a deal with your partner so that you each get a decent stretch of sleep every night. Your baby may wake cheerful and bouncy at 5.30 a.m.: take it in turns to handle the early-morning shift. Many babies will sleep again after a couple of hours of playfulness – you can sleep as well, especially in the early weeks.
- gratefully accept any offers of help.
- get some practical support if you are exhausted: someone to shop, clean, cook, or take the baby for a walk in the carriage if he or she doesn't sleep in the daytime so that you can have a nap.
- get help with other children. Find someone to deliver and collect children to and from school or the childminder or to give practical help with a toddler.
- persuade older children to help out.
- read undemanding books and magazines.
- talk about anything that is bothering you. Your midwife, health visitor, doctor, homeopath or breastfeeding counsellor may be able to help, with sympathy or practical advice. You may need to talk some more about your birth experience: it is exhausting continually to hold on to anger, regret, sadness or any strong emotion.
- take gentle exercise, which will help create energy. If it doesn't, take the appropriate homeopathic remedy and get help.
- ask your partner or a good friend to give you a face, foot or back massage. Some masseurs will visit your house: a good post-natal present for you could be a wonderful massage.
- seek the help of an osteopath (especially a cranial osteopath) if you feel stiff and achy after the birth. The gentle art of cranial osteopathy (without manipulation) will help you to heal and rebalance.
- introduce the odd bottle from early on if you are breastfeeding so that you are not on call 24 hours a day for an unlimited period of time. You can express your own milk or give some formula, unless you have a history of asthma, eczema, hay fever or milk allergies, in which case breastmilk is preferable.
- do one thing every day to give you a sense of accomplishment. This may be a walk to the shops, writing a letter to a friend, having a bath and washing your hair, visiting a friend or having one visit you.
- get out and about. Find another mother or two with babies of a similar age so you can do some swaps.
- do something wonderfully self-indulgent once a day.
- be quiet and boring during night feeds. Put double diapers on the baby so you don't have to do a change and risk really waking them up.
- get a lot of support and sympathy if your baby is a poor sleeper: use a post-natal support group (see Organisations, p. 305) to meet other women, reassure yourself and pick up some tips on how to get your baby to sleep better.
- remind yourself that this is a short phase in your baby's life. Rearrange your routine as necessary and *enjoy it* while it lasts!

Don't
- breastfeed through the night if you turn into a demented monster after being woken from deep sleep more than once.
- isolate yourself.
- wake your baby for a feed before you go to bed in the hope that it will help him or her to sleep through the night. It won't.
- change your baby in the night, unless *absolutely* necessary.

HAIR FALLING OUT

(See also p. 90.)

After childbirth your hair may lose its shine and/or its curl, and it may fall out in handfuls for what seems like ages, especially if you are breastfeeding. If self-prescribing doesn't help, do seek the advice of a professional homeopath.

Do

• look after *yourself*, resting as much as you can, and eating well and regularly, including plenty of mineral-rich whole grains.

HEALING AFTER LABOUR

Childbirth is incredibly stressful physically, which some women find easy to cope with and also they heal well afterwards. For others, healing may be slow and arduous. Homeopathy can speed this up and prevent complications developing.

The common physical injuries include stitched wounds from a tear, an episiotomy or a Caesarean scar; bruising of the vagina, cervix and uterus, and the bladder, the hand or arm (if a drip was used); strained muscles and ligaments anywhere; general muscular aching and soreness; back pain after a backache labour or an epidural. Avoid the likelihood of further strain on pelvic-floor or back muscles by taking particular care of yourself post-natally, using the suggestions given below. The more care you take, the quicker you will heal. (See also Pain in Pregnancy, pp. 96–9.)

The speed of physical healing is closely related to how you are feeling emotionally. If your stitches are taking a long time to heal and you are feeling resentful, angry and let down by your experience of childbirth then you must prescribe on your emotional state *and* your physical symptoms: *Staphysagria* may be called for.

Many remedies may be indicated after birth to aid healing including *Arnica* or *Bellis perennis* for aches and pains in the muscles caused by bruising; *Hypericum* or *Nux vomica* for pains in the sacrum or coccyx after an epidural or forceps delivery; *Staphysagria*, *Calendula* or *Hypericum* for severe pains in tears, episiotomies or Caesarean section scars; *Kali carbonicum* for backache after a posterior labour; *Calcarea sulphurica*, *Hepar sulph.*, *Lachesis* or *Silica* for sore or lumpy scars that are slow to heal; *Rhus toxicodendron* or *Ruta* for strained muscles or joints. List your symptoms and repertorise them carefully to choose a remedy that fits as much of your picture as possible, bearing in mind that you may need a change of remedy as your symptoms change – in the days after the birth you may need different remedies every day. (See also Afterpains, p. 117.)

Do

• take as long as you need to rest and recover, especially to avoid a prolapse (see p. 131).
• whatever will help you recover from any injuries: indulge in hot baths, massage, sleep, gentle exercise, etc.
• start with gentle physical exercise and build up slowly. It is important to include some exercise in your daily life from as soon after the birth as is practicable – you'll both benefit from the fresh air if you go out for a walk with the carriage. And you can exercise with your baby, for example, lifting her gently on your legs when you are lying or sitting down . . . remembering to do only what you can without straining yourself.
• keep wounds clean and encourage healing by: wiping or washing your genitals from front to back after you have passed a stool to minimise the risk of infecting a wound; 'bottle washing' (see p. 85) and then drying yourself thoroughly after you've urinated (pat dry with soft toilet paper or use a hair-drier if you are very sore); using soft sanitary towels and making sure they are held firmly in place so they don't rub. Change them frequently.
• see a cranial osteopath to help your body heal and rebalance you, especially if you have a sore back.
• look at your genitals as soon as you feel able to if you feel anxious about your anatomy. You can do this with your midwife or your partner, asking them to tell you what has changed. It is important that you reconnect with your body for healing to take place.
• use *Calendula* lotion on your episiotomy scar (see p. 61).

Don't

• be impatient or critical of yourself if your healing takes longer than other women you know.
• strain your pelvic, back or stomach muscles by lifting or carrying heavy weights (you can cuddle small children on the floor or get them to climb on to a bed or sofa and snuggle up to you).

INCONTINENCE

See Urinary Difficulties, p. 132.

INSOMNIA

The hormonal high often experienced after childbirth can make sleeping impossible for the first night and difficult for a while after that. Choose between *Coffea cruda* and *Kali phosphoricum* for sleeplessness, unless you have other symptoms that would lead you to another remedy. You might, for example, have missed prescribing the first two nights and be suffering from irritability due to loss of sleep as well as excitement, indicating *Nux vomica*.

Do
- enjoy the elation and express it – joy, happiness and excitement deserve and need to be expressed.
- write copious notes in your diary or journal about your birth experience.
- use the extra energy to have special nice times with your partner and baby.
- relax in a warm bath at night and take boring books to bed (see also p. 93).
- nap with your baby in the day. This will help you get into the habit of being able to sleep.

Don't
- drink tea, coffee, hot chocolate or Coca-Cola because the high caffeine content will further overstimulate you.
- drink alcohol or take sleeping pills if you are breastfeeding because it will pass into your milk.
- invite crowds of relatives and friends around just because you feel good as this can over-excite you.

LOCHIA

You will bleed for a while after the birth until the wound left by the detached placenta has healed and the uterus has fully emptied itself. The discharge is referred to as lochia and the amount is noted: your midwife and/or your doctor will check it regularly because heavy bleeding after the first week may lead to anaemia or, especially if there are clots or an unpleasant-smelling discharge, indicate a uterine infection or some remaining fragments of the placenta. Lochia is bright red for a few days after the birth, then turning reddish brown for a while before becoming brown and petering out. It lasts for anything from two to six weeks. As you get up and about you may find that it turns back to red for a few hours or even a few days.

If you decide not to breastfeed your baby then it will usually stop after your next period, which will come about four weeks after the birth.

Arnica will help your uterus to contract and the site of the placenta to heal. I have included some additional remedies to help speed up this process if, say, you stop discharging lochia then restart, or it becomes smelly without there being an infection. Choose between them based on the whole symptom picture.

Do
- observe a rigorous cleanliness: change your pads frequently; wash after urinating and/or passing a stool; 'bottle wash' (see p. 85), shower or use a bidet, if you have one.
- add a handful of sea salt and/or a teaspoon of *Calendula* tincture to the bath to promote healing.
- use only sanitary pads, not tampons, until discharge of lochia has ceased: it isn't advisable to push anything up against your cervix while it is closing and healing.

Don't
- worry if you start to bleed again once the lochia has more or less stopped.

Seek help if
- you carry on bleeding heavily or notice clots after the first week.
- you stop bleeding and then it restarts suddenly and heavily after the fourth day.
- the lochia smells unpleasant.
- you are having to change your pads every hour for longer than 3 hours.
- your temperature rises.

LOSS OF A BABY

The loss of a baby is devastating whether it is before birth (a miscarriage), at birth (a still birth), or in infancy (a cot death, illness or an accident). It leaves a great, gaping wound, a hole which can hurt more than anything has ever hurt before. Some of the feelings that surface after such an event can be hard to understand. They can come with great force, be fleeting or pass and then return unexpectedly. They can last for days, months or years.

Death is still a taboo subject. People often don't know what to say. We have very few rituals to help people through this time except for the cremation or burial, after which the bereaved are often expected to carry on with their lives, especially if they have other children to care for.

The feelings that follow the tragedy of a child's death run strong and deep and need to be expressed. Their healthy expression will help you through this time, however painful it is, while suppression will lead to ill-health. Some common emotional responses are shock with numbness (no feelings), denial, rage, resentment, shame, guilt, great overwhelming sadness, depression, a terrible blaming – a wanting to find someone or something to blame for what happened (including yourself and/or your partner) – hopelessness, suicidal thoughts, despair about the future and a hatred of people with live babies.

I have included several remedies for the acute shock and grief of a still birth (or miscarriage) but it is essential to seek the advice of a homeopath if your health suffers and home prescribing hasn't helped. Don't prescribe on yourself after the death of your own child: ask a close friend or your partner to do this for you. Minor physical symptoms after a bereavement are common: headaches, back pain, difficulty in sleeping, loss of appetite, nausea, tension, inexplicable pains, overwhelming lethargy and so on. If you need a remedy to help you sleep and ease the acute emotional pain, they should prescribe carefully taking all your symptoms into account. Emotional symptoms to look up in the Repertory may include: apathy (numbness); shock; complaints from anger, suppressed anger, grief, shock or suppressed emotion; denial of suffering; tearful; tearful, with difficulty crying, cries alone; dislikes consolation or better for consolation; depressed.

The following suggestions are to help you begin to work towards healing this wound, effectively and healthily.

Do

- what feels right to you, whatever that may be. Express the feelings that surface: cry if you feel sad, rant and rail if you are angry.
- remember that you *will* learn to live with this hurt, *and* you'll never get over it – however much people (kindly but misguidedly) tell you that you will.
- name your child if he or she was stillborn. It is important that you see and touch and even hold the baby so that you can in a small but important way have a memory of the little person you were never able to know properly. Take a photo if possible so that you have a record of him or her in your album and/or cut a little of his or her hair if there is some – it can be even more devastating to have nothing. Go straight home if you delivered in hospital: the sound of other mothers with their babies is hard to bear at a time like this.
- hold and touch your baby if he or she died in infancy. However painful this is it will help you come to terms with it.
- ask your doctor for reassurance. If your baby's death had no known cause ask him or her to tell you as often as you need to hear it that your baby's death was not your fault, that there was nothing that you could have done to prevent it.
- talk with your partner about your feelings and his feelings – over and over and over again, until you both feel the pain healing. The more you talk to each other about it the closer you will feel. Don't allow yourselves to grieve independently. If you feel unable to talk to him, consult a psychotherapist either as a family or with your partner.

The apparently irrational feelings that surface after the death of a baby can drive parents apart if they aren't expressed and dealt with or if they become acrimonious and blaming. It is normal to feel alienated from your partner at a time like this.

- talk to your older children about what has happened and share your feelings with them. Don't hide your sadness but find a way of sharing your feelings that doesn't overwhelm them and use language appropriate to their age and maturity.
- give yourself permission to take as long as you need to grieve.
- contact the organisations that give support to parents who have lost children (see pp. 305–8). They will put you in touch with others who have suffered a similar loss, who can talk with you, listen to you, and help you through this period of mourning.
- seek the support of a bereavement counsellor who will help you come to terms with your baby's death.
- plan the funeral carefully and take an active part in it. Use it as an opportunity to express your grief.
- write your baby a letter. Writing is surprisingly healing. As you write down the first things that come to mind your deeper thoughts and feelings will surface. Share them with your baby, and tell him or her what has happened to you and the family's life since she died. Tell your baby how and why you miss him or her and as you write let your feelings flow.

Don't

- be put off by your friends' or relatives' embarrassment and suppress your own feelings so that they will feel OK.
- put up with people who find your feelings difficult until you feel ready and able to cope again.
- let others tell you what to do or how to behave. If your family suggests that the time to grieve is over, gently tell them to mind their own business, that your grieving will be over in your time, not theirs.
- feel pressured to get through this grieving period as quickly as possible. Unresolved grief always returns, on the back of another loss, and can then be overwhelmingly difficult to cope with.
- worry if you 'go off' your partner and lose your libido. Your interest in each other and in sex will return once your sadness and your spirits lift, when you and your partner have come to terms with what has happened.

NB The recent successful cot death prevention campaign in New Zealand advised parents to put their babies to sleep on their side or back (and never on their front). Be reassured that babies lying on their backs always turn their heads sideways so there is no danger of choking if they posset or vomit in their sleep. This campaign grew out of a research project that also found a worrying correlation between cot deaths and mothers who smoked, so try not to start smoking after the birth if you gave it up when you became pregnant. Avoid smoky places while your baby is small and ask visitors not to smoke in the house.

Also, don't let your baby get too hot *or* too cold – during the day or at night. Once your baby is about a month old he or she is good at keeping warm. To check – feel the tummy (not the head, feet or hands) – it should be warm, not hot. If you have been outdoors take some clothes off your baby so that he or she doesn't overheat (hats, gloves and blankets for a start). And remember, sick babies may need fewer clothes, not more. Ask your health visitor for help with this and with up-to-date information.

LOSS OF LIBIDO

It takes time for the vagina to heal after birth and for the nerves, muscles and ligaments of the pelvis to return to normal. If you didn't tear or have an episiotomy, if your muscles snap back quickly and you have a baby that sleeps reasonably well, and if your relationship with your partner is close, your libido may well return within a few weeks of the birth. You may even find that your sex life will improve.

The more stress you experience around childbirth, however, the longer it can take for your sex drive to return. An episiotomy or a large tear can take anything from several weeks to several months to heal. If you feel tense or ill at ease or upset – either physically or emotionally – you are likely to find it difficult to express much interest in sex. Any of the following can contribute to this: drugs taken during childbirth, an unexpected Caesarean, unresolved feelings dating to the birth (including the shock of having been such public property during labour), a difficult homecoming, a baby who has colic and doesn't sleep, pain, sore nipples and piles. Some women find that it can take the best part of a year to begin to feel the familiar sensations again, to 'regain' their bodies after childbirth, and to get used to the new mother-shape – the more rounded abdomen and fuller breasts.

Some women discover that breastfeeding stimulates their interest in sex, while others find that the close physical relationship they have with their babies satisfies their need for contact. Others, or their partners, struggle with unconscious messages from their own childhood that 'mothers don't have sex'.

This is a time of adapting to change, when great sensitivity is needed between partners. Take your time to process it and integrate sex back into your own life in your own time and in a way that feels healthy and satisfying to you.

When self-prescribing on loss of libido, you must be sure to treat the root cause – the episiotomy scar that is still painful, the backache, the colicky baby who won't sleep at night. The main remedies are *Causticum*, *Natrum muriaticum* and *Sepia*.

Do

- be patient and accepting and allow your libido to assert itself in its own time.
- find some time each day to be alone – to have a bath, read a book or go for a walk – even if only for 15 minutes.
- be intimate and affectionate with your partner. Find ways of being close from the very beginning without worrying about it leading to sex. (See also Loss of Libido in Pregnancy, p. 94.)
- be sensitive to your partner's needs at a time when he may be feeling jealous – unconsciously – of the special relationship you are developing with your baby.
- familiarise yourself with your body to get used to the changes: notice the differences as you wash in the bath or shower, while you smooth on body lotion or talcum powder. Look at yourself in the mirror. Does what you see match what you feel? Get a mirror and look at your vagina if you want to; ask your midwife to reassure you that all is well but ask her about anything that looks unfamiliar or peculiar. Talk about the ways your body has changed with your partner and ask him to tell you what he thinks and feels. Ask him to massage you. Tell him which bits are sensitive and be explicit about how you would like to be touched.
- exercise your pelvic-floor muscles as this will bring a healing blood-flow to your pelvic area.
- keep talking: communicate clearly, openly, honestly but sensitively about how you are feeling.
- wait until your episiotomy scar has fully healed before you try to make love.
- choose a time when you know the baby will sleep to make love.
- be prepared to be interrupted.
- go slowly, there's no rush; the slower the better. Start at the beginning again – with kissing, cuddling, exploratory touching and masturbation.
- use KY-Jelly (not a petroleum-based jelly) as you may find your vagina dry while you are breastfeeding.
- stop if it hurts – from as yet incompletely healed wounds, cervix or sore abdominal ligaments.
- try making love in positions where your partner is

not on top of you, which will enable you to be in charge of how deep he penetrates.

- use contraception if you don't want to become pregnant. Even if you are breastfeeding you can ovulate before your first period.
- seek the help and advice of a sex therapist or counsellor if you can't sort out any problems between you and your partner.

Don't
- force yourself to have sex. This will only create more problems and resentments.
- be goal-orientated about sex: there are many ways to make love other than penetration.
- worry if your breasts spurt milk during lovemaking. This is common, especially in the early months after the birth.
- worry if you go off sex for what seems like a long time. This will pass.

Seek help if
- the above self-help measures haven't helped and one or both of you is becoming resentful.
- sex is consistently painful.

PAIN

See Healing, p. 127.

PHLEBITIS (superficial thrombosis)

Troublesome varicose veins can become inflamed after childbirth. This is known as phlebitis (or superficial thrombosis) and is not as serious as it sounds. It is an irritating but not dangerous complication of childbirth. The vein of the inner thigh or inner calf becomes tender over an area of, usually, around 2 inches (5 cms) in diameter. It is painful to touch as well as on standing and walking. The benefit of this unpleasant symptom is that it cures the affected varicose vein. (See also Varicose Veins, p. 103, and treat phlebitis in the same way.)

Do
- inform your midwife/doctor or homeopath if phlebitis develops.
- bandage the area with a Tubigrip (elastic bandage).
- rest as much as possible until the inflammation has subsided.
- keep the leg elevated, preferably higher than your heart. Raise the feet of your bed with a block or bricks under the legs.
- soak the area of the bandage over the vein in

Hamamelis lotion (or undiluted witch hazel) three times a day, use separate compresses and leave them on for an hour or so while you are resting.

Don't
- stand when you can sit and try to sit with your feet elevated.
- sit when you can lie down.

PILES

If piles have developed in the rectum during pregnancy, they will be pushed out at the same time as the baby. They take a variety of shapes and sizes from a single small one the size of a large pea to a 'bunch of grapes'. The pain of piles after a good birth really feels unfair: it can make sleeping, sitting and walking difficult. Remedies for piles after childbirth are *Ignatia*, *Kali carbonicum*, *Pulsatilla* and *Sulphur*. If another piles remedy is strongly indicated in other ways but not for the post-natal period, like *Nitric acidum* or *Staphysagria*, take it if your whole picture matches.

Do
- see Piles, p. 99.
- try pushing back protruding piles, or ask your midwife to do so. Wash with a non-scented soap and smear with a little Vaseline before pushing them gently back up the rectum where they will no longer be painful – if they stay there. If they keep falling out then do not persevere.
- push your piles back after you pass a stool if you can do so easily and painlessly and if they will stay up.

Don't
- squat as this is the worst position for encouraging piles to pop out.

Seek help if
- they protrude, are painful and haven't shrunk by the time your baby is six months old.

PROLAPSE

A prolapse of the uterus, vagina, bladder or rectum occurs when the muscles or ligaments of the pelvis are either damaged or weakened by a long, difficult childbirth or by subsequent births. They become unable to hold the organs of the pelvis in place with the result that the bladder can push back into the vagina; the rectum can push forwards into the vagina; the uterus can fall down into the vagina pushing against the rectum and the bladder, causing discomfort; or the vagina itself can prolapse with the walls becoming weak and floppy. You may feel a dragging-down sensation in the pelvis, at its worst as if everything will fall out of the vagina, lower backache, pain or discomfort on urinating, stress incontinence and/or discomfort when passing stools.

Prevention is the best cure. It is absolutely essential to exercise generally in pregnancy and to do your pelvic-floor exercises religiously both during pregnancy and after the birth. Either *Calcarea fluorica*, *Pulsatilla*, *Rhus toxicodendron* or *Sepia* may help but prescribe according to your whole symptom picture. Seek professional help if it doesn't help your symptoms quickly.

Do
- lie flat or with the legs elevated – this will always relieve the unpleasant symptoms.
- take care not to strain yourself further: squat down to older children; ask someone else to carry heavy shopping.
- exercise your pelvic-floor muscles at every opportunity.

Don't
- lift or carry anything.

Seek help if
- the measures outlined in this section don't help. Homeopathic treatment may help to prevent surgery.

RETENTION OF URINE

See Urinary Difficulties, below.

URINARY DIFFICULTIES

Incontinence

Your bladder may feel bruised along with your pelvic-floor muscles and it can take a while to get the hang of peeing again – knowing when to go, being able to go and to retain urine without leaking. A sore bladder is most likely after a long or posterior labour or a forceps delivery. If you had a Caesarean (see also p. 58), you will have had a catheter during the operation and for some time afterwards. After it is removed your urethra may be sore and you may have difficulty in controlling your urine.

If you can't control your urine or your pelvic-floor muscles, *Arnica*, *Arsenicum*, *Calcarea fluorica* or *Sepia* may help. If homeopathic remedies and self-help

measures don't work, seek the advice of a professional homeopath or your GP.

Do
- avoid constipation (see pp. 83 and 123).
- exercise your pelvic-floor muscles religiously (see p. 43). You can also exercise these muscles when you are sitting down in a chair leaning forward slightly (or flopped right over). Tighten the muscles around your vagina – you may only feel a flicker after the birth but keep persevering – even if you only feel a little tightening try to hold it for up to four seconds and repeat it three more times. Do this at least 10 times a day – they will begin to feel stronger in a month although they can take up to six months or longer to regain their former strength.
- pee frequently.
- practise stopping and starting your urine midstream every now and again to check you can do it and to strengthen the muscles.
- cut out, or down, food or drink which irritates the urinary tract, such as tea, coffee and alcohol.
- see a cranial osteopath who will help rebalance the lower spine: it houses the nerves that supply the pelvis.

Don't
- stress your bladder by holding on when it feels full, even if you can only pass a little urine when you go.
- cut down on the amount of fluids you drink. You can still 'leak' even if you have just been to the toilet. Cutting down on fluids can cause your urine to become strong which will irritate your bladder and cause other problems.

Seek help if
- you can't control your bladder and you have a bearing-down sensation in or around your vagina. You may have a prolapse (see p. 131).

Retention of Urine

Immediately after childbirth you may feel sore and bruised and have difficulty in identifying a full bladder. It is important that you pee regularly so that your bladder doesn't become weakened or strained as this can lead to stress incontinence (see opposite).

Your doctor or midwife will intervene if you aren't able to pee within a few hours of the birth and will insert a catheter (see p. 60). If you have had a forceps or Caesarean delivery, you may already have one in place.

You can avoid a catheter with speedy homeopathic prescribing. The two remedies that are strongly indicated for this condition are *Arsenicum* (with the accompanying anxiety and panic) and *Causticum*. Other remedies, such as *Arnica*, *Nux vomica*, *Opium*, *Pulsatilla*, *Staphysagria*, or *Stramonium*, might be better indicated depending on your emotional state.

Do

- make sure you are as private as you need to be. Some people can't urinate in front of others – they may feel inhibited if the door doesn't lock or if there are people standing around outside (see *Natrum muriaticum*).

- use tricks to get yourself weeing again like running a tap while you are sitting waiting to pee – the sound of running water is an unconscious incentive as far as your body is concerned; 'bottle washing' (see p. 85): pour a bottle of warm water slowly over your genitals as you sit on the toilet. The fear of peeing can be worse than the actual pain caused by urine contact with the sore or stitched area. If you pour warm water over the area while you pee the urine will be diluted and won't sting, and the warm flowing water will encourage your muscles to relax; urinating in a warm bath (see p. 115). This may be the only place you *can* pee for a day or so after the birth, or you can pee in the shower or even in the bidet if you have one.

- tense your pelvic-floor muscles a little if you can and then slowly relax them while breathing deeply and evenly.

- gently bear down as you did when you were pushing your baby out.

- imagine yourself peeing – shut your eyes and relax the muscles and sphincters of your pelvis.

Don't

- build up tension and anxiety as this will only make it worse.

COMPLAINTS – BABY

ACCIDENTS

See Injuries, p. 151.

BIRTH INJURIES

Modern methods of delivery are designed to minimise the risk of injury or death to both mother and baby but some birth injuries are fairly common:

Bruising:

1. to the baby's head after a long labour where the cervix has dilated slowly and the pressure against the head causes it to swell, sometimes in an unsightly lump;
2. to the head after a forceps delivery where the pressure of the forceps can leave bruises around it (and sometimes the face). With vacuum forceps there is a circular swelling where the cap was applied, usually on the scalp;
3. to the head from monitoring electrodes;
4. to the buttocks (or scrotum in boys) after a breech birth.

Fracture or dislocation of the shoulder or collarbone if the baby is very large.

Arnica is the remedy that will deal with all these injuries in the initial stage and as you will probably be taking it after the birth for yourself, it will pass through to the breastmilk from which your baby will also get a dose.

If the injuries are severe and do not resolve with *Arnica* alone then you should repertorise carefully and prescribe, say, *Symphytum* if there is fracture, *Rhus toxicodendron* for dislocated shoulder, *Sulphuric acid* or *Ledum* if the bruising doesn't clear up quickly – swelling and bruising should disappear within 24–48 hours with *Arnica* alone.

Do

- use external creams where appropriate, such as *Arnica* for bruising and *Calendula* for the heel prick.

Don't

- worry. The above injuries will heal given time, however awful they look. Your midwife will be monitoring them daily so ask her for reassurance should you be at all concerned.

BIRTHMARKS

Birthmarks are caused by discolouration of the skin (pigmentation) or by collections of blood vessels (naevi or 'strawberry' marks). Some are flat and others are raised, most are soft and some have hairs growing in them.

Coffee-coloured birthmarks are irregular patches or spots of darker skin browner in colour than the owner's skin. They are usually permanent although they may fade over time. Port-wine stains are dark red patches that appear on the face. They also usually fade a little over time. Strawberry marks are small red patches that usually disappear within a year or two. If they are raised, they will initially grow bigger, reaching their maximum size by the time your baby is 9–12 months old. They may take up to three years to fade. Mongolian spots are bluish-grey patches resembling bruises which appear on the back, buttocks and, sometimes, the arms and thighs. These usually fade within about five years. Stork marks, reddish patches on the back of the neck at the base of the skull, on the eyelids or the forehead, will usually fade within a year or two.

Moles usually develop as children grow older. They can be prevented from 'multiplying' once they start to appear by constitutional homeopathic treatment.

Birthmarks sometimes respond to homeopathic treatment. Give a short course of *Thuja 6* three times daily for up to 10 days or *Thuja 12*, twice daily for up to a week. Apply *Thuja* tincture twice daily for up to a month. It is worth seeking the advice of a professional homeopath before resorting to surgery if *Thuja* hasn't helped as there are other ways of treating birthmarks homeopathically that are beyond the scope of the home prescriber.

Do
- ask your doctor to tell you what sort of birthmark your baby has and whether or not it will fade, and if so when.
- ask for advice about surgery if your child has a permanent birthmark in a prominent place such as the face.

BLOCKED TEAR DUCT

A tear duct is situated in the inner corner of each lower eyelid. The eyes are bathed with fluid tears all the time, not just when we cry, and the tear ducts drain these tears down into the nose. In babies, ducts become blocked either because they are so small or because they have not fully developed. The result is constantly watery eyes. Sometimes the discharge becomes sticky, an indication that the eye is infected. A blocked duct usually clears itself by the time the baby is a year old.

Silica will help clear a blockage so give this in a low potency (6 or 12) two to three times a day for up to a week. Then wait a week and repeat if there has been an improvement. If *Silica* doesn't help at all and you suspect that the duct has not fully developed, give *Baryta carbonica* in the same dosage as *Silica*. If the eye becomes infected see Sticky Eyes, p. 157.

Do
- gently massage the corner of the eye (or eyes) beside the nose every two or three hours. This helps to clear a blocked duct.

Seek help if
- these measures have no effect and your baby's tear duct is still blocked at a year old. If homeopathic treatment and massage have not helped, your doctor may suggest a minor operation to clear it.

BREATHING DIFFICULTIES

Babies usually breathe for the first time within a minute of birth, but breathing problems in newborn babies are not uncommon, resulting from such circumstances as the cord having been wrapped around the neck at birth; or a long and/or difficult labour in which the baby suffered severe distress; or if the mother had a general anaesthetic, or pethidine late in labour. Premature babies are also vulnerable because their lungs may not have had time to develop to their full size and strength. Doctors, nurses and midwives are all thoroughly trained in getting babies to breathe.

If babies up to six months old develop a viral infection affecting the lungs, pneumonia can develop or (rarely) a small baby can suffer heart failure. Danger signs to watch out for are: blueness of the face or of the area around the mouth; difficulty getting air in; wheezy breathing; baby refuses to feed.

You can prescribe while you wait for emergency help to arrive. The main remedy for the first-aid treatment of babies who have difficulty in breathing is *Carbo vegetabilis* – the baby is collapsed, limp and cold to the touch. If the breathing difficulty accompanies an infection and the baby is making very noisy efforts to breathe then give *Antimonium tartaricum*. If you have nothing else to hand Rescue Remedy may help the baby *and* you: a drop or two every five minutes or so.

These are emergency prescriptions only – it is essential that you seek expert medical help immediately.

Do
- get emergency help.
- keep your baby warm and very close to you.
- talk reassuringly and constantly to him or her.

CHILDHOOD ILLNESSES

(See also Fever, p. 149.)

Babies are born with a temporary protection from or immunity to the infectious diseases that *you* have had, passed from you to the baby through the placenta. The colostrum in breastmilk adds to this immunity. It was thought to last for about the first three months but recent studies are showing that fully breastfed babies are protected for much longer (see *The Art of Breastfeeding* by La Leche League, 1974), until their own immune system begins to develop. Even if you decide to bottle-feed do try to breastfeed for the first couple of weeks so that your baby has the full benefit of this protective colostrum.

Homeopaths believe that childhood illnesses (such as chickenpox, mumps, measles, etc.) are not necessarily a 'bad' thing: they provide children with the opportunity to develop resistance and strength, and to clear inherited weaknesses. Those who have come through a childhood illness without medical interference and without complications are seen to be stronger afterwards and often have a growth spurt, either physically or mentally or both.

A sick child must be nursed through a childhood illness. This may seem obvious, but it is becoming increasingly common to give children antibiotics and analgesics and to encourage them to carry on a normal life, including going to school or visiting friends. If you are a working parent you should prepare yourself for the fact that your children will fall ill from time to time and need nursing, either by you or with the help of a reliable carer. If you are unprepared for this, you will feel harassed and resentful when it happens.

If you have more than one child they will tend to fall ill one after the other rather than all at once. Your role as nurse/mother will probably seem interminable so try to set up a support network that will give you some time off in each day.

Before prescribing a remedy assess how well your child is coping with the disease and whether he or she *needs* a remedy. It is not worth giving one if she is getting through it with ease unaided. Should the symptoms become distressing, however, remember to prescribe on the whole picture including the general symptoms and the emotional state as well as the specific symptoms of the illness.

A child who doesn't recover quickly from a childhood illness always needs constitutional treatment from a professional homeopath.

For general warning symptoms see Cause for Concern, p. 23, and Fever, p. 149.

Do

- offer extra fluids to sick babies, especially if they are feverish. Give water or diluted freshly squeezed lemon or orange juice with honey (not to babies with mumps; these drinks are too acidic for sore salivary glands), either warm or cold, or herb teas.
- continue to breastfeed as often as your baby asks. The breast will comfort her at a time when illness is making her feel awful.
- give babies that are on solids small, easily diges-

ted, nutritious meals if they are hungry, such as fruit or vegetable purées, soups and porridge.
- encourage a sick baby to sleep or rest as much as possible.
- keep a hot, feverish child cool and a chilly, feverish child warm.
- lie down with your baby and stay while he or she sleeps if necessary. Some babies, when sick, will only sleep well if their mother's body is close to theirs. Use this time to catch up on some sleep or reading.
- let your baby sleep with you at night if you want to – or on you if you are able to. The comforting sound of your heartbeat will often help.
- put your baby's cot or crib next to your bed so that you can reach out a comforting hand at night or talk soothingly.
- sing to your baby and/or play music.
- carry your baby around in a sling while you do the things you have to do.
- sleep or rest in a rocking chair or comfortable armchair with your baby held upright if a cough is preventing sleep while lying down. Wrap a duvet or enough blankets to be warm around both of you and use one of those inflatable airline cushions for your neck (to stop your head lolling if you drop off) so that you can sleep sitting upright. They really do work.
- talk reassuringly to your baby about what is happening. The sound of your voice is comforting.
- engage the help of neighbours, friends or family to look after older children so that either you can rest *with* your baby in the daytime, or cook or shop or just have a break doing something completely different – and enjoyable.
- laugh at anything and everything, a sense of humour is a great bonus at times like these.
- be careful that your child does not overdo things in the convalescent stage of a childhood illness, as relapses are common at this time.

Don't

- overstimulate sick babies by taking them out or by having lots of visitors.
- encourage sick babies to eat.
- take any child with a fever out and about.
- worry if sick babies regress emotionally by becoming clingy or whiny. This behaviour may also be the first sign that they are not well. It will pass as they recover.

Incubation and infectious periods vary, so the information regarding them in the individual illness entries below should be used as a rough guide only.

Never give a child aspirin in any form during or after a childhood illness as this can cause serious complications.

Chickenpox

Incubation period 7–21 days.
Infectious period from a few days before onset until the last spot or blister has formed a scab.
Chickenpox generally occurs in a mild form in young babies – the younger they are the milder it is, some babies have only a couple of spots. Homeopathic treatment will help with the spots if they are very itchy or if they take a long time to heal.

Don't worry about elderly friends or relatives getting shingles (caused by a virus identical to that of chickenpox) as a result of contact with your 'poxy' child. It is rare for the chickenpox virus (herpes zoster) to be passed on to adults as shingles.

Do
- dab dilute cider vinegar on very itchy spots (one tablespoon to a pint/½ litre of water) or put a cup of cider vinegar in a tepid bath and let your baby soak in it as often and for as long as it helps. An alternative to cider vinegar is bicarbonate of soda (a handful in the bath/a tablespoon to a pint (½ litre) of water).
- dress your baby in loose cotton clothes to prevent further irritation.
- cut the baby's fingernails or try mitts on the hands to prevent scratching, which will leave scars.

Seek help if
- the spots become badly inflamed (infected), that is, if there is redness or swelling around them, or pus oozing from them.
- the itching is severe and not alleviated by the above self-help measures and home prescribing.
- the spots affect the eyes (not just the eyelids).

German Measles

Incubation period 14–21 days.
Infectious period 5 days before and 7 days after the rash appears.
German measles, or rubella, is generally a short-lived, mild infection. A faint pink rash of tiny spots starts behind the ears or on the face and spreads down the body. It may be accompanied by watery eyes and swollen glands at the back of the neck and/or behind the ears, under the arms or in the groin.

Your baby will probably feel unwell for a few days before the rash comes out, will be more demanding and may have a fever with no other symptoms.

Homeopathic treatment is rarely needed for babies who contract German measles. However, if your child is miserable with, say, a fever and an itchy rash, then you can prescribe to help him or her through it.

Do
- avoid contact with pregnant women while your baby has German measles because the infection can damage the foetus, especially in early pregnancy. For the same reason, notify pregnant women with whom you were in contact in the three-week period before the spots came out (when your baby was incubating rubella).

Seek help if
- you suspect you are pregnant.
- there is a high fever, marked drowsiness and your baby is crying in that particular way that you know indicates pain.

Measles

Incubation period 8–21 days.
Infectious period 4 days before and 5–10 days after rash appears.
If you suspect your baby is incubating measles – if he or she has become unwell with, say, a fever, sore eyes, cough and irritability or clinginess within three weeks of having been in contact with another child with measles – look for small spots like grains of sand in the mouth, inside the cheeks. These spots, known as Koplik spots, confirm measles before the characteristic red rash appears, usually a day or two later. The rash starts behind the ears and spreads down the body. It is a blotchy rash with raised spots in the blotches.

Don't be tempted to suppress the fever, even if the temperature is high (see Fever, p. 149), as it is essential that the disease 'burns' itself out naturally. Some complications are thought to be caused by suppression of the fever and include ear infections, respiratory problems, pneumonia and (rarely) inflammation of the brain or encephalitis. Children need careful nursing through measles to reduce the possibility of these complications developing.

Homeopathic treatment will help at all stages but especially with the cough and sore eyes and in avoiding the development of more serious complications.

Do
- resign yourself to looking after a measly baby for at least a week.
- encourage a baby with measles to sleep and rest as much as possible. Stay around and read aloud or stock up on story tapes from the library.
- keep a baby with sore eyes out of bright light, with

curtains partially closed and lights dimmed, and bathe the eyes with *Euphrasia* lotion to ease soreness (see p. 163).

Seek help if
- your baby under six months old contracts measles.
- there is a cough that lasts longer than 4 days and doesn't respond to home prescribing.
- the measles is accompanied by severe earache.
- your baby is no better 3 days after the rash has come out.
- your baby begins to get worse after a period of recovery.

Mumps

Incubation period 12–28 days.
Infectious period 2 days before the swelling appears until it has gone.
Mumps usually occurs as a mild childhood infection, especially in infants. The most common (and often the first) symptom is the swelling of one or both of the salivary glands (in front of the ear and just above the angle of the jaw), which gives a hamster-cheeked appearance. The glands under the tongue and jaw may also swell.

Homeopathic treatment will ease the pain caused by eating and give relief from earache, both of which are common in mumps, and it will speed recovery. Again, you'll need to take the whole picture into account when prescribing.

Do
- encourage your baby to drink plenty of fluids – cold drinks may be easier than warm ones.
- give drinks through a straw or from a bottle if it is painful to open her mouth.
- avoid acid juices such as lemon, orange or grapefruit, as these will hurt the salivary glands.
- be understanding if breast- or bottle-fed babies are fussy about feeding, as sucking may hurt.
- give liquidised foods to babies on solids – soups, purées and ice creams.
- wrap a hot-water bottle in a towel and let your older baby lie on it to soothe painful swellings. Hold a heated towel against the face of a younger baby and repeat if it is obviously helping.

Seek help if
- your baby doesn't seem to hear you – doesn't turn round to your voice as usual.

Roseola

Incubation period 5–15 days.
Roseola is a mild, infectious illness which rarely needs treating. It is very similar to German measles, and the two are sometimes confused. The rash will distinguish between the two: in German measles it is more likely to appear with the fever and in roseola it appears when the fever has come down. The fever usually lasts for about 4 days and then the rash that appears is characteristically pink with small spots like that of German measles.

Scarlet Fever

Incubation period 2–7 days.
Infectious period 7 days after the rash comes out.
This highly infectious disease is caused by the streptococcus bacteria, and, although it is rare nowadays, when it comes, it can sweep through whole neighbourhoods or schools.

The symptoms are a sore throat, followed a day or two later by a rash of tiny spots which begins on the neck and chest and spreads over the whole body, giving the skin a texture like sandpaper; vomiting; and fever and a flushed face (though the area around the mouth may be pale). The tongue may also have a red and white 'strawberry' appearance.

It responds extremely well to homeopathic treatment and patients usually recover without any complications. Prescribe on each stage as necessary: different remedies for the fever, the vomiting and the rash may be appropriate.

Whooping Cough

Incubation period 7–21 days.
Infectious period up to 3–4 weeks after the illness appears.
The first signs of whooping cough are a slight fever and runny nose. This is followed by a loose cough. The mucus then thickens and extended, uncontrollable coughing fits occur to bring it up, after which the child draws air convulsively back into the lungs resulting in the characteristic whoop. Whooping cough may be accompanied by other symptoms such as nosebleeds, vomiting and blueness of fingers.

The danger of whooping cough in young babies is that they may not be able to breathe in properly after a coughing fit and may also find feeding difficult if they vomit frequently. If you have decided not to immunise against whooping cough I strongly recommend that you 'sign on' with a professional homeopath so that if your infant contracts this unpleasant illness, you can get effective help if home-prescribing does not produce a quick response.

Whooping cough can last from three weeks to four months and is a long and tiring infection for both child and parent. Complications are rare in children over a year old. In babies or children who are prone to coughs and colds whooping cough can recur with every cough or cold for up to a year after the first attack.

Do
- follow the general advice for coughs (see p. 142).
- keep your child away from other children until the infection has ceased.

Don't
- give proprietary cough medicines to reduce the coughing – your child *needs* to cough to expel the mucus.

Seek help if
- you suspect your baby has whooping cough.

CIRCUMCISION

The removal of the foreskin of the penis is a religious ritual which was originally performed on grounds of hygiene, mainly by Jews and Muslims. It has now become a widespread custom, particularly in America and Europe even though there are now no medical grounds for it. Many people are questioning this practice because of the physical and emotional trauma to the baby.

No local anaesthetic is used for ritual circumcisions, which are performed a week after birth. The foreskin is simply cut off the penis with a sharp knife or razor blade and the penis is wrapped tightly to prevent bleeding. A plastic device is used where the circumcision is out of choice (rather than on religious grounds) – it is tied on to the foreskin and falls off (with the foreskin) after three to four days. This is a painless and less emotionally traumatic procedure.

The penis will usually be slightly inflamed and swollen for a few days afterwards, whichever method is used, which may cause pain or soreness on urination. Some babies are distressed afterwards, waking at night more often, crying more during the day, wanting to be carried around more, wanting to breastfeed more frequently and so on.

Prescribe on your baby after the circumcision according to his reaction: *Arnica*, if he has gone into delayed shock, *Aconite*, if he is severely shocked, *Staphysagria*, if he is enraged, *Ignatia*, if he becomes hysterical and inconsolable or *Stramonium*, if he is shocked and wakes screaming in the night as if from a terrible nightmare when he was formerly a good sleeper.

Use *Calendula* externally to help the wound to heal quickly (see p. 162). Give *Hepar sulph.* if the wound becomes infected and follow it with *Silica* if it takes a long time to heal. Seek professional advice if the self-help measures outlined in this book don't help and your baby remains distressed.

Do
- keep your baby very close to you afterwards: he has suffered an injury and he may be more clingy.
- breastfeed your baby frequently if it soothes him.

Seek help if
- your baby's penis bleeds for longer than a day after the circumcision.
- your baby is in great distress and the remedies outlined above do not help.
- his penis is still swollen or inflamed after a week.

COLIC

Colic simply means sharp, intermittent abdominal pains or cramps and occurs commonly in babies as their digestive systems mature. Babies with colic usually pull up their legs (see *Colocynthis* in the Materia Medica) or stretch them right out (see *Dioscorea*) and in some you will notice a change in the colour of their stools, which may become greenish (see *Chamomilla*). Sometimes colic is accompanied by constipation (see p. 140), in which case you should treat that as well.

Mothers of breastfed babies with colic should consider their own diet, as many foods are known to affect some babies through the milk; these include cow's milk and all dairy products, alcohol, tea, chocolate, coffee, spices (including chillies and pepper), onions, garlic, broccoli, cabbage, cauliflower, Brussels sprouts, peppers (especially raw green peppers), strawberries, oranges and grapes. Occasionally egg or wheat products are to blame or even fruit with stones (cherries, apricots, etc.). A breastfeeding counsellor will help you sort out which foods may be responsible for your baby's colic. Some bottle-fed babies are allergic to cow's milk and will usually do well on soya milk, although that is acidic for some. Seek advice if you are concerned. If the colic starts within the first week after birth, consider whether it might have been precipitated by the syntometrine injection (see p. 114) and if so, give *Secale*. Otherwise, differentiate between the colic remedies to find one that fits your baby best.

Some babies swallow air with their feeds which can cause colic if they can't bring it up easily. This can happen with bottle-fed babies if the teat is too big for new babies and too small for older ones, or breastfed babies if the flow is too strong. If your baby is gulping milk *and* air then experiment with different feeding positions or a teat with a different size hole.

Do

- help your baby to pass a stool, if the colic precedes the passage of one. Massage the abdomen very gently in gentle clockwise circular movements or hold the baby in a semi-squatting position, back to your tummy, legs pulled up a little, again very gently.
- place the baby face-down on your lap over a rolled-up towel, as pressure sometimes eases colic.
- place your baby over your knees so that there is no pressure on the abdomen: pressure sometimes aggravates colic. (You can use these symptoms as a part of your prescribing picture.)
- give your baby some dill- or fennel-seed tea. Simmer a teaspoonful of seeds in a pint (½ litre) of water for 10 minutes. Strain and cool and give it to your baby in a bottle or on a spoon.
- offer a bottle of boiled and cooled water instead of a breast- or bottle-feed as there are times when babies are thirsty, especially in hot weather or if they are inclined to be sweaty, and need something thirst-quenching. Do this to check whether your baby is thirsty and only if she is plainly thriving (gaining weight and producing lots of wet diapers).
- burp your baby after a feed or carry her around upright (over your shoulder) until she settles down.
- relax when breastfeeding a colicky baby.
- take a break from your baby if you are at the end of your tether and suspect that your own irritability is affecting her.
- self-prescribe on your own exhaustion (see p. 125).
- eliminate suspect foods from the diet of a baby who has just started on solids and give small meals of bland, easily digestible foods.
- offer your baby a finger or dummy to suck if she is distressed. Some babies will feed almost continuously when colicky but the extra milk may overload the stomach and aggravate the colic when she just wanted to comfort-suck. Even with demand feeding it is possible sometimes to offer the breast too often when it isn't needed.

Don't

- let your baby get desperate for a feed as she may gulp and take in air which may cause her discomfort.
- give gripe water as this can contain a worrying amount of alcohol.

Seek help if

- the colic persists – especially if the baby screams inconsolably.
- the colic is accompanied by persistent vomiting, diarrhoea, constipation or absence of urine.

COMMON COLD

Some babies seem to have a constant cold from fairly soon after the birth. This chronic catarrh is beyond the scope of the home prescriber and should always be referred to a professional homeopath.

Wait and see if a basically healthy baby throws off a mild cold in a day or two. A runny nose in one who is otherwise happy and contented, feeding well and sleeping at night is no cause for concern. However, a snuffly nose may interfere with feeding – a baby with a blocked nose will find it difficult to suck and breathe at the same time – and sleeping, causing some babies to wake frequently at night. Once the cold starts to affect your baby's energy, moods, sleep patterns or appetite then you should prescribe as neglected colds can turn into more serious chest infections.

In the Repertory see Common Cold and Snuffles: it is the type of runny nose that will help you prescribe. Observe whether the discharge from your baby's nose is clear and watery, thick and clear like egg white, yellow or even green, whether it produces crusts inside the nose or whether there is no discharge but you know there is congestion because your baby can't breathe properly with her mouth shut (see also the sample case on p. 27).

Do

- take sensible precautions to prevent a cold developing into a chest infection. Don't take the baby outside if it is cold and/or windy; don't bath him or her until the cold has passed as they may easily get chilled afterwards; encourage plenty of sleep and rest; and ensure that a baby on solids has lots of fruit and vegetables.
- breastfeed a nursing baby more often: babies who have started on solids may go back to breastfeeding fully until the cold has passed. This is normal.
- keep your baby away from polluted environments such as smoky rooms and traffic jams as far as possible.
- take the baby out for some fresh air if the weather permits to see if this helps (and use the response as a symptom to repertorise).
- use a vaporiser, filled with plain water, to humidify a dry, centrally heated atmosphere. Don't add strong-smelling substances as they may affect the action of the homeopathic remedies you give.
- use a little lavender and/or rosemary oil (essential oils) in the vaporiser at night to help clear the nasal passages, or put a drop of each on a piece of cotton wool and place it under the sheet. You can also mix a drop of the essential oil with a little almond

oil and massage a little in clockwise circles into your baby's chest and back.

- clear your baby's nostrils gently with a tissue or a cotton bud, being careful not to push it in, before a feed so that sucking and breathing are not difficult. Use a drop of water or oil or a little breastmilk in a blocked nose to make it easier to clear.
- put a pillow underneath one end of your baby's mattress.
- cut cow's milk and all dairy products from your baby's diet for a day or two, if you can, as they encourage mucus production.

Don't
- use decongestants. These only irritate the nasal membranes and make matters worse as soon as the effect wears off.

Seek help if
- your baby's cold goes to the chest and your prescribing doesn't help within a day or two.
- the runny nose is more or less continuous as your baby may have a mild allergy.

CONGENITAL DISORDERS

A congenital disorder is a defect present at birth rather than one that develops later. Many early miscarriages are of fetuses whose development is not as it should be. The number of babies born with an abnormality is relatively small. The most common include cleft palate, hare lip, club foot, dislocation of the hip, hole in the heart, hydrocephalus, obstructions of the rectum or small intestine, pyloric stenosis (projectile vomiting), sickle-cell disease, Down's syndrome, haemophilia, cystic fibrosis and spina bifida. These range from disorders that clear with a little help in a relatively short time, such as a dislocation of the hip, to those which produce severe disabilities and are not curable, such as Down's syndrome.

Although homeopathic treatment cannot 'cure' most of these disorders, good constitutional treatment will help by boosting the immune system, and therefore improving vitality and general health, and helping children with emotional stress. Babies who need surgery can be prescribed on both pre- and post-operatively to speed their recovery. I suggest that you give *Aconite* before the operation – just one dose. Afterwards, choose between *Aconite*, *Arnica*, *Phosphorus*, *Staphysagria* and *Stramonium*. You may find that Rescue Remedy is good for *you* (administer frequently!) and you can also massage a few drops into the forehead of a distressed baby at any time while you are in hospital.

Do
- seek genetic counselling before or during pregnancy if you know or suspect you or your partner has an inherited weakness.
- read up thoroughly on the disorder your baby is suffering from and ask your GP, consultant and homeopath to explain in detail what your child has and why.
- ask (if appropriate) what are the chances of recovery with an operation, the potential risks, what will happen (how long it will take, which bits will be cut, stitched and bandaged, and how long recovery will take) so that your shock afterwards is lessened.
- go with your partner, a close friend or family member to all visits to the GP or hospital and ask them to take notes and go over them with you afterwards.
- create a network of support for yourself (including contacting any organisations that represent your child's disorder) to help you cope.
- seek the advice of a counsellor to help you adjust to this new circumstance – a disabled baby requires more care and time, and some disabilities are more of a strain than others. Coming to terms with reality is essential for you.
- make contact with other parents in a similar situation.

Don't
- feel guilty.
- isolate yourself and your child.

CONJUNCTIVITIS

See Sticky Eyes, p. 157.

CONSTIPATION

The first day after the birth babies pass meconium (a sticky, greenish-black substance) which gradually changes to normal stools. In breastfed babies these will be liquid, mustard yellow, sweetish-smelling, curdy stools (like half-cooked scrambled egg); and a more formed, conventionally smelly brown stool in a bottle-fed baby. Babies will settle quite quickly into their own pattern of passing stools and it is the variation from this pattern that may be significant.

Very young babies vary enormously in the number of stools they pass. Some open their bowels with every single feed; others happily pass one large mass every three to seven days. Babies with this latter pattern are simply absorbing most of their food.

Constipation in a baby is defined not by the

number of stools that are passed but by whether the stools themselves are hard and painful and/or difficult to pass. Some babies become constipated when they start on solids. Introduce one food at a time initially so that you know which is the culprit. When you introduce starch give rice rather than wheat as the gluten in wheat can cause the digestion to slow down. Bananas are a favourite first food and if they are unripe (with yellow or green skins) they commonly cause constipation because they are very starchy. The skins need to have gone black, indicating that the starch has turned to sugar, for babies to be able to digest them more easily.

Like adults, some babies become constipated when they travel away from home.

Constipation in breastfed babies is rarer than in bottle-fed babies. Some bottle-fed babies are sensitive to the protein in cow's milk and benefit from a change of formula to a different cow's milk or even one made from soya. It is essential that you seek the advice of your health visitor or GP when changing formulas. If the formula mix is too rich (not diluted enough) it will cause constipation.

Babies with fevers can become constipated unless they drink more than usual as their need for fluids increases. (See also Colic, p. 138.)

Although I have included a few remedies for treating acute constipation, it is not a complaint for home prescribing if it becomes chronic. A tendency to constipation should be referred to a professional homeopath.

Do
- give a little prune juice to a constipated baby. Pour boiling water on to a handful of organic prunes and soak overnight. Give the strained juice on a spoon or in a bottle.
- give your baby a little strained and diluted freshly squeezed orange juice.
- repeat the above measures as and when they are needed, if they work.
- make sure that there is plenty of water and fibre in *your* diet if you are breastfeeding, and that *you* are not constipated.
- give your baby some extra water, especially if the weather is hot. Some babies need more fluids than others and will take water greedily if they need it.
- add more water to formula (bottle) feeds.
- massage the abdomen gently if the baby strains to pass a stool.
- smear *Calendula* ointment gently around the anus if your baby has a tendency to pass large stools to avoid a tear.
- cut out solids introduced at the time the constipation started and if it clears but returns when you

reintroduce them, wait until your baby's digestion is stronger before trying again.
- wait until your baby is a year old before introducing egg, as it has a 'binding' effect on the bowels.
- give home-made foods for a while if you have weaned your baby on to tins, bottles or packets. Prepared foods are usually cooked in aluminium containers; some babies are sensitive to the very small quantities that dissolve into the food, which may be the cause of the constipation.

Don't
- boil the water or milk you give to your baby in aluminium saucepans or kettles as aluminium, even in very small amounts, can cause constipation. The same goes for any cooked solid food.
- give laxatives.
- give enemas to babies or any children: as the walls of the rectum are very thin and delicate and easily torn or damaged. It is a highly invasive procedure that is no longer accepted medical practice.

Seek help if
- your baby cries when passing a stool.
- there are streaks of blood in the stools or diapers.
- the constipation lasts longer than a week.
- the constipation is accompanied by severe, unusual pain.
- the constipation alternates with diarrhoea.
- the stools are an unusual colour, either very dark or very pale, or have changed in colour from their norm.

CONVULSIONS

Convulsions usually occur in children up to the age of about five and commonly accompany a fever, although children who are teething or who have worms or who have been recently immunised may also experience them. It is not uncommon for a child to have a single convulsion and then no more.

Convulsions are often preceded by a sudden rise in temperature and cause a temporary loss of consciousness often with a vacant expression, blueness of the face, stiffness, usually of the whole body, noisy breathing rather like snoring and uncontrollable twitching. They usually last a matter of seconds and never longer than a few minutes, although it can seem like for ever. The child is usually tired afterwards and will sleep. Convulsions are not as dangerous as they look: the fever affects the part of the brain that controls muscles which is why convulsions are accompanied by twitching. It is the danger of inhaling vomit after a convulsion which can kill rather than the fit itself, which is relatively innocuous.

Children who become delirious with a fever will not necessarily convulse even though their delirious state can be alarming (see Fever, p. 149); a tendency to have convulsions can be inherited. It is important to watch your baby carefully if she produces a fever.

Should your baby or small child have a convulsion, *telephone your GP or homeopath immediately*. You can prescribe from among the remedies included in this book while you wait for assistance to arrive. Constitutional homeopathic treatment will help to reduce the occurrence of convulsions in children who have them with fevers.

Do
- lay your baby flat and stay with him or her.
- loosen clothes or take them off if the baby has a fever (see p. 149).
- turn the baby on to the side in case of vomiting.
- lift his or her head up if they start to vomit so that it runs out of the mouth and not down the throat.
- telephone for help once the convulsion has passed.

COUGH

If the cause of your baby's cough is very clear, for example if it occurs with a chill, then by all means prescribe. Some children suffer from coughs while they are teething: the teething does not cause the cough except indirectly because it can be stressful in itself. If the baby's lungs are a vulnerable area too, a cough will be more likely to develop at that time, or at any other when vitality is low.

You can prescribe for coughs but watch your baby's response, checking that moods and energy remain good. If the cough recurs or doesn't clear in spite of careful first-aid prescribing then do seek professional advice, rather than confuse the case by prescribing several remedies that only work to a limited extent.

However, repeated coughs and colds which don't respond to constitutional treatment may be an indication of an inherited weakness and, if this is so, a professional homeopath should prescribe on the underlying miasm (see p. 7). Coughs and colds are also common after vaccination: if the timing of the cough leads you to suspect that this is the culprit, seek the advice of a homeopath.

Do
- follow the advice for Common Cold and Childhood Illnesses (see pp. 139 and 134).
- make sure your baby has enough rest and sleep.

- offer extra fluids, such as water and diluted freshly squeezed juices (with a little honey if needed) as they will help to loosen the mucus.
- use a humidifier or vaporiser in the bedroom to fill the room with steam (see also Croup, p. 143).
- keep the room temperature constant so that your baby doesn't have to adapt to either heat or cold.
- stay with your baby during coughing fits to reassure and watch for breathing difficulty. Stay calm: if you both panic, it will be even harder for the baby to breathe.
- encourage your baby to bring up phlegm by sitting him or her on your lap and holding them leaning slightly forwards; or lay them over your knees with the knee slightly raised under the baby's bottom with the head lower. Pat the back gently while he or she coughs. Have a bowl positioned to catch any expelled phlegm or vomit. Clean the bowl out afterwards with boiling water to prevent the infection from spreading.
- prop up the baby's head with a pillow *under* the mattress which may ease the cough where lying down makes it worse.
- offer your baby small meals at frequent intervals if the cough is accompanied with vomiting. Try giving a small snack immediately after a coughing fit.
- distract the baby from coughing with entertainment: amazingly, this does work for limited periods. It is important, however, not to let excitement get out of hand, as that too can bring on a coughing fit.
- sleep in the same room as your baby so that you can help if a coughing fit erupts in the night.
- take it in turns with your partner to be on 'night duty' so that you get a reasonable amount of sleep each night.
- cuddle and comfort your baby if he or she is distressed by the coughing. If you are still breastfeeding then offer a feed when you are sure the coughing fit is over.
- avoid environmental pollution, in high streets with a lot of traffic, or car journeys where you are likely to get stuck in traffic.

Don't
- let your baby get chilled, as this will aggravate the cough. Bathing is unnecessary, especially if the weather is cold. If you have to go out, carry him or her in a sling close to you.
- forget, some coughs are aggravated by breathing in cold air. This applies to babies as well as adults: don't take your child out unless you know that fresh air is a magic cure.
- suppress the cough routinely with a cough medicine. This may prevent your baby from coughing

up mucus, and if mucus is not expelled a more serious infection may develop.

- give cod-liver oil regularly to babies: they may 'prove' it, constant coughs and colds may be brought on in a previously healthy child (see p. 10) or an existing cough or cold may worsen and cause them to go off their food.
- smoke or take your baby into a smoky atmosphere.

Seek help if

- your baby is keeping neither fluids nor solids down but coughs and vomits everything up almost immediately. Small babies need careful nursing through bad coughs and may need hospitalising if self-help measures and home prescribing don't help *and* you don't have a professional homeopath to turn to. (See also Diarrhoea p.146 for advice on dehydration.)
- there is difficulty in breathing and/or wheezing and/or chest pain.
- the cough seems severe and doesn't respond to self-prescribing within 48 hours.
- the breathing is unduly rapid.
- your baby has a bluish tinge around the face, mouth and tongue.
- your baby is abnormally drowsy and unable to speak or make the usual sounds.
- your baby deteriorates suddenly and *you* feel concerned.

See also Cause for Concern, p. 23.

NB Pneumonia (especially in babies) is not always accompanied by a cough. Seek urgent medical help if your child has a fever, is breathing rapidly and seems unwell – is limp and pale.

CRADLE CAP

Cradle cap ranges from flaky patches of white scales mainly on the top of the scalp to a thick, yellowish scaling which covers the whole scalp like a swimming cap. It may be smelly. It is caused by the glands in the hair follicles overproducing oil (sebum). Homeopathic treatment will prevent it from recurring.

Do

- rub your baby's head generously with almond or olive oil at night, comb it very gently the next day to encourage the softened scales to detach and then wash them off with a very mild shampoo.

Don't

- pick it off.

Seek help if

- the skin around or under the cradle cap looks irritated or inflamed – red or sore or itchy.
- it looks infected and begins to ooze.

CROUP

Croup is a frightening-sounding cough that usually occurs in children under four years old. It starts with hoarseness and fever and develops into a loud, barking, ringing, harsh cough that wakes the child at night. The breathing may also be noisy. *Aconite, Calcarea sulphurica, Hepar sulph., Kali bichromicum, Lachesis, Phosphorus* and *Spongia* are all indicated for croup. If it recurs it is essential you seek the advice of a professional homeopath for constitutional treatment.

Do

- follow the guidelines for Common Cold and Cough (see pp. 139 and 142).
- stay with your baby all the time.
- try steam as this can alleviate the symptoms relatively quickly. Go into the bathroom, close the doors and windows, fill the bath with very hot water, and sit with your baby in the steamy atmosphere until the cough eases. Or boil an electric kettle in the baby's bedroom until the room is filled with steam.

Seek help if

- steam doesn't relieve the symptoms within half an hour.
- the cough is accompanied by a blue tinge to the lips.
- your baby is having trouble breathing.

CRYING

Some babies cry rather a lot in their first year. It is their first 'language' and as you get to know your baby you will be able to distinguish between a cry that means 'I'm hungry', one that signals pain and another that says 'Please pick me up, I want a cuddle, I'm bored'.

All babies have different cries: some have a cry that is impossible to ignore and all parents have different levels of tolerance to their own baby's cry. Most mothers become so tuned into it that they wake even before the first whimper.

The human cry is one of nature's loudest sounds. At eighty to eighty-five decibels, it is as loud as an unmuffled truck, not far below the pain threshold.

It is understandable, then, that parents of fussy kids tend to see nothing but a sea of tranquillity outside their home . . . for most (but not all) fussy babies, heavy crying begins at about two weeks, increases to a crescendo at six to eight weeks, and comes back down to manageable levels around three to four months. (Diana S. Greene, *70 Ways to Calm a Crying Baby*, Sphere, 1988: an excellent book, full of useful tips and tricks to soothe fretful babies.)

Babies cry when they are wet or cold and hungry; if they are sickening for an illness such as chickenpox or even a cold – when they will cry more, perhaps more feebly, sounding out of sorts; and if they are having a growth spurt – if you are breastfeeding, feed your baby more often to increase your milk supply (see p. 120). If you are miserable then your baby will cry more.

I have included several homeopathic remedies for fretful babies including *Borax*, *Chamomilla*, *Lycopodium*, *Pulsatilla*, *Rheum* and *Stramonium*. You will need to observe your baby carefully and match its picture withone in this book. If you can't or if the remedy you give doesn't work, then see a professional homeopath who may well be able to help by prescribing at a deeper level.

See also 'Difficult' Babies, p. 146.

Do
- respond to your baby's cries without fussing anxiously.
- try all the obvious things, like feeding, changing, cuddling, putting more clothes on if you suspect he or she is cold or vice versa. Offer the breast or bottle, even if your baby has just had a feed because it may be comfort sucking that is needed. Sometimes babies suck with a light, intermittent, at times barely perceptible sucking for up to half an hour. Finally when they let go they are drowsy, blissfully content and ready for their cot or crib. If your baby has had a full bottle and still wants to suck offer a pacifier or your little finger (see p. 76) so that she can finish sucking.
- feed your baby in a quiet room: some babies will cry if there are distractions like television, radio or people talking and laughing.
- cuddle your baby – lying down or sitting up, or walking around. Each baby has a favourite position for cuddling.
- develop a repertoire of 'tricks' that *your* baby responds to – be inventive, creative and flexible.
- put your baby outside in a stroller or carriage under something interesting, like a tree, protected from cats and insects with a fine-gauge net. Fresh air and outside noises work like magic for some.

- go out for a walk in the fresh air with the baby either in a sling or a carriage.
- face the baby forward in the sling or the pram as soon as she is old enough and can hold up her own head – some babies scream unless they can see where they are going, when they will gurgle and smile happily.
- place interesting things for your baby to look at in and around the cot: mobiles and pictures and anything brightly coloured. Change them if interest wanes!
- sit your baby in front of a front-loading washing machine with a glass door when it is in action: many are mesmerised by the clothes going round and round, or soothed by the sound. A tumble-drier or spinner is equally effective.
- sit the baby in front of the mirror once he or she can focus that far or 'chatter' to each other when you're both reflected *in* the mirror.
- try putting your baby into a cot with bars. Some babies won't sleep in a cot with rigid sides as they seem to need to be able to see out.
- try playing music: invest in several music boxes of the kind where you pull a cord and it plays a tune, experiment with putting it fairly close to your baby's head; play a tape of soothing womb noises (commercially available); play your baby the music you listened to when you were pregnant; experiment with types of music – orchestral, choral, opera, really loud rock music or Wagner, quiet folk music or Chopin.
- invest in a lambskin – some babies find them incredibly soothing.
- make your baby's room a little warmer: newborn babies are easily chilled as they have been used to a constant temperature of 97°F (36°C) in the uterus. They can also feel too hot – if the forehead feels hot, the baby will *be* too hot: take off her top layer of clothes.
- keep bright lights, and that includes sunlight, out of your baby's eyes: some babies are sensitive to bright light and will cry if it shines directly in their face.
- carry your baby around in a sling (if your back will take it) while you do some of your household chores – remember that your baby was carried 24 hours a day before birth and some find the separation more difficult than others.
- give the baby a bath – or better still, have one together!
- rock in your rocking chair with the baby snuggling on your belly. Wrap yourselves up in a blanket, duvet or shawl and sing silly songs.
- try rocking gently, vigorously or fast, or jiggling in your arms. Be creative – every baby has a favourite, soothing movement.

- place your baby in a reclining chair in front of the television – your baby may find the afternoon horse-racing compelling viewing, which will give you enough space in a day to prepare a meal or take a break.
- take all your baby's clothes off in a warm room. Some children hate clothes and love to be naked.
- swaddle your baby tightly. This is especially effective for babies up to about two months old.
- try noise. The vacuum cleaner or food processor can soothe a hysterical baby (and freak out a calm one, so watch out!).
- let him or her cry for a short time. Some babies need this and it does help discharge tension. Don't let it go on for too long (longer than half an hour or longer than *you* can bear it): if the crying continues, try something else.
- put your baby in her cot, on the sofa or your bed or your lap and pat gently and rhythmically, either slowly or fast, on the back, bottom or tummy.
- place one hand on the baby's tummy and the other on his or her head or under the neck, and just whisper sweet nothings while he or she is lying in the cot.
- lie your baby on the floor on a blanket (with something interesting nearby to look at) and get on with doing things in the same room. Some babies like to be left alone at times – but not quite alone (see *Lycopodium*).
- consider a ride in the car. Some babies hate this – but not many – so only do it if it works. They usually fall asleep – but, frustratingly, wake up again when the car stops!
- visit a friend – some babies, and many more mothers, become cranky when bored.
- go easy on visiting if your baby prefers a quiet, ordered life.
- take your baby to a cranial osteopath if the birth was long, difficult or fast, or if she was delivered by forceps. The physical tension induced by this can cause a whole host of problems including sleeplessness and irritability.
- ask other mothers – of any age! – for ideas and their favourite tricks.
- settle the baby in the cot if he or she has been fed and changed, it is a long time since the last sleep, and you have been trying for what seems ages to stop the crying.
- respond to your own needs. Your baby's crying may make you feel frustrated and incompetent and like howling as well. Let yourself have a good cry – it will help to release physical and emotional tension.
- make sure your other child (or children) know how to carry a baby well supported. Small children can 'haul' babies around too roughly and

actually cause minor stress to the spine – enough to cause the baby discomfort.
- go out for the evening. Leave the baby with a trusted friend or relative who is calm and confident and has the telephone number of where you will be in case they can't cope. Some babies just need a change of company and will settle with someone else if you have become tense and anxious. An evening out will help restore some of your own equilibrium.
- seek the advice of a psychotherapist if you overidentify with your baby's crying, if you end up howling too often or if you take the crying as a personal statement that you are a bad mother.

Don't
- leave a very distressed baby to cry – the distress will only get worse – *unless* you are at the end of your tether and in danger of snapping. In that event, put him or her safely in the cot and let your anger out in another room, by having a good scream yourself. Vent your anger safely by kicking a cushion, punching it or even biting it. Then you may feel like crying. Congratulate yourself on choosing not to be angry with the baby and resolve to get some support as soon as possible. Go back to your baby when you feel calmer if he or she is still crying.
- expect methods that have worked to work again. Some will only work once and others will only work for a short time.
- give up.
- do anything that doesn't work. For instance, some babies hate baths – they just cry and cry. Don't bath them: sponge them down, limb by limb, from time to time instead. The time will come when baths will suddenly be fun: do try them occasionally but don't push it.
- listen to those who say you must let your baby 'cry it out' and that you will 'make a rod for your own back' if you respond to the crying. Recent studies have shown that the rapid response decreases the amount of crying (Dr Bruce Taubman, *Pediatrics* 1984). 'One very important study showed that counselling parents on more effective responses to crying reduced crying in fussy babies by 70 per cent, down to the same level as the average baby! So the most important question to ask is not what starts the crying but what will stop it.' (Diana S. Greene, *70 Ways to Calm a Crying Baby*, Sphere, 1988).
- feel guilty if you feel angry with your child – everyone does from time to time.
- wait until you have hit your child to ask for help. Ring your partner, a friend, a close and trusted relative, or even one of the organisations dedi-

cated to helping desperate parents in times of need if you find yourself on the edge of snapping. It's never too early to ask for help.

- feel bad if you throw your baby rather roughly down on the bed in exasperation. Every parent has a tale to tell of violence acted out on their child. Try to make sure that it doesn't happen again.
- blame yourself for your child's crying.
- let every visitor handle the baby if he or she seems unsettled by being passed around relatives and friends.

Seek help if
- you want reassurance that there is nothing wrong with your baby.
- you 'know' that your baby's crying is signalling that something is wrong, even if your doctor checked recently and could find nothing amiss.

DIARRHOEA

First stools after the birth (meconium) are greenish-black and sticky, changing to greenish-brown, for a day or two and then, in breastfed babies, becoming mustard yellow with a sweetish smell. Variations in the colour, from yellow to green, and in the smell can signal teething, a reaction to something you have eaten, a cold or a stomach upset. Bottle-fed babies have a formed, brown stool.

Diarrhoea, characterised by frequent, watery stools, is a cause for concern in small babies who can become easily and quickly dehydrated.

I have included several remedies for acute diarrhoea as well as for the tiredness (loss of vitality) and loss of appetite that can follow a bad attack. Repertorise carefully at each stage to find the remedy that is indicated.

Do
- watch out for signs of dehydration in babies under six months old, and especially in those who are refusing to drink or are drinking less than usual: mouth and eyes are dry (no saliva/tears); skin tone is poor – if the skin is pressed it does not spring back; the eyes look sunken; the fontanelle (soft spot on your baby's head) is sunken; the urine is scanty and smells strong (there are fewer wet nappies).
- limit the intake of food.
- continue to breastfeed a nursing baby.
- encourage the intake of liquids: breastmilk, water, diluted freshly squeezed fruit juices, vegetable broth (simmer a selection of chopped vegetables in water for 15–20 minutes and strain), or rice water

(rice cooked in double the amount of water for slightly longer than usual and strained).
- give a wet flannel or sponge to an infant of more than six months who refuses drinks, or an ice cube, either of water or fruit juice.
- put a not-very-sick child in the bath – not many children can resist drinking bathwater!
- give a rehydration mixture (available from the chemist) if your infant is becoming dehydrated or make up one of your own by simply mixing a teaspoon of sugar or glucose with ½ teaspoon of salt in 1 pint (½ litre) of water (boiled and cooled) and offer at regular intervals. Some babies will take small amounts on a spoon and others will prefer to suck it from a bottle.
- cut out liquids that obviously aggravate the condition.
- introduce food carefully to a baby on solids: start with white rice, toast, very ripe, black-skinned, bananas or low-fat (live) yoghurt.

Don't
- give rich foods that are difficult to digest.
- encourage eating if there is no appetite – a few days without food will do no harm.

Seek help if
- the diarrhoea persists and fluids are not being tolerated.
- there is exhaustion and loss of skin tone.
- there is acute pain in the abdomen that doesn't respond to first-aid prescribing within 2–12 hours (depending on the severity) or that is getting steadily worse.

'DIFFICULT' BABIES

(See also Crying, p. 143.)

Some babies feed well and quickly, are healthy, responsive when awake, sleep for what seems like most of the time, quickly learn to sleep through the night . . . These, in my experience, are the exceptions.

Babies, like adults, have their own characters, their own individual responses, and this, combined with the inability to talk, can make life very difficult for them and therefore for you! You can help them to adjust with homeopathic treatment or with the self-help measures that follow.

A combination of the types of baby I describe below can make life hell for their parents: for example, a baby who is shocked, distressed *and* clingy or one who is bad-tempered *and* wakeful will be a real challenge. You won't be able to change someone's character with homeopathic treatment, whatever their size or age. However, you can heal the effects of emotional stress. The right remedy will help your baby back into balance, to feel better and more at ease.

If *Borax* is indicated, a jumpy baby will calm down and sleep more easily, though will probably relapse under stress so you may need to repeat it when, for example, teething starts, if the baby gets chilled or has a bad fall *and* produces the typical *Borax* emotional state again. If the baby's emotional state changes – if he or she becomes irritable and demanding instead of nervous and jumpy – you will have to decide whether to choose another remedy based on the new symptom picture. You must take into account the whole picture when you prescribe on a difficult baby, carefully repertorising the emotional state as well as the general symptoms.

In the case of temperature, a baby's response is only significant if he or she is chilly, and feels the cold. Most babies are warm-blooded and it is only if they are markedly worse for hot, stuffy atmospheres that this symptom counts.

If there isn't a picture in this book that fits, seek the advice of a professional homeopath, who will have a much larger choice of remedies. If you are at your wits' end, not enjoying being a parent because of your baby's behaviour and perhaps even beginning to feel like a bad one, a homeopath will delve in great detail and prescribe on both of you to ease the passage of this difficult time in your lives.

Do
- resolve any emotional stress in your own life if you suspect that is what is affecting your baby.
- get support from sympathetic friends and family or counsellors.
- call one of the crisis numbers if you feel you are close to battering your baby – every single parent I have ever talked to has wanted to hit, bite or otherwise hurt their baby more than once. Your feelings are normal. Do not respond to them except by doing to a cushion (or inanimate household object) whatever you want to do to your baby. The organisations listed on pp. 305–8 are all trained to deal with parents at the end of their tether and will offer sympathy *and* practical advice and support. Do not go through this on your own. Remember, asking for help is a sign of strength not weakness or failure.
- try to find something good about your difficult baby. An active baby will almost certainly develop faster – after all they have been awake for longer!

Don't
- feel guilty or blame yourself if you have a difficult baby.

- compare your baby to the boy- or girl-wonder next door.

Bad-tempered Babies

Some just come out wanting a fight and carry on as they started. They wake angry from a sleep or a nap and you have the distinct feeling that almost nothing you do is right. Some babies respond to pain with anger so that, for example, colic or teething can set off a *Colocynthis* or *Chamomilla* state. And some babies are angry because they are impatient. They are hungry, they want to eat *now* and they tell you so in no uncertain terms. Symptoms to look up in the Repertory are: angry; biting; capricious; dictatorial; dislikes being touched or examined; hitting; impatient; irritable; tantrums; rage; moaning/complaining; stubborn; tearful when they can't have what they want.

Clingy Babies

Some babies are insecure and want to be constantly close to you. They won't let you put them down even for a minute. This might be part of their character but if you suspect that birth trauma may have caused this, add shock to your repertorising. Other symptoms to look up are: affectionate; anxious; aversion to being alone; clingy; desires to be carried; fear – of falling/of strangers/of downward motion; tearful/tearful at least little thing.

Discontented Babies

Some babies don't respond, don't smile or laugh much, if at all. They *look* miserable and make their parents feel that this job is very hard work. There are fewer rewards with these babies because it is the blinding smiles that keep us going. Symptoms to look up are: discontented; resentful; serious.

Distressed/Nervous Babies

Some babies just cry a lot (see also Crying, p. 143). A horrible noise, a grating scream, a constant whining, miserable crying which drives their parents mad. They wake with a shriek instead of a gurgle. Others are sensitive to almost everything – they jump at the smallest of noises, don't like to be thrown about (as many babies do) and are almost over-responsive. Some are so sensitive to downward motion that they will startle and wake on being laid down gently in their cot. Some scream inconsolably at unexpected noises, like the telephone ringing or an aeroplane flying overhead. These babies need careful handling. Some are traumatised at birth, by a too-fast birth, a long difficult one, a forceps delivery, or separation afterwards. They look shocked. Their little bodies may feel tense. Some of the symptoms to look up are: anxious, and particularly with strangers; expression is anxious or frightened; fearful, especially at night; jumpy; screams on waking or in sleep; sensitive to noise, light, pain; shock.

Quiet Babies

Some babies are shy by nature. They prefer a quiet life and are unhappy or distressed in company. This can be very difficult for mothers who are naturally gregarious and derive their comfort and energy from being with others. Symptoms to look up are: sensitive; shy/timid; dislikes company; introspective; play – babies don't want to play.

Sleepy, Floppy Babies

These babies have to be woken for feeds. You keep wondering if yours is OK in spite of all reassurance that nothing is wrong. They sleep more than is recommended and, like the discontented baby above, don't seem particularly interested in anything. Symptoms to look up are: apathetic; dreamy; indifferent; slow; sluggish.

Wakeful Babies

Some babies simply do not need much sleep: they have eight hours at night, a short nap in the day and are otherwise content. There is nothing you can do except to make sure that each day you have some time to yourself.

Some babies become temporarily wakeful. They are sensitive to being over-stimulated, missing sleep and can become marginally hyperactive, being more difficult to put down at night and waking in the middle of the night wanting to play – for hours, quite happily!

Wakeful babies fall neatly into two categories, those who are happily awake and those who are unhappily awake. If your baby is wakeful *and* bad-tempered, distressed or jumpy, then you will need to add in the appropriate symptoms from the other categories above. Symptoms to look up include: cheerful; excitable; exhilarated; hyperactive; lively; wants to play at night; restless and better for being carried; tearful.

EAR INFECTION

Earache often occurs during a cold and results from the build-up of catarrh in the middle ear, which presses against the eardrum, causing great pain. This is not necessarily a cause for concern, and the indicated homeopathic remedy will usually give speedy pain relief. The only reliable symptom of earache in a baby may be fever and inconsolable crying; they sometimes rub their heads seemingly randomly or one or both ears.

It is not the end of the world if the eardrum perforates with a subsequent discharge from the ear. It will give instant relief from pain, and, provided your baby is in a clean environment, the eardrum will heal well in a couple of weeks with no troublesome consequences. Recent studies have shown that antibiotics are rarely effective for the treatment of earaches, that they will resolve in the same length of time whether antibiotics are given or not. Children who have had antibiotic treatment, however, will then suffer side effects from the drug treatment, which can include diarrhoea, thrush, loss of appetite and glue ear (a chronic condition in which catarrh in the middle ear causes some hearing loss and a tendency to repeated infections).

Do
- suspect earache and a possible infection in babies with a fever who cry and rub their heads.
- ask your GP to have a look in your baby's ears – it is important that you get a diagnosis for your own peace of mind.
- nurse a baby with earache conscientiously so as not to stress the immune system further.
- make sure he or she drinks plenty of fluids.
- use a hot-water bottle (well wrapped up) or an ice pack to relieve the pain.

Don't
- be tempted to clean the ears. The pain is never the result of wax.
- take a baby with earache out into a cold wind.
- let water get into the ear while it is healing.
- bath your baby or wash hair until a few days after the ear has recovered.

Seek help if
- a baby has a depressed or bulging fontanelle.
- there is swelling, redness, tenderness or pain behind the ear.
- the earache doesn't respond to first-aid prescribing within 24 hours.
- the pain is very severe.

See also Fever, p. 149, and Cause for Concern, p. 23.

EYE INFLAMMATION

See Sticky Eyes, p. 157.

FEVER

A fever can be a helpful and necessary healing stage of an acute disease, during a cold, perhaps, or 'childhood illness' (see p. 134) – something positive, to be encouraged rather than suppressed. By understanding that fever is a symptom and not a disease in itself, you can come to see it as an ally rather than an enemy. Fevers that recur, possibly for years, after illnesses like glandular fever or malaria are not to be confused with the type of fever we are discussing here and should always be referred to a professional homeopath.

When our bodies become stressed by external or internal events we become susceptible to disease. Typical examples of external stresses are overwork, lack of sleep, an accident, environmental pollution, becoming chilled, overheated or wet through, over-indulgence in rich foods or alcohol, etc. Examples of internal or emotional stresses are shock, the death of a close relative or friend, boredom, fear, resentment or any strong feeling which isn't expressed. Where a person is under continued stress, a cold or flu may well surface as the body's way of saying, 'Help! Please take some rest so that I can recharge my batteries and heal myself.'

A high temperature generally indicates that the body's defence mechanism is fighting an infection and temperature variations indicate how it is coping. The healing reactions of the body are speeded up, by approximately 10 per cent for each 1°C rise in temperature: the heart beats faster, carrying the blood around the body more quickly; breathing speeds up, increasing oxygen intake; perspiration increases, helping the body to cool down naturally; and hormones are released which stimulate the body to fight disease. Fever is the body's first-line defence against infection and therefore attempts to 'control' it artificially with paracetamol, vitamin C, or even with inappropriate homeopathic remedies, can suppress the body's natural efforts to heal itself.

Hippocrates said, 'Give me a fever and I can cure the child.' A weak child may be endlessly 'sick', neither very ill nor very well, but with no significant rise in temperature. A more robust child whose temperature soars may look and feel very ill, therefore giving more cause for concern, but is usually ill for a shorter time and recovers more quickly.

Each person has their own pattern of falling ill and will experience different fever symptoms. You may feel hot with a high fever, or you may feel chilly and shiver. You may be irritable, intolerant of any disturbance and need to be kept warm, or you may be aching and restless, may moan and complain. You may sweat profusely, be thirsty and slightly delirious; you may want company or prefer to be alone. Each person with a fever will respond to an individual homeopathic remedy depending on their emotional state and general symptoms.

The average normal temperature in a healthy human is said to be 98.4°F (37°C), but this can vary quite markedly. Most people, adults and children, can run a fever of up to 104°F (40°C) for several days with no danger. It is normal for healthy infants and children to throw high fevers (103°F (39.5°C) and over) with an infection. A temperature of 105°F (40.5°C) is serious cause for concern, but it is only when it passes above 106°F (41°C) that there is a risk to life.

Fevers usually peak towards night-time and drop by the following morning, so that a temperature of 104°F (40°C) registered in the evening may recur on subsequent evenings. A drop in temperature in the morning does not mean that the fever is past its peak. It can rise and fall several times over several days before finally returning to normal.

Small children who develop a fever, especially infants under six months old, must be watched carefully because they are vulnerable to becoming quickly dehydrated. Delirium and tantrums in children sometimes accompany high fevers and, although these are distressing, they are not dangerous.

Do

- take the temperature with a thermometer, placed under the tongue or tucked tightly under the armpit for 5 minutes, for an accurate reading. A temperature taken by tucking the thermometer tightly under the armpit will read about a half degree Fahrenheit lower than that taken under the tongue. A fever strip (for the forehead) is a rough guide only and a hand held on the forehead is next to useless. The newer digital thermometers are much easier for young children and give a quick and accurate reading. (Always keep a spare battery in the house.)
- provide a calm environment for your feverish baby. This is not a time to go visiting!
- encourage a feverish patient to drink plenty of fluids or at least sips of water at frequent intervals. Water, lemon and honey or diluted fresh fruit juices, warmed or cold as desired, are best. Breast-milk is fine for a nursing baby and is probably all that will be wanted. Older babies and young children who are reluctant to drink will often suck on a wet sponge or flannel, especially if the water is warm, or try an ice cube or frozen fruit juice.
- immerse a feverish but not desperately ill child in the bath from time to time to bring down the fever. Thirstless children will often drink the bathwater as an added bonus!
- sponge down with tepid water if the fever goes

above 103°F/104°F (40°C) and your patient feels uncomfortable (hot and sweaty). Expose and sponge one limb at a time until it feels cool to the touch. Dry and replace it under the covers before going on to the next limb. This will help the temperature to drop by 1 or 2°F (up to 1°C) and can be repeated as often as necessary. Sponging the face and forehead alone can also give relief.

- undress a feverish baby especially if either the weather or your house is very hot. Small babies can throw a fever if they become overheated and will quickly revert to normal with undressing and/or a tepid sponging down.
- respond to your patient's needs. Keep a hot, feverish baby lightly dressed and a chilly, feverish child (who feels cold to the touch and shivers) well covered.
- prescribe homeopathic remedies where the fever is one of a number of symptoms, for example, where the patient is clearly suffering from, say, earache or a sore throat *and* a fever. If the first symptom to arise is a fever then wait a while for other symptoms to surface before prescribing for the whole picture. Contain the fever, again if necessary, by sponging down (see above).
- suppress the fever with Calpol (paracetamol) in an emergency, that is, where the fever rises above 105°F (40.5°C), or if your child is in severe pain, from say, teething in the middle of the night, and homeopathic first-aid prescribing isn't helping. Ring your homeopath or doctor in the morning or during the night if you are anxious.
- watch for signs of dehydration in infants under six months old, and especially in children who are refusing to drink or who are drinking less than usual (see p. 146).

Don't
- encourage a sick child to eat. Many children with a high fever will not wish to eat. This is a good sign: fasting encourages the body further to eliminate toxic wastes and helps it focus on recovery. Encourage a hungry patient to eat light, easily digested dishes such as vegetable soup, raw or stewed fruit with honey.
- give any homeopathic remedy at the first sign of a rise in temperature as this can confuse the symptom picture. Any attempt to interrupt the body's own healing processes is unwise. Wait until a fuller picture develops when other symptoms emerge.
- suppress a fever in children with any form of aspirin. This has been known to lead to dangerous, although rare, complications, in particular Reye's syndrome, which affects the brain and liver. Calpol (paracetamol) may be used in an emergency but *never* exceed the recommended dose.

Seek help if
- a baby under six months old has a fever.
- an older baby has a fever of over 104°F/40°C that doesn't respond to sponging and homeopathic treatment within 24 hours.
- your family has a history of convulsions accompanying fevers – keep a close eye when your baby throws a fever. It is the rapid rise in temperature that can cause a fit. (See also p. 141.)
- the baby or older child is also refusing to drink (is thirstless) as dehydration can occur.
- there is a lack of reaction (listlessness and limpness), which can imply that a serious illness such as pneumonia or meningitis has developed. (See Cause for Concern, p. 23.)

If you are worried contact your GP and/or homeopath immediately.

HERNIA

A hernia is a swelling in the abdomen caused by muscular weakness. The most common type in babies is an umbilical hernia, where the navel sticks out, especially when the baby cries, coughs or sneezes. It is not painful and the weakness in the wall will usually repair itself by the time the child is five years old. If it doesn't it may need surgery.

An inguinal hernia (weakness in the muscles of the groin) needs more urgent attention because part of the bowel can become trapped in it. In boys an inguinal hernia is sometimes associated with undescended testicles.

Although I have included a few remedies for hernias in babies they are mostly beyond the scope of the first-aid prescriber. You should consult a professional homeopath if your doctor has advised you to wait and see if your baby's hernia will heal in time.

HICCUPS

Some babies hiccup a lot, even while still in the uterus – audibly. They may hiccup every time they feed, laugh, get excited or anything. There is nothing to worry about and the hiccups will decrease over time. If your baby's hiccups are associated with colic you should prescribe on the whole symptom picture.

Do
- place your hand gently over your baby's nose to reduce the amount of oxygen taken in, being care-

ful not to cut off the air supply altogether. Leave it there for a minute or two, but no longer.

- offer a little cold water on a spoon or in a bottle as this sometimes helps to stop them.

Don't

- prescribe if your baby's hiccups are mild and you are charmed and amused by them!

INFLAMMATION

In newborn infants the navel (umbilicus) may become inflamed after the cord drops off. A baby's penis can become sore, sometimes for no apparent reason. Treat an inflamed navel as you would a cut that has become infected, by giving *Hepar sulphuricum* in the initial stage where there is some redness around it and bathe it with *Calendula* lotion or smear on a little *Calendula* cream and keep it lightly bandaged until it heals. If *Hepar sulph.* doesn't help within two or three days give a short course of *Silica*.

Treat an inflamed penis with *Arnica* and bath your baby frequently in water to which you have added a handful of sea salt and 40 drops of *Calendula* tincture. If you have inadvertently pulled your baby's foreskin back and it has become 'stuck' to the head of the penis (the glans) and can't be pulled back at all because scar tissue has formed, wait until he is older (at least five) and then give him *Thiosinaminum* tincture, 5 drops twice daily in a little water. This will dissolve the scar tissue and enable the foreskin to be pulled back freely. I suggest that you give the drops for 7 days at a time with 10-day gaps, repeating it if the foreskin is still stuck in places. It can take up to 3 months to work.

Don't

- automatically use antibiotic powders or creams on your baby's navel – explore other options for helping it to heal first (see External Materia Medica and Repertory, pp. 161–8).
- pull your baby's foreskin back to clean it if he has one until he is at least five years old – it won't retract until then and has a seal of its own that keeps it free of dirt. It will be fine just as long as you don't mess with it. If you do try to force it back you can cause it to become inflamed and then stuck. It is only when a child is able easily to move it back that he should be taught how to wash underneath it.

INJURIES

The combination of a tired or sick baby with a tired or distracted mother can lead to accidents. One qualifi-

cation for the job of parent is the possession of a revolving head with antennae that sense what is happening to a baby or child even when they are out of sight. It is often an unnerving quiet which alerts many mothers to the fact that something is wrong – otherwise the terrifying shriek of pain.

Prevention is the best cure for accidents and many are preventable – but unfortunately injuries to babies are common because small people are awkward for a long time after they start to move. They also stubbornly refuse to learn the lesson of cause and effect when they really need to: if you throw yourself off a high surface you won't fly and you might break a leg; if you touch a hot surface you will burn yourself . . . Their need to explore and find out about the world is intense and unbounded. All parents learn to be vigilant and to anticipate the direction their offspring will take, and to distract them from danger.

Use a combination of common sense and skill to deal with accidents. Always follow your instincts and take a badly injured child to the casualty department of your local hospital where they will be seen fairly quickly (unless it happens to be a children's hospital). The tests, X-rays and medical treatment, if needed, as well as the reassurance are all invaluable.

Act quickly if your baby starts to choke on a small object – a button or stone or even a fishbone. Thump her between the shoulder blades, hard and sharp with the flat of your whole hand. The object should fly out of her mouth. If it doesn't, hold her upside down by her ankles and thwack her again in the same place. Remember: **you are saving her life, don't hold back.** Comfort her mightily afterwards.

If your child sustains a burn which doesn't warrant a visit to hospital then immerse it in running cold water for as long as it takes for the pain to ease off, then prescribe.

Don't let a child who has banged their head badly go to sleep just in case delayed concussion is lurking. Keep him/her awake, prescribe on the injury and observe closely until you are sure the danger is over.

Teach your child how to approach animals of all shapes and sizes. Strange cats and dogs should always be avoided. Dogs of friends and family should be approached with an outstretched hand which can be fully sniffed before being accepted and then the animal stroked gently with an adult supervising. Children often rush at dogs and try to pat their heads, which is interpreted as an aggressive gesture by the animal who may then bite in retaliation.

You can, of course, first-aid prescribe for any minor and inevitable accidents, such as burns, cuts, bruises, bumps, shocks, bites, stings and splinters, but remember to take into account the whole picture when doing so.

Do

- be careful when away from home. Most houses are not childproof and are full of traps of the sort that you have removed from your own house and possibly forgotten about.
- check that equipment conforms to the safety standards.
- check second-hand equipment thoroughly.
- store plastic bags, plastic wrap, all cleaning fluids and powders, all medicines, razors, cosmetics, your rubbish bin and sharp kitchen knives out of reach. Invest in babyproof safety locks for cupboards.
- keep electric cords short on appliances like toasters and kettles or buy coiled ones.
- fit a guard around your stove pilots. Turn pan handles so that they don't dangle temptingly over the edge of the guard.
- fit locks on your fridge and freezer.
- put hot drinks, pans and dishes with hot food and kettles, etc., at the back of kitchen surfaces or in the middle of a table. Give up using tablecloths for a while as they can be pulled with dire consequences.
- fit safety catches on all windows above the ground floor.
- change your baby's nappy on the floor or on your lap but only on a high surface if you are *not* going out of easy reach, even for an instant. Keep the talcum powder out of reach as it can cause severe choking if accidentally shaken out over the face.
- use straps in all chairs – prams, pushchairs, highchairs, bouncing chairs – at *all* times.
- fix fireguards in front of all open fires and heaters.
- cover unused electric sockets with dummy socket covers, plug-guards or strong insulating tape.
- keep cigarettes, matches, alcohol, sewing equipment, money and all other small objects out of reach.
- get rid of glass-topped tables.
- make glass doors safer by covering them with a plastic film that makes them shatterproof.
- fix a gate at the bottom and top of all stairs, unless your baby is well co-ordinated and learns to crawl safely up and down stairs.
- make sure your banisters are safe and that the gaps between them are too small for a baby to squeeze through.
- make sure the catches on the front and back doors are too high for the baby to reach.
- put house-plants out of reach.
- supervise your child in the garden. Store all gardening equipment and chemicals in a locked shed.

- dig up poisonous plants and pull up fungi if they appear.
- secure play equipment on grass or sand (not a hard surface) and check it frequently.
- cover the sandpit when your child is not playing in it to protect it from fouling by cats or other animals.
- use childproof locks on car doors so that they can't be opened from the inside and don't let your child play with the window. *Never* leave your baby or child alone in a car, whether or not you can see them from where you plan to be.
- put a net on your baby's carriage when unattended outside as cats are drawn to the warmth and have been known to smother babies.
- train your dog to be 'handled' by your child without responding aggressively. Get professional help from a dog-trainer if your dog is jealous of the baby or if it growls or nips once the baby becomes mobile.
- keep your pets dewormed and defleaed.
- train your dog *not* to lick faces, especially the faces of your children, as this can spread disease.
- use the word 'no' for things that really matter, that are dangerous so that your baby will listen when you say it.
- take a basic first-aid course so that you can deal with accidents and injuries confidently.

Don't

- leave a baby of any age on a table or bed or high surface of any kind without constant supervision. If you have to go and fetch something (even across the room) take the baby with you. Far too many babies have suddenly rolled over and dropped off high surfaces on to their heads.
- leave your baby unattended in a room with the family pet, either a cat or a dog.
- let older, but not old enough, children carry the baby up or down stairs.
- leave older, but not old enough, children on their own in a room with the baby until they have proven their responsibility and capability over and over again. It is all too easy for a crawling baby to put a small object in his or her mouth. It takes the skill of an adult to spot it in the first place and then to prevent choking if necessary.
- let your baby travel unharnessed in the stroller. The *one* time you do it, your pushchair will engage with a piece of uneven paving and catapult your precious bundle head first on to the pavement.
- let your baby travel unharnessed in the car. Make sure that car seats are rigidly fixed: if it is loose, your baby's life will be at risk in an accident. Have the straps or seat fixed in by an expert such as your garage mechanic.

- leave your baby unattended in the car, a room with an open fire or in the bath even if he or she can sit up on their own apparently quite safely.

Seek help if
- your child has a serious accident of any description.
- your child falls unconscious even for a few seconds.
- your child has trouble breathing or stops breathing even for a few seconds.
- you are concerned for your child even if you don't have anything concrete to go on.
- your child is extremely distressed after an accident or conversely becomes apathetic.

See also Cause for Concern, p. 23.

INSOMNIA

See Sleep Difficulties, p. 154.

JAUNDICE

Many babies develop jaundice 2–4 days after the birth. The skin (of white babies) and the whites of the eyes turn yellow. It is not harmful and will disappear within about a week, although it can last longer with no ill effects. Jaundice occurs in babies whose livers have not matured fully by the time they are born. Phototherapy for babies is being thoroughly questioned as a treatment for jaundice. The majority of babies are much better if *not* separated from their mothers and only very severely jaundiced babies will benefit from this treatment.

Some jaundiced babies become lethargic and feed less often but the condition rarely causes any complications unless there is a more serious medical problem such as a (very rare) congenital abnormality of the liver or ducts leading from it, or Rhesus incompatibility (see p. 50) in which case the baby will be yellow within a few hours of the birth. Jaundice is more common in premature babies or if a baby is badly bruised during birth. Most cases will clear up quickly and effectively if you give *Chelidonium 30* – one dose every two hours for a day. If it doesn't help and your baby has a number of other symptoms, such as colic, irritability, constipation or whatever, prescribe on the whole picture taking into account all the symptoms.

Do
- breastfeed your baby frequently.
- expose your baby to sunlight if the weather is fine.

You can go out for a walk well bundled up but with his or her face exposed to the sun's rays.

Don't
- give water if you are breastfeeding. This may discourage the baby from breastfeeding and extensive research has shown that extra water does not affect the jaundice. (*The Art of Breastfeeding*, La Leche League, 1974, p. 210)

MILD RASH

See Spots, p. 157.

NAPPY RASH (DIAPER RASH)

Diaper rash has many causes: a chemical reaction between the urine and stools creating ammonia which burns the skin if diapers are left unchanged for too long; irritating chemicals in the stools; residues of soap or detergent (especially biological soaps) in diapers; teething or a general infection. The area around the genitals looks red, spotty and sore and your baby's diaper may smell of ammonia. In boys the foreskin may also become red and sore-looking, making peeing painful. It can itch (your baby will tear at the rash when you take the diaper off) or sting or burn (he or she will cry when passing urine). It may become painful and, at its worst, sores may develop so deal with it as soon as you notice it.

It is important to differentiate between stubborn diaper rash and thrush. Thrush will spread above the navel which diaper rash won't. If you are breastfeeding and have had antibiotics, or if your baby has, diaper rash can develop into thrush (see p. 158).

Try home prescribing for a mild or non-recurrent diaper rash, but seek professional advice if it fails to clear quickly or recurs frequently.

Do
- change diapers frequently (more frequently if a rash develops) and use almond or olive oil, or *Calendula* or *Symphytum* ointment after every change if your baby has a tendency to nappy rash.
- wash and rinse your baby's genitals and bottom thoroughly with water only (not soap) paying special attention to all creases, wiping from front to back in girls (but do not clean inside their inner vaginal lips).
- dry the area *thoroughly*. A hair-drier on a very gentle heat (at a safe distance) is ideal as no further moisture will remain on the skin, but test the heat on your own skin first (on your inner forearm) and remember that a baby's skin is much more sensitive than an adult's.

- leave your baby's bottom without a diaper for as long as possible (overnight if practical), making sure that the room is warm enough. Lay her on several thicknesses of towel (with a plastic sheet underneath) to soak up the urine.
- stop using plastic pants if a rash starts. They make diaper rash worse because they stop air getting to the skin.
- try a different type of liner or disposable diaper, preferably a more absorbent brand.
- wash towelling diapers in soap powder instead of biological powder and put a little vinegar into the final rinse to neutralise the acids in urine.
- change to disposable diapers until the rash has cleared up.
- cut out all fruit juice. It makes urine acidic, which stings in contact with the rash when the baby pees. Give plain water instead.
- smear a coating of raw egg white on the skin after washing and drying. This makes an effective waterproof seal over a mild but stubborn diaper rash. Don't apply it to broken skin and apply it cautiously if your baby is allergic to eggs.

Don't
- use zinc and castor-oil cream or petroleum-based products. The chemicals in them are absorbed through the skin and can cause minor health problems as zinc can affect the nervous system.

PRICKLY HEAT

Prickly heat occurs in babies if they are too hot, either from the weather or because they have been over-dressed. It starts as small red patches, usually on the neck, chest and upper arms, and itches and prickles which can make small babies restless and distressed.

Do
- remove the top layer of clothing or bath the baby in a tepid or cool bath, or sponge him or her down and let them dry in the air.
- avoid direct exposure to the sun.

Don't
- use bubble bath, oils or scented soap until the rash has cleared up.
- use talcum powder as this can block the pores and aggravate the condition.

Seek help if
- the itching is intolerable and homeopathic treatment and self-help measures don't work.
- your baby becomes lethargic and floppy.

RETENTION OF URINE

A baby can take up to 36 hours to pee after the birth and the first urine may be red because of urate crystals, which are completely harmless. A baby may also find it difficult to pee after a fright or getting chilled.

Most babies pee at every feed although others do so less often. You will automatically become familiar with your baby's pattern from how often diapers need changing. It is a variation from the normal pattern that is significant. If there are no wet diapers for an unusually long time *and* the baby is drinking as normal something may be wrong.

If your baby takes longer than 24 hours to urinate for the first time *and* still seems shocked from the birth, choose between *Aconite* and *Opium*. The right remedy will help with shock *and* get him or her peeing. Otherwise, repertorise carefully if the retention is linked to something else.

Do
- encourage a baby (not necessarily a newborn) to pee by: putting them in a warm bath; taking off the nappy, putting the baby on a towel in the bathroom and running the tap as an added encouragement.

Seek help if
- your baby hasn't passed any urine for 15–20 hours.
- urine retention accompanies a fever.
- you suspect the baby is in pain – is crying as if distressed.
- the baby is vomiting.

SLEEP DIFFICULTIES

Babies need differing amounts of sleep. Some fall into good sleep patterns very early on while others take a lot of persuading. Sleeping is a skill which some find easier to acquire than others!

You may choose to have the baby sleep with you in your bed. If he or she sleeps peacefully and you are able to sleep well with them in the bed, this is fine. In countries where cot deaths are virtually unknown babies traditionally sleep with their parents for at least the first year of life, which has its advantages. For parents who work, it is one way for them and the baby to be together, a means of bonding. If you are breastfeeding it is easy to let your baby feed while you are half asleep. Parents do not roll on to their babies if they sleep with them – unless they are drunk. A breastfed baby will tend to wake more frequently: a feed is digested in about two hours because the fat content in human milk is lower than that of cow's milk so being able to feed and fall asleep again straight away will help you avoid the exhaustion experienced by someone who has to get up several times a night.

However, some people cannot sleep deeply when their babies are in bed with them. Some mothers are light sleepers and wake with every whimper. Some babies sleep restlessly, or jerk and wriggle during the night and always end up with their feet in your face no matter what you do. Some women cannot breast-feed happily lying down or cannot breastfeed and sleep at the same time. Some parents do not want that sort of relationship with their babies. Fine.

Decide what will work and is right for you. If you try it and it doesn't work you can always try something else. Do not be persuaded to take your baby into your bed if you don't want to. Conversely, do not be told that you are making a rod for your own back if your baby is sleeping with you and you are all enjoying it. If you suspect that your family might be scandalised if they knew, don't tell them. It's not worth it.

You can be creative and flexible about night-times. If you decide that your baby will sleep separately, you may make a proviso that you will sleep with him or her when they are ill. You can put a largish bed or mattress on the floor of the baby's room so that you can feed lying down in the night, which is more restful for you, but not in your bed. You may both end up sleeping the rest of the night together or you can pop the baby back in the cot and go back to your own bed. You could put the cot next to your bed so that you can reach out a comforting hand in the night if the baby whimpers and wakes you.

The following guidelines apply to all babies, whether they are sleeping in your bed or not. If you want your baby to sleep well and easily at night, start by trying to establish a convenient sleeping pattern as early as you can; you should adopt some of the following ideas wherever you all sleep. Symptoms to consider when you repertorise if you decide to prescribe are insomnia, jerking on falling sleep, jerking during sleep, screaming on waking and screaming during sleep, but seek the advice of a homeopath if your baby persists in waking frequently at night, especially if distressed, or you find it impossible to cope with being woken every two hours every night, even though the baby is perfectly well.

Do

- make sure a baby has done all the sucking she needs before you tuck her up for the night. Some need a lot of sucking, whether they are breast- or bottle-feeding. Get a teat with a smaller hole for your bottle or let your baby suck your nipple until

he or she lets go of their own accord, or offer a dummy.
- try moving the cot into another room if the baby wakes frequently during the night, especially if a light sleeper. Some babies are disturbed by a parent moving about, or grunting or snoring.
- set your own priorities first. If you are someone who needs plenty of sleep, try to settle your baby's sleeping pattern to suit you straight away. Start as you mean to go on. Be clear and determined.
- establish a bedtime routine or ritual: choose a time that suits you and your partner, bearing in mind that babies who go to sleep early wake up early!; always use the same room and the same cot or crib for the night-time sleep not the pram or carrycot used for day-time naps. You can put the Moses basket in the cot in the early days; bath or sponge the baby down, making sure that this is a pleasure, that he or she isn't too tired, that you only do it if they enjoy it; give a soothing massage with a light oil or talcum powder; dress him or her in 'night' clothes – a nightie, which makes changing nappies easier, a sleep suit or pyjamas, which you have warmed on the radiator (only night clothes get warmed!); swaddle a jumpy baby firmly, which may help one who jerks in their sleep not to wake up (some babies hate being swaddled – yours will let you know if he or she doesn't like it); lay the baby down to sleep in the position they prefer (you will get to know which it is) place a rolled blanket or cushion against the feet and head so that he or she feels secure all around as they were in the uterus. If she sleeps better on her side put a rolled-up blanket along her back so that she can't roll on to her front. Turn the lights down and draw the curtains if it is still light outside; make sure that the bedtime routine occurs quietly and calmly; always do the same reassuringly relaxing things – play a certain tape, sing certain songs, arrange the animals in the cot, tell a bedtime story in a bedtime tone of voice; warm the cot with a hot-water bottle, which you can remove just before you put the baby in; give the last feed in a special bedtime chair; make sure he or she is *awake* when you put them to bed after the last feed of the day, and at some other times during the day. Falling asleep is a learnt skill. You provide the environment and the encouragement and they do it; tuck them up with a special night-time blanket and/or cuddly toy; say the same goodnight words every night and then, instead of walking straight out, potter about tidying up for a few minutes; leave a night-light on and a music tape or a tape of womb sounds.
- go to the baby if he or she wakes in the night, but make your visits short and boring. Feed, change if

absolutely necessary and, again, put him or her down awake so that they fall asleep on their own.

- soothe a distressed baby at bedtime by rocking or rubbing for a bit until they calm down; then put them in the cot, preferably still half-awake.
- let other people put your baby to sleep at night from the beginning – your partner if willing and able, or a friend or neighbour who wants to babysit. If you are breastfeeding express your milk so that someone else can do the night-time feed.
- make your baby's cot attractive: hang a mobile above it, out of reach; string some interesting, colourful objects across it some of which make noises, such as bells, when they move and change them regularly. Hang them so that the baby can touch them as soon as he or she is able to but make sure they are absolutely safe. Clip an 'activity centre', a mirror or colourful pictures, to the cot bars or tie a soft toy to them.
- buy a specially treated lambskin for your baby to sleep on.
- encourage thumb-sucking from early on: many babies will comfort themselves like this if they need to in the middle of the night. You may prefer to use a pacifier but this needs putting in every time it falls out.
- take it in turns with your partner to get up in the morning for your baby so that one of you can have an extra few hours' sleep.
- cut out caffeine (tea, coffee, chocolate, Coca-Cola), especially after midday if you are breastfeeding as the caffeine passes through to your baby in your milk.
- anticipate your baby's needs when you travel so that you take, for instance, a night-light, the mobile from the cot, favourite toys, a tape-recorder and tapes, as well as bedding so that the bedtime routine can be similar wherever you are.
- give a bottle of formula milk last thing at night if you are frazzled and your milk supply seems low. It tends to decrease through the day, especially if you have been super-busy; if the last feed you give is a small one then your baby will wake after a relatively short time and before long you will both be desperate. Seek the advice of a breastfeeding counsellor if you want to avoid this (see also pp. 305–8).
- be careful not to cut out day-time naps for babies who sleep badly at night: you may inadvertently over-stimulate them so that they find it difficult to fall into a deep sleep, waking more frequently at night. If your baby regularly wakes to play in the night then he or she may be 'hyped-up'. Encourage them to sleep more, not less and bring bedtime forward.

Don't

- always breastfeed your baby to sleep or let him or her fall asleep on the bottle. If you help them to fall asleep they won't learn to do it alone: you may end up spending 2 hours a night putting the baby to bed and although this is acceptable occasionally, it becomes a trial if it happens routinely.
- always rock or walk your baby to sleep for the same reasons as above.
- let babies under the age of two sleep with a pillow, as it could smother them.
- make your house specially quiet so that the baby can get to sleep. Small babies will sleep through all levels of noise and should be encouraged to do so. Otherwise, you will find yourself creeping around for years to come.
- worry if you can't get back to sleep after a night feed. Be philosophical and catch up on some reading, write a letter or even do some housework. Catch up on your sleep the next day when the baby has a nap.
- let an older baby suck fruit juice from a bottle at night. They become addicted to it and it will ruin their teeth when they come through. It is better to offer water in a bottle to quench thirst if a feed isn't due or being demanded.
- put your baby on solids too early, without consulting your doctor and/or health visitor, because you think waking at night means hunger.

SORE THROAT

A sore throat is hard to diagnose in a small baby. The voice may become either a little hoarse or lower in tone. They may cry when they try to take either solids or liquids or both, because swallowing is painful, and the cry may have a hoarse ring. On examination your doctor may find that the glands in the neck and tonsils are swollen. If an ear is inflamed, the pain on swallowing will be felt there as well as in the throat.

If you decide to prescribe, it is important that you observe whether the pain is worse for swallowing or better for it and whether hot or cold drinks ease the pain. A child with a sore throat *and* earache will almost certainly have a fever so you should have a number of symptoms to hang your prescription on. Take into account anything that happened before he or she fell ill, such as getting cold and wet, having a fall, or starting with a new childminder. If the illness coincides with an inoculation, up to 2 weeks later, you should consult a professional homeopath who will prescribe carefully to clear any ill effects from the inoculation, which is beyond the scope of the home prescriber.

Do
- offer plenty of fluids, breastmilk if you are still nursing, a little honey and freshly squeezed lemon or orange juice with boiled and cooled water in a bottle, on a spoon, or in a feeder beaker.

Seek help if
- there is excessive dribbling, difficulty in breathing and great pain with swallowing.
- your child is very distressed, obviously in pain and not reacting to home prescribing quite quickly, within a day or two at the most.

SPOTS

Most newborn babies go through a spotty phase. The spots come just when you are beginning to feel like showing the baby off, when both of you have recovered from the birth. The most common rash is neonatal (newborn) urticaria which occurs a week or two after birth. It can range from a few reddish spots on the face which clear up quite quickly to a bad attack of 'acne', red spots with yellow centres that spread on to the body and last for a week or so. One theory suggests that the baby's body is clearing out the toxins from the birth.

Another common rash, 'milk rash', manifests as tiny white spots usually over the nose and sometimes on the cheeks. They can last much longer but are not as unsightly and will disappear in their own time.

If the spots are particularly severe give a short course of *Sulphur* or *Silica* – choose between them by reading the pictures in the Materia Medica – or *Carbo vegetabilis* if your baby is also windy.

Do
- keep your baby's face clean with water only. Don't use oil or talcum powders as these will further clog the pores.

Don't
- squeeze your baby's spots as you may cause an infection.

STICKY EYES

See also Blocked Tear Duct, p. 133.

A sticky eye, which discharges or in which the lids are stuck together after sleep, is not necessarily infected. A sticky eye in a small baby needs professional help if it doesn't clear quickly and easily within 3 days.

A sticky eye will usually clear up with external

bathing alone so avoid using an antibiotic cream without trying an alternative method first.

Do
- be scrupulously hygienic in dealing with your baby's eyes. Wash your hands before and after touching them: eye infections spread all too easily.
- when bathing or cleaning your baby's eyes do one at a time using a clean piece of cotton wool for each eye.
- bathe the eyes with *Euphrasia* (p. 163) or *Hypercal®* (p. 163) and give the indicated internal remedy as well.
- bathe the eyes with a saline solution (1 teaspoon of sea salt in a glass of warm, boiled water) or herb tea – chamomile or eyebright (*Euphrasia*).
- bathe your baby's eyes with a little freshly expressed breastmilk – this can act miraculously quickly in clearing up a mild sticky eye.
- wipe from the inner corner of the eye to the outer corner.

Don't
- let your baby rub his or her eyes as this can make it worse.
- ever use antibiotic or hydrocortisone drops in the eye unless prescribed for a specific complaint.

Seek help if
- the eyelids become red and puffy, the eye becomes bloodshot and the discharge is yellow.
- the symptom persists, especially in a newborn baby. Ask your doctor to check that the discharge is not serious.

STOMACH-ACHE

See Colic, p. 138.

TEETHING

Some children produce teeth without any fuss or discomfort whereas others become a nightmare for their entire teething period, suffering great pain from sore, swollen gums, as well as producing colds, coughs, earache, diarrhoea, mood swings and sleeplessness with every tooth that comes through.

Homeopathic treatment can ease teething pain as well as helping to push out teeth that are having difficulty in erupting of their own accord. If the remedy you prescribe fails to help, consult a professional homeopath.

Do

- rub your baby's gums with your finger as pressure sometimes helps.
- give something hard to chew on: a teething ring which has been kept in the fridge (not the freezer) is ideal. If you give a piece of cold carrot or celery remember to watch carefully to prevent the baby choking on little bits. Home-made rusks (hunks of bread baked hard in a slow oven) are also good for teething gums to chew on.

Don't

- resort to giving Phenergan or other sedatives.
- give gripe water as it is always high in sugar and sometimes alcohol. The maximum recommended daily dose for an 8½-pound (4-kg) baby is the equivalent to five tots of whisky drunk by an 11-stone (70-kg) adult.
- give too much chamomile tea. It is easy for a baby to 'prove' it (see p. 10), becoming irritable and sleepless, the symptoms it was supposed to cure. If it does help, use only while it has a soothing effect.
- give chamomile tea if you have prescribed *Chamomilla* in potency (see p. 195).

THRUSH

Thrush is an infection caused by a yeast that ordinarily lives quite harmlessly in the mouth and intestines. It can, however, get out of control, especially if either mother or baby has recently had antibiotics, producing white patches that are usually sore and/or itchy. It is not serious and is relatively common in young babies.

Genital Thrush/Yeast

Genital thrush in babies is often confused with diaper rash (see p. 153). The main difference is that thrush is more likely to start around the anus and spread outwards whereas diaper rash tends to start in the creases, where the urine-soaked nappy rubs against the skin. Thrush tends to spread up to the navel whereas diaper rash won't.

Do

- change the baby's diaper frequently and wash his or her bottom in water or *Hypercal®* lotion (see p. 163). Don't use soap and dry it well, using a hair-drier on a low setting.
- let your baby lie diaperless as often and as long as is practical.
- add half a cup of cider vinegar (always useful in combating fungal infection) to the bathwater.

- wash towelling diapers and muslin liners in non-biological soap powder or unscented soap flakes and rinse well, putting some cider vinegar into the last rinse.
- apply live yoghurt to ease itching and discomfort.
- use separate towels for yourself and your baby to avoid spreading the thrush further.

Don't

- use plastic pants over your baby's nappies until the rash has cleared up as they will stop air from circulating and aggravate the problem.
- use bubble baths or oils in the bathwater.
- use talcum powder.

Seek help if

- pus forms.
- the thrush doesn't respond to home treatment within a few days.

Oral thrush

Thrush in the mouth is characterised by white patches on the tongue or the inside of the cheeks, which resemble milk spots but don't come off if wiped gently with a clean cloth. It may be sore and/or itchy.

Do

- give bland foods that are easy to eat to a baby who is on solids, such as soups, liquidised foods, ice cream, and yoghurt – which is also helpful in combating yeast infections.
- give all foods cold or cooled as hot food can aggravate the soreness.
- avoid strong-tasting or acidic foods, including fruit and fruit juices, as the acid can make the thrush patches sting.
- give drinks from a bottle, feeder beaker or straw.
- sterilise pacifiers and teats very carefully.
- buy a specially soft teat for bottle-fed babies.
- wash your own nipples thoroughly after each feed if you are breastfeeding as it is possible for them to become infected. Use water only, not soap.
- wipe the inside of your baby's mouth with a cloth soaked in a solution of water and cider vinegar or bicarbonate of soda (¼ pint/125ml of boiled and cooled water to a teaspoon of vinegar or bicarb). You can use this on your nipples too.

Don't

- wear breast pads if you are breastfeeding.
- use a medicated mouthwash as this can destroy healthy bacteria and further upset the balance in the mouth.

Seek help if

- pus forms.
- the infection does not respond to home treatment and your baby is miserable.
- your nipples become infected.

TONSILLITIS

See Sore Throat, p. 156.

TRAVEL SICKNESS

Although most babies are magically tranquillised by car journeys, some hate them – I suspect because they feel sick. If your baby usually (or even occasionally) vomits in the car *and* screams when put in it, travel sickness may be the reason.

I have included the following remedies for simple travel sickness: *Borax, Cocculus, Nux vomica, Petroleum, Sepia, Staphysagria,* and *Tabacum.* If you can fit your baby into a particular type – say *Borax* or *Nux vomica* – then, fine. Otherwise it will be pot luck, I'm afraid, with *Tabacum* or *Petroleum* being the two main car-sickness remedies.

Do

- set your baby's car seat facing towards the back (instead of the front) and tip it so that he or she is lying with their head back.
- try putting the seat in the front where the baby can see you.
- play story tapes or music (try very loud music) as a distraction to the baby.
- give a pacifier or a safe toy to a young baby as sucking can help. Give a bottle of milk or water to an older baby.
- open the window next to your baby's seat as fresh air sometimes cures travel sickness.
- talk reassuringly.
- drive smoothly, stopping and starting gently as jerky driving can make the most stalwart feel nauseous.
- make frequent stops.

Don't

- smoke in the car.
- get upset with your baby if he or she vomits in the car as it will only make them worse the next time.

VACCINATION

It is beyond the scope of this book to go into the issue of vaccination. Alternative health care practitioners are mostly cautious about their supposed benefits, observing that the health of children and adults who have been heavily vaccinated is often very poor. Every homeopath has seen formerly healthy children become chronically ill after certain vaccinations.

However, all parents take a risk, whether they choose to immunise their children or not. Our responsibility as parents is to weigh up those risks to minimise the trauma to our children. You will need to research the issue thoroughly by reading through some of the literature now available. You may also choose to seek the advice of a homeopath who offers vaccination counselling – not all do. In any case, it is essential that you get alternative medical support for your child or children should you decide not to immunise in some or all instances.

If you do vaccinate you can prescribe on your child if the vaccination itself is distressing. Give *Aconite* if there is shock, *Arnica* for bruising at the site of the injection, *Staphysagria* if there is anger, betrayal and hurt resentment, or *Stramonium* if your child suffers from nightmares afterwards.

Seek help if

- you suspect or *know* instinctively that your child's health has suffered as a result of immunisations. It is beyond the scope of the home prescriber to treat these effects: a professional homeopath will be able to help your child regain his or her former vitality. Report any symptoms that develop as a result of vaccination in writing to your doctor.

VOMITING

See also Diarrhoea, p. 146.

Small babies frequently 'posset' (throw up) small amounts of their feeds. This is normal and is not classified as vomiting. Very rarely, babies suffer from pyloric stenosis, an unpleasant congenital disorder which is projectile vomiting, when the stomach contents are hurled violently across the room. You must not attempt to deal with this condition yourself.

Babies up to a year old can have a mild stomach bug which lasts for 24 hours without any serious side effects. If your baby is vomiting frequently and throws a fever, gastro-enteritis, or food poisoning, is likely. This is rare in breast-fed babies. Babies who are bottle-fed or who have been weaned and contract it are seriously at risk from rapid dehydration.

Do be particularly careful when weaning your baby on to solid foods by introducing bland, easily digestible foods first. Avoid meat until you are sure that his or her stomach can take it.

Do

- hold your baby while he or she is vomiting as it

can be frightening. You can hold the stomach with one hand and the forehead with the other.

- place a bowl or bucket nearby.
- once the vomiting is over cuddle the baby re-assuringly.
- sponge his or her face if they find it soothing.
- encourage the baby to take a little water, firstly to rinse the mouth and then to drink, to replace some of the lost fluids. Don't let them take too much until you are sure it is staying down.
- encourage your child to drink, if old enough, by being creative about how you offer it. Let them choose a favourite drink, offer it in a small cup – an egg cup or even a doll's tea-set cup; try a straw; offer a bottle if he or she has just given it up; freeze a favourite juice or juices and offer it in the form of ice cubes or an ice lolly.
- encourage rest. You may need to carry a small baby around for much of the day, or at least lie down with him or her.
- avoid all food until vomiting stops. Most babies won't eat until they feel better.
- carry on breastfeeding if you are still nursing your baby and don't worry if a lot of each feed comes up. The usual number of wet diapers means the baby is getting enough fluids.
- encourage a baby who is vomiting a lot to take as much as 2–3 pints (1½ litres) of fluids a day. You can give diluted formula for a day or two until the vomiting has stopped or cut it out altogether and give rehydration fluid (see p. 146).

Seek help if
- your baby shows any signs of dehydration: dry mouth and lips; dark, concentrated urine; dry diapers, no urine for longer than six hours; sunken eyes; sunken fontanelle; abnormal drowsiness or lethargy.
- your baby is screaming inconsolably.
- your baby is vomiting incessantly.
- there is blood in the vomit or if it looks dark in colour.
- your baby vomits after a fall on the head.
- your baby is vomiting a fair amount without being ill *and* is not gaining weight.

WEIGHT GAIN

Babies vary greatly in the rate at which they gain weight. I have seen fat breastfed babies and thin bottle-fed babies.

Some brands of formula do not agree with some bottle-fed babies. Some are sensitive to lactose in cow's milk, and usually produce some physical symptoms such as iarrhoea (frothy, acidic stools), constant coughs, colds, snuffles, colic or eczema. If you suspect that your baby is sensitive to cow's milk do seek the advice of a professional homeopath, who will help build up your child's immunity through constitutional treatment, which, in the long term, may enable them to tolerate lactose. Consult your health visitor about other brands of formula or the possibility of feeding soya milk.

In breastfed babies, a low weight gain is more complicated. Some women produce a smaller volume of milk; some may have a delay in the let-down reflex so that their babies only get the foremilk and not the fat-rich hindmilk. I have included some remedies and guidelines for increasing the volume of breastmilk (see Repertory and p. 120).

Sometimes a bowel infection can be the cause of a low weight gain: your doctor or hospital consultant will check for this. Older babies are sometimes unable to digest the gluten in wheat cereals or rusks, so if you are concerned, see your doctor or health visitor.

Unless the baby is otherwise fit and healthy, low weight gain usually needs the attention of a professional homeopath. However, if one of the remedy pictures in this book matches your own baby, including the general symptoms, physical complaints and emotional state, give it in a low dose, repeating it from time to time if it is truly effective. Remedies for children who have difficulty in gaining weight are *Baryta carbonica*, *Calcarea phosphorica*, *Silica*, *Calcarea carbonica* and *Magnesium carbonate*, the last two also being indicated for children who have difficulty in digesting cow's milk.

Do
- take into account the weight and size of both parents. Babies of small parents, or of parents who were small babies, will tend to inherit this characteristic.
- change a bottle-fed baby's brand of formula – try one made with soya if you have been giving cow's milk.

Don't
- worry if your baby is thin, healthy and developing normally in all other respects.
- let yourself be persuaded into believing that you are a bad parent.
- give your baby cow's milk if you or the baby's father are known to be sensitive to lactose.
- introduce wheat until you are sure your child's digestion can cope with it. Many doctors are recommending that parents wait until their babies are a year old before introducing it. Give cereals made from oats, millet, corn and rice instead.

· 6 ·
THE MATERIA MEDICAS AND REPERTORIES

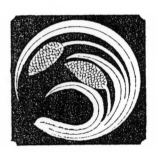

EXTERNAL MATERIA MEDICA

INTRODUCTION

External remedies are not true homeopathic remedies; they have not been proved, or tested, on healthy individuals to establish their symptom pictures, and they have not been potentised. They are basically plant extracts and the indications for their use have developed out of herbal lore over thousands of years. I have chosen the remedies I have found most effective from my own experience.

The remedies are listed in alphabetical order, and precise instructions are given for using each one. The symptoms, or complaints, for each remedy are also listed alphabetically within each entry.

External remedies come in various forms (see below) and next to each symptom are instructions for the most appropriate form to use. In the entry for *Arnica*, for example, I suggest you use *Arnica* oil or ointment for bruised muscles and *Arnica* tincture for a wasp sting.

Tinctures, oils, ointments and creams are sold by homeopathic pharmacies (and sometimes stocked by ordinary chemists). Lotions are usually made up at home by diluting tinctures, and instructions for these are given below.

Tinctures

A tincture is a solution of the plant in alcohol – usually a 1 in 10 dilution. It is prepared by homeopathic pharmacies.

Lotions

A lotion is simply a dilution of tincture in water, used for burns, gargling or douching. Lotions do not keep so you should keep a stock of tinctures and make up lotions as and when you need them.
Basic lotion: Dilute 5 drops of tincture with 1 tablespoon of cooled, boiled water, or for a larger quantity use 40 drops to ¼ pint (40 drops = approximately ½ teaspoon).
Strong lotion: Dilute 10 drops of tincture with 1 tablespoon of cooled, boiled water, or 40 drops to ⅛ pint. Use only where indicated in the External Materia Medica.

Eyebaths

Add 2 drops of tincture to an eyebath of cooled, boiled water and use in the normal way.

Ointments

To make an ointment, the tincture is incorporated into a lanolin base, which serves to seal cuts from dirt. Ointments are not water-soluble and so do not wash off easily. Some people are allergic to lanolin (particularly those sensitive to wool), so it's worth testing it overnight on a small patch of skin. If this produces any redness or irritation, avoid using ointments.

Creams

A cream is a tincture in an aqueous (water-soluble) base, which washes off easily and isn't sticky. It is easily absorbed by the skin and is good for areas that are not going to get wet, and for people who don't like sticky ointments.

Oils

The plant material is crushed and macerated in oil and allowed to stand for a period of time before being strained ready for use. I have indicated in each instance where an oil might be more useful than, say, a cream or a lotion.

NB Before prescribing for any complaint it is essential to read the general advice.

AESCULUS AND HAMAMELIS (Aesc./Ham.)

Piles

A combination of these two herbs in an ointment or cream provides relief from painful piles, but you should seek professional help so that they can be treated 'from the inside' to prevent their recurrence.

ARNICA (Arn.)

Warning: *never* apply *Arnica* externally to open wounds, cuts or grazes – that is, to broken skin – as it can cause a nasty rash.

Bruises

Apply the ointment, cream or lotion directly to the affected part (remembering to use it only on *unbroken* skin) as soon as possible. If you can do this before the bruise has started to discolour (even if it has already swollen), it will simply be reabsorbed by the body,

especially if you take *Arnica* internally as well. Rub ointment or cream in gently, or if you are using lotion apply it on a piece of lint or gauze and keep in place until the swelling has subsided – usually a matter of several hours.

Sore muscles

Rub *Arnica* ointment or oil into sore, bruised muscles after exertion (such as gardening or skiing) and take the appropriate internal remedy if your symptoms are severe.

Sprains/strains (first stage)

Rub in *Arnica* ointment or cream, or wrap the sprained joint in a lotion-soaked bandage. This will deal with the initial swelling.

Wasp stings

Dab the wound with neat tincture immediately after being stung.

CALENDULA (Calen.)

Warning: *Calendula* helps the layers of the skin (the epithelium) to 'knit' back together and will mend a clean wound in a matter of hours. It heals so rapidly that it can seal dirt *into* the body, so always clean the wound very carefully before applying *Calendula*.

Burns/scalds (second degree)

Use *Calendula* cream or lotion for the later stages of a burn once the pain has passed. *Calendula* will promote new skin growth and is especially useful where blisters have broken.

Childbirth

Massage *Calendula* oil into the perineum during labour to soften the area and to help make an episiotomy unnecessary.

Cracked nipples

If *Phytolacca* has failed to help, apply *Calendula* ointment, or cream if sensitive to lanolin, to heal cracked, painful nipples.

Cuts/wounds

Apply ointment or cream to minor cuts, and bandage

if necessary. For serious wounds apply lotion on a piece of lint or gauze and keep in place. Use a plant spray filled with lotion to keep the dressing damp but do *not* remove the dressing until the bleeding has stopped and healing is well under way.

Eczema/rashes

Calendula lotion or cream is especially useful for soothing eczema or rashes where the skin has cracked or been scratched raw. It will not treat the underlying cause of the eczema; you should seek professional help for this.

Handcream

Calendula cream makes a marvellous handcream especially where there may be little cuts in the skin.

Mouthwash

Use a strong lotion after dental treatment, or for bleeding gums.

Nappy rash (Diaper rash)

Use ointment or cream several times daily, making sure that the whole area is clean and dry first (wash with water and a mild, unscented soap). See also *Symphytum*.

Sunburn

Use the lotion or cream (see BURNS, p. 162).

Thrush/Yeast infection

For vaginal thrush douche with the following mixture to relieve soreness and itching: make 1 pint of chamomile tea (1 pint of boiling water to 1 tablespoon of dried chamomile leaves or one chamomile teabag). Leave to cool, strain, add 40 drops of *Calendula* tincture and douche twice daily for up to a week only. You can buy a reusable douche from larger chemists (not the disposable type which comes with its own solution). Douching will not cure the complaint; it will only help during the acute phase (see p. 102), and you should seek professional help.

EUPHRASIA (Euphr.)

Eye infections/inflammations/injuries

Use *Euphrasia* whenever the eye needs bathing – whether it is sore after the removal of dirt or grit, after swimming in a chlorinated pool, when irritated by hayfever or when actually infected or inflamed.

If *Euphrasia* doesn't help, use *Hypercal* tincture (see below). Some people find it more effective, especially in the case of infection.

It is essential to use cooled, boiled water in an eyebath, and to clean the eyebath itself with boiling water after *each* eye is bathed to prevent the spread of infection.

HAMAMELIS (Ham.)

Hamamelis, or witch hazel, is widely sold in chemists as distilled witch hazel, but it is neither as astringent nor as effective as the tincture available from homeopathic pharmacies. Use the distilled form if this is all you can find.

Bruises

Hamamelis is useful for bruises where the skin has been broken (*Arnica* is for use on *un*broken skin). Use *Hamamelis* in the same way as *Arnica*, as an ointment, cream or lotion.

Piles

Apply a compress of the lotion (you can use a small sanitary towel or a strip of cotton wool) to provide instant relief from pain. Keep in place for a while (up to an hour, twice daily) to reduce inflammation.

Aesculus and *Hamamelis* ointment or cream may be applied as often as necessary. It is also important that the correct internal homeopathic remedy is given so that the piles are treated from the inside and real healing can take place.

Varicose veins

Apply the lotion to varicose veins, especially painful ones, by wrapping the leg in lotion-soaked bandages. Leave in place for as long as possible, until the discomfort eases and then use only when needed. An elastic (tube) bandage over the top will keep bandages in place.

HYPERCAL®

This is a mixture of *Calendula* and *Hypericum*; the combined healing qualities of the two plants make it especially effective in soothing and healing wounds.

Childbirth

After childbirth *Hypercal®* will help to heal a cut or

torn perineum. Apply a strong lotion on a small pad or compress to the affected area, keeping it in place for up to an hour at a time, and repeating every four hours for several days.

Cold sores

Dilute one part tincture to three parts cooled, boiled water and apply this strong lotion frequently to cold sores as soon as they appear, or use ointment. Take the appropriate internal remedy at the same time.

Cuts/wounds

Use ointment, cream or lotion to heal wounds just as you would use *Calendula* or *Hypericum* on their own.

Soak cut fingers, toes or elbows in a basin of water into which a teaspoon of *Hypercal*® tincture has been added and gently remove any bits of dirt. The clean wound can then be dressed with a smear of the cream or ointment.

Eye infections/inflammations/injuries

As an alternative to *Euphrasia*, use 2 drops in an eyebath to help clear inflammation caused by dust, foreign bodies, infection or injury. Seek professional help if the soreness persists.

Mouth ulcers

Use the mouthwash below frequently, as well as taking the appropriate internal remedy.

Mouthwash

This mouthwash is good for mouth ulcers, inflamed, sore or spongy gums. Make a strong lotion by diluting 40 drops of tincture in ⅛ pint and swoosh it well around the mouth after brushing your teeth, then massage it into the gums with your fingers.

Sore throat

Dissolve 1 teaspoon of sea salt in ¼ pint of hot water. Add 40 drops of *Hypercal*® tincture and gargle as frequently as necessary.

HYPERICUM (Hyp.)

Hypericum soothes and heals wounds, especially where nerves have been damaged and the injury is painful. The pains of a 'Hypericum wound' are typically shooting and/or severe.

Burns (second degree, with blistering)

Soak gauze strips or lint in *Hypericum* lotion, wring out and lay over the burned area. Keep the bandages damp by spraying the area with the lotion. Do not remove the cloth until the pain has ceased. *Hypericum* is also useful in the first stage of a burn on a nerve-rich and therefore very painful part. Give the appropriate internal remedy.

Cuts/wounds

Use lotion to bathe and clean dirty cuts/wounds, and apply ointment before bandaging. *Hypericum* is especially good where there are shooting pains in or around the wound and for injuries to nerve-rich parts (crushed fingers and toes). If a compress is applied to a crushed finger or toe and kept damp for a few days, a damaged nail can be prevented from taking an odd shape once healed.

Insect bites

Use neat *Hypericum* tincture on any insect bite. If swelling persists, apply the lotion as a compress, and keep in place for as long as it takes for the swelling to diminish.

Piles

Use a compress of *Hypericum* lotion (or ointment if preferred) for bleeding piles with severe shooting pains. Repeat as necessary, but seek professional help.

Sunburn

See BURNS above.

LEDUM (Led.)

Insect bites/stings

Use *Ledum* tincture neat on insect bites and stings to prevent swelling and itching.

Many homeopathic pharmacies have their own preparations for relieving bites and stings. These are generally mixtures of a number of remedies and are applied neat as above.

If you are often bitten and are sensitive to insect bites, you will benefit from constitutional homeopathic treatment (see pp. 6–7), especially if your response is extremely severe.

PHYTOLACCA (Phyt.)

Sore throat

Use a strong lotion as a gargle (40 drops to ⅛ pint of cooled, boiled water to which a teaspoon of sea salt can also be added). Take the appropriate internal remedy.

PLANTAGO (Plant.)

Earache

Dilute a few drops of tincture with equal quantities of warm almond oil (or cooled, boiled water) and drop into the painful ear. Follow these guidelines:

1 Heat a spoon by dipping it in boiling water, then pour the oil and the tincture into it and wait 30 seconds for the spoon to cool and the oil to warm.
2 Tip the head on one side.
3 Drop the liquid into the ear.
4 Pull the lobe of the ear down and round and out very gently so that the liquid goes right into the ear.

Some children will not allow anything to be put into their ears when they are in pain. Do not force this on them. Offer instead a warm hot water bottle wrapped in a soft towel for them to lie on; if that doesn't help try an ice pack (crushed ice in a plastic bag in a thin, soft towel). Or wrap the head tightly with a scarf. One of these measures might offer temporary relief and also guide you to the correct internal remedy.

NB Seek professional help if pain is severe.

Toothache

Apply neat tincture to the affected tooth or swoosh the mouth out frequently with a strong lotion (40 drops tincture with ⅛ pint cooled, boiled water).

PYRETHRUM (Pyreth.)

Insect repellent

Apply the lotion to all exposed areas of skin, and carry a spray bottle of the lotion with you to renew the applications. Some pharmacies sell *Pyrethrum* in a spray, otherwise buy the tincture and make a fresh batch of lotion daily. Some homeopathic pharmacies also produce their own 'anti-bite lotion' which can be diluted and used as above. Experiment to see which suits you best.

RESCUE REMEDY (RR)

This wonderful all-purpose 'remedy' is based on flowers and comes in a cream or as a tincture. It has been known to help anything from bruises, cold sores, cracked nipples, eczema, insect bites and stings, diaper rash and piles to sunburn. If Rescue Remedy is all you have then use it.

Rescue Remedy is a combination of five of Edward Bach's Flower Remedies and is not, strictly speaking, homeopathic. Bach was a homeopath who devoted his energies to finding plants which would act on negative emotions alone, and by so doing restore peace of mind which would lead to physical health.

There are few complaints that are not helped, even temporarily, by Rescue Remedy, including shock (after an accident, bad news, the dentist, etc.); panic; emotional upset or distress of any sort; sunburn; travel sickness; fear (stage fright, birth nerves, sleeplessness through anxiety or fear, fainting from fright); childbirth (before, during and after); headaches from emotional stress, and so on.

Take a few drops on the tongue and repeat this as often as needed – once for a minor injury and every few minutes for a serious situation. The drops can be added to water and sipped frequently, or added to a bath (7 drops) and soaked in for a good quarter of an hour, or applied neat externally as a cream for rashes, bruises, cracked nipples, etc – as often as needed.

RHUS TOXICODENDRON (Rhus-t.)

Joint pain

Rhus toxicodendron ointment rubbed into joints can provide relief for sufferers from rheumatism and arthritis.

Sprains (second stage)

After the swelling has subsided (with applications of *Arnica* ointment or cream), apply *Rhus toxicodendron* ointment twice daily to the sprained joint, and bandage tightly. Use the joint/limb as little as possible and keep it elevated to give it a chance to heal. *Rhus-t.* is especially useful where ligaments are torn.

Strains

After lifting or over-exertion, the ointment can help

enormously, especially if you have the typical *Rhus-t* symptoms: stiffness on beginning to move (on getting up, for example), improvement with continued movement, but a return of the painful stiffness if you overdo it or sit down again.

RUTA GRAVEOLENS (Ruta.)

Bruises

This is for when bony parts of the body are sore after a knock, after *Arnica* has reduced the swelling, but the soreness persists. Shinbones, elbows and kneecaps are all parts that have little protective muscle and the covering to the bone can take longer to heal. *Ruta* can speed up the process. Apply the ointment two or three times daily until the pain eases.

Eye strain

Dilute two drops of *Ruta* tincture with an eyebath of cooled, boiled water, to help eyes strained by too much study, reading, or working at a VDU.

Sprains

Use *Ruta* where *Rhus-t.* hasn't helped and the covering to the bone may have been damaged. I have found a mixture of *Rhus-t.* and *Ruta* in an ointment wonderful for sprains and strains.

Tennis elbow

Apply ointment or cream as necessary to relieve the pain. Do not further stress the joint by more strenuous activity.

SYMPHYTUM (Symph.)

Cuts/wounds

Symphytum is a good all-purpose ointment or cream. Use on minor cuts once you have cleaned them.

Nappy rash

Where *Calendula* hasn't helped, *Symphytum* ointment often will. If it doesn't, your baby will need constitutional treatment from a professional homeopath.

Sprains

Apply *Symphytum* ointment to sprains that don't respond to *Ruta* or *Rhus-t.* within 48 hours. Also take *Symphytum* internally, as there may be damage to the bone itself.

TAMUS (Tam.)

Chilblains

Apply the ointment two to three times daily *before the chilblains break* to stop itching and to speed up healing. **Warning**: *never* apply to a chilblain where the skin has broken.

THIOSINAMINUM (Thios.)

Scars

Thiosinaminum reduces the swelling of a badly healed scar – where there are lumps and bumps (keloids) – as long as it is used soon after the event (within three months), but it is still worth trying on older scars. It is useful for lumpy scars following a Caesarian, episiotomies, and so on. Massage the cream into a scar three times daily for several weeks – longer if it is helping but hasn't quite healed. A professional homeopath can also treat these types of scars with internal remedies.

THUJA (Thu.)

Warts/verrucas

Neat *Thuja* tincture can be applied twice daily and *Thuja* 6 taken orally for up to ten days.
Warning: if this remedy has no effect seek the advice of a professional homeopath. The continued use of *Thuja* is not advisable as the symptoms from the proving are unpleasant and difficult to get rid of. It is a deep-acting remedy that should not generally be used in a first-aid kit for self-prescribing. However, since it is part of the range stocked by many chemists I have included the minimum indications for safe administration.

It is now accepted that you do not 'catch' verrucas in swimming pools as was commonly believed until recently. Homeopaths believe warts and verrucas are part of an overall symptom picture and need to be treated with respect. They are cured successfully with constitutional homeopathic treatment, so do not suppress them with acids from the chemist or have them cut out. Homeopaths have found that suppressing warts in this way can lead to the development of more serious complaints.

URTICA URENS (Urt-u.)

Bee sting

Dab on neat tincture and take the appropriate internal remedy.

Burns (minor)

For minor burns with redness but no blistering, apply cream, ointment, or a compress soaked in lotion. Take the appropriate internal remedy if needed.

Eczema/rashes

Urtica cream or lotion can relieve the itching of eczema or any rash, especially if it itches *and* stings and then burns. It is essential to seek professional help for this condition.

Sunburn

Apply lotion or cream to sunburned areas, repeating according to the severity. Use a mixture of *Hypericum* and *Urtica* tinctures in the lotion if there are severe shooting pains (20 drops of each tincture in ¼ pint of water) and take the appropriate internal remedy.

VERBASCUM OIL (Verb.)

Earache

Drop the warmed oil into the ear to relieve pain and promote healing. Follow the instructions under *Plantago* (p. 165).

EXTERNAL REPERTORY

The External Repertory is an index of the symptoms listed in the External Materia Medica.

Bee stings   see **Stings**
Bruises
   on unbroken skin   *Arn.*, RR
   on broken skin   *Ham.*
   to bones   *Ruta.*
Burns/scalds
   minor   *Urt-u.*
   second degree (with blistering)   *Calen.*, *Hyp.*
Chilblains   *Tamus*
Childbirth   *Calen.*, *Hypercal*®
Cold sores   *Hypercal*®, RR
Conjunctivitis   see **Eye infections**
Cracked nipples   *Calen.*, RR
Cuts/wounds   *Calen.*, *Hypercal*®, *Hyp.*, RR, *Symph.*
Earache   *Plant.*, *Verb.*
Eczema/rashes   *Calen.*, RR, *Urt-u.*
Eye infections/inflammations/injuries   *Euphr.*,
   Hypercal®
Eye strain   *Ruta.*
Gargle   see **Sore throat**
Handcream   *Calen.*
Herpes   see **Cold sores**
Insect bites   *Hyp.*, *Led.*, RR
Insect repellent   *Pyreth.*

Joint pain   *Rhus-t.*
Mouth ulcers   *Hypercal*®
Mouthwash   *Calen.*, *Hypercal*®
Nappy rash (Diaper rash)   *Calen.*, RR, *Symph.*
Piles   *Aesc./Ham.*, *Ham.*, *Hyp.*
Pink eye   see **Eye infections**
Scars   *Thios.*
Sore muscles   *Arn.*
Sore throat   *Hypercal*®, *Phyt.*
Sprains
   first stage (with swelling)   *Arn.*
   second stage   *Rhus-t.*, *Ruta.*, *Symph.*
Stings
   bee   *Led.*, RR, *Urt-u.*
   wasp   *Arn.*, *Led.*, RR
Strains   *Arn.*, *Rhus-t.*
Sunburn   *Calen.*, *Hyp.*, RR, *Urt-u.*
Tennis elbow   *Ruta.*
Thrush   *Calen.*
Toothache   *Plant.*
Ulcers   see **Mouth ulcers**
Varicose veins   *Ham.*
Warts/verrucas   *Thu.*
Wasp stings   see **Stings**

INTERNAL MATERIA MEDICA

ACONITUM NAPELLUS (Aco.)

Other name: common aconite

General symptoms

Complaints from cold, dry wind; fear; getting chilled; shock. **Face** red. **Likes** cold drinks. **Onset of complaint** sudden. **Pains** unbearable. **Palpitations** of pregnancy. **Sweat** hot; on covered parts of the body. **Taste** mouth tastes bitter. **Thirsty**.
Better for fresh air.
Worse at night; for touch.

This remedy works best at the beginning of an acute illness – within the first 24–48 hours. Fright, shock or exposure to draught, or cold, dry wind can cause a wide range of symptoms (colds, coughs, cystitis, etc.) which respond to *Aconite* if the accompanying general symptoms are present – the thirst, the sudden onset of symptoms which are worse at night. The pains are intolerable and drive people to despair.
    Babies needing *Aconite* are fine on going to bed but wake around midnight (usually just before) with a cough or earache. They resent interference, don't want to be touched or examined and are better for fresh air.

Emotional state

Anxious when chilled; generally; during a fever; during pregnancy/labour. **Expression** anxious; frightened. **Fearful** in a crowd; of death during pregnancy/labour. **Moaning/complaining. Restless sleep**, during labour. **Screaming** with pain. **Sensitive** children; to noise. **Tearful** during a fever.

Is extremely distressed, anxious and fearful (the opposite of *Arnica*). Looks anxious and may have shocked, staring, glassy eyes. The pupils may be dilated. May be inconsolable and scared of going into a situation where there are crowds of people.
    In childbirth, pains are severe. Goes from being afraid of dying to saying 'I want to die'.

Physical complaints

Bleeding (vaginal) in pregnancy

With ANXIETY.
Cause fright.

Chickenpox

First stage. With FEVER.

With *Aconite* general symptoms and emotional state.

Common cold

With HEADACHE.
Cause shock; getting chilled; cold, dry wind.

Give *Aconite* at the first sign of a cold if it comes on suddenly after a shock or getting chilled.

Cough

Barking; dry; irritating; short; tickling. BREATHING fast. With VOICE HOARSE.
Worse at night; during fever; for dry, cold air.
Cause cold, dry wind.

Air passages are irritated. Often worse at night after being out in a cold, dry wind (especially north/east).

Croup

See COUGH (above) for symptoms.

Cystitis

PAINS pressing.
Cause getting chilled.

Earache

PAINS unbearable.
Cause getting chilled; cold, dry wind.

Eye inflammation

EYES sensitive to light; whites of eyes red. PAINS aching; burning. With a COMMON COLD.
Worse for cold dry wind.
Cause getting chilled; foreign body in the eye.

Fever

HEAT alternating with chills at night; burning; dry at night. PULSE fast; strong. With ANXIETY.
Better for uncovering.
Worse at night; in the evening.
Cause getting chilled; teething in babies.

Feels hot inside and chilly externally. Babies' cheeks alternate between being hot and red and pale and ghostly. Colour may drain from the face on getting up. One cheek may be hot and red and the other pale and cold, especially in teething babies. Clothed parts of the body become sweaty; babies kick off their covers. Fever is accompanied by a burning, unquenchable thirst; everything tastes bitter except water and even that tastes bad.

Headache

PAINS burning; bursting; throbbing.
Cause fright; shock; getting chilled.

Injuries

CUTS/WOUNDS bleed freely. With SHOCK (see below). *Aconite* helps with wounds that bleed excessively where the characteristic shock is present.

Insomnia

In PREGNANCY. Restless SLEEP. Anxious DREAMS, VIVID.

Labour

PAINS severe. Labour too fast; LATE with fear of labour.

For those short, sharp labours, violent and terrifying, often accompanied by a fear of dying. This remedy eases the fear and slows the roller-coaster down to manageable proportions.

Measles

ONSET sudden. SKIN RASH itches; burns. With FEVER; COUGH.

Sudden onset with restlessness, fever, cough, thirst.

Mumps

ONSET sudden. With FEVER.

Retention of urine

In NEWBORN BABIES; in BABIES WHO CATCH COLD.

For newborn babies who don't pee, who have been shocked by the birth (especially a fast labour).

Roseola

See MEASLES (above) for symptoms.

Shock

Cause injuries; surgery; childbirth.

Accompanied by the extreme *Aconite*-type fear and

anxiety. Useful during or following operations and for shocked mothers and/or babies either during or after labour, especially a fast labour. The mother may feel shaky with the shock, whereas the baby may be very still, with an anxious or fearful look in its eyes.

Sore throat

PAINS burning; stitching.
Cause getting chilled.

Teething

CHEEKS hot and red. With symptoms of FEVER (see p. 169). PAINFUL in babies; with restless sleep.

Babies toss and turn in their sleep and bite their fists and scream.

AESCULUS HIPPOCASTANUM (Aesc.)
Other name: horse chestnut

General symptoms

Heavy or **full** feeling.
Worse for movement; walking.

Useful in pregnancy if there are constipation, piles *and* backache: bowels become sluggish causing piles. Subsequent congestion in pelvic area, with feeling of fullness and/or heaviness, causing backache.

Physical complaints
Backache

In PREGNANCY. With CONSTIPATION (see below).

Lower back feels sore and bruised.

Constipation

In PREGNANCY. STOOLS large, hard. With INEFFECTUAL STRAINING. With PAIN AFTER PASSING A STOOL.

Passes stool with difficulty because it is large and hard – feels as if sticks are being passed. Little if any bleeding.

Piles

In pregnancy. Painful; BLEEDING; EXTERNAL, LARGE, ITCHING. With BACKACHE and CONSTIPATION (see above).
Better for bathing in warm water.
Worse for standing/walking.

AGARICUS MUSCARIUS (Agar.)

Other name: toadstool

General symptoms

Clumsy trips easily while walking. **Trembling. Twitchy.**
Worse for cold.

Specific remedy for chilblains, especially of feet and toes. Used with Tamus ointment, will cure most straightforward cases.

Physical complaints

Chilblains

Burning; itching; red.
Worse for cold.

On hands and feet, or very occasionally ears, but worst on feet; most painful with cold hands or feet.

ALLIUM CEPA (All-c.)

Other name: common red onion

Physical complaints

Common cold

Eyes streaming. Discharge from eyes, watery. Nasal catarrh: burning; one-sided; profuse; watery. Nose streaming. With eye inflammation; headache; sneezing; sore throat.
Better for fresh air.
Worse in a stuffy room.
Cause cold wind; getting feet wet.

Nasal discharge may be one-sided. Cold symptoms, especially the sneezing, generally worse in a warm room. *Euphrasia* is similar in that it too produces streaming colds but in *Allium cepa* nasal catarrh burns and eye discharge doesn't.

Cough

Hacking; irritating; painful. Larynx tickles. Voice hoarse.
Better for being in a warm room.
Worse for cold air.

Eye inflammation

Symptoms of common cold (see above). Discharge: bland, non-irritating; profuse. Eyes watering.

ALUMINA (Alu.)

Other name: aluminium

General symptoms

Discharges white. **Food cravings** for strange things, such as chalk, coal, in pregnancy.

Typical *Alumina* state is extreme exhaustion with feelings of faintness on standing and exhaustion on walking or talking. In pregnancy there may be strange cravings for dry 'foods' like raw spaghetti and rice or even chalk or coal. Small amounts of metal from aluminium pans dissolve into food cooked in them, especially if those foods are acidic (like spinach and some fruits). Some people are sensitive even to tiny traces of this metal, which may cause exhaustion and constipation. Don't expose your baby to risk: get rid of aluminium pans and be careful when weaning as many commercially prepared baby foods contain minute quantities.

Emotional state

Apathetic. Depressed on waking, doesn't want to be bothered. **Desires to be alone. Squeamish. Feels faint** at the sight of blood.

Becomes depressed and indifferent to everybody and everything.

Physical complaints

Constipation

In pregnancy. In babies. Stools soft. Straining ineffectual; desire to pass stool absent.
Cause bottle-feeding (cow's milk or soya); weaning.

Babies (or adults) have difficulty in passing soft stool and become pale and wan. Some babies are very sensitive to the aluminium in some powdered milks or in commercial baby foods. Change the brand if you suspect this may be the problem.

Exhaustion

During labour; nervous during pregnancy. With faint feeling; desire to lie down.
Worse for physical exertion; talking; standing; walking.

Exhaustion is extreme.

Thrush (genital)/Yeast infection

In pregnancy. Discharges like egg white; burning; profuse; white.

Usually accompanied by characteristic exhaustion.

ANTIMONIUM CRUDUM (Ant-c.)
Other name: sulphide of antimony

General symptoms

Complaints from overeating. **Cracks** on corners of mouth/nostrils. **Eyes** sunken; dull. **Headache**. **Lips** dry. **Nausea** in pregnancy. **Sluggish**. **Thirstless**. **Tongue** white-coated.
Worse for getting overheated; for sun; swimming in cold water.

Those who need *Antimonium crudum* often eat too much becoming sluggish, irritable and sick, developing weak stomachs and frequently upset digestive systems. Thirstlessness is often present with nausea or indigestion. The white coating, like whitewash, on the tongue must be present in any complaint if remedy is to work well. Cracks may recur around nostrils and corners of the mouth.
Antimonium crudum types are sensitive to sun, or being overheated, which exhausts them and causes them loss of voice or aggravates any complaint they may have. Swimming in cold water on a hot day may bring on a cold.

Emotional state

Angry babies. **Aversion** to being looked at or touched. **Irritable. Sentimental. Stubborn. Sulky.**

Sick adults needing this remedy may behave in sulky, morose way, not wanting to speak or be spoken to, especially if suffering from gastric problems.

Physical complaints
Chickenpox

With COUGH.

With typical emotional state and general symptoms.

Cough

Worse in stuffy rooms.

Diarrhoea

STOOLS small, hard lumps; watery.
Worse for getting overheated.
Cause overeating.

Exhaustion

With SLEEPINESS.
Worse in hot weather; late morning.

Fingernails split

Cause injury to nail.
Injured or crushed fingernails grow back with splits (see also *Silica*).

Indigestion

BELCHES empty; tasting of food just eaten. ABDOMEN/STOMACH feels bloated; empty; full.

Nausea

CONSTANT. VIOLENT during pregnancy. BELCHES empty; tasting of food just eaten.
Worse after eating acidic and/or starchy foods.
Cause pregnancy.

May be accompanied by headache.

Vomiting

Of bile; of curdled milk; during pregnancy. In breast-fed babies.
Worse after drinking milk.
Cause measles.

For nausea and vomiting during pregnancy where there is the characteristic white tongue and an intolerance of milk and/or bread. Also for babies who vomit breast milk after a feed, who get cross and refuse the breast next time it is offered, or who don't tolerate formula milk well.

ANTIMONIUM TARTARICUM (Ant-t.)
Other name: tartar emetic

General symptoms

Exhaustion. Face pale. **Sweat** cold, profuse. **Thirstless. Tongue** white-coated.

Antimonium tartaricum and *Antimonium crudum* are similar – both are thirstless, irritable and have coated tongues. *Antimonium tartaricum* also has profuse cold sweat, mostly during the night; face is pale and sunken and lips may go blue. Particularly useful for babies and may be called for during chickenpox or measles if a chest infection sets in.

Emotional state

Angry babies. **Apathetic. Clingy. Irritable. Screaming** if touched.

Typically, babies are irritable, drowsy; they whine, complain and are clingy; do not want to be examined, will scream if touched in a way they don't like.

Physical complaints

Breathing difficulties

In babies after birth.

Newborn babies have trouble breathing, are full of mucus which rattles audibly.

Chickenpox

SKIN RASH slow to appear. With symptoms of COUGH (see below). The rash may begin to come out and disappears again.

If *Antimonium tartaricum* is indicated but doesn't work, give *Antimonium crudum*.

Cough

COUGH loud; rattling; whooping. BREATHING asthmatic; abdominal; difficult; fast, rattling. MUCUS difficult to expel. With SLEEPINESS; VOMITING.

In a chest complaint that will respond to this remedy, there is a characteristic loud rattling which can usually be heard *before* entering room, whether chest infection is simple cough, bronchitis or whooping cough. Bringing up phlegm is difficult and provides only temporary relief. Anger can aggravate the cough which may alternate with yawning.

Fever

HEAT, alternating with chills. With intense HEAT DURING SLEEP.

Often accompanies chest or gastric complaints.

Nausea

INTERMITTENT, VIOLENT during pregnancy. **Better** for belching; for vomiting.

Felt in the chest or as a weight on the chest, and is as intense as that associated with *Ipecacuana* but not so persistent. Vomiting and belching provide only temporary relief. Desire to vomit may be accompanied by ineffectual retching.

Vomiting

VOMIT sour. VOMITING difficult. With FEVER. **Worse** for coughing.

May be aggravated by eating and drinking, and may be worse if there is fever (the higher the temperature, the stronger the vomiting). Vomiting is difficult with ineffectual retching.

APIS MELLIFICA (Ap.)

Other name: honey bee

General symptoms

Clumsy drops things. **Face** red; puffy. **Lips swollen**. **Oedema** (swelling) of ankles/feet or hands/fingers. **Pains** burning; stinging. **Symptoms** right-sided: move from right to left. **Thirstless**. **Tongue** fiery red.

Worse for heat; for touch; at 3–5 p.m.

These are warm-blooded types who are better for fresh air; although generally thirstless they are better for cold drinks, and having painful parts bathed in cold water. If there is fever or localised inflammation, the body surface is sore and sensitive, as if bruised, and is worse for touch (pressure of heavy blankets will aggravate, for example).

Emotional state

Apathetic. **Fearful** of being alone; of death. **Irritable**. **Jealous**. **Restless**. **Tearful**. **Whiny**.

Generally, *Apis* types are jealous. This may be seen in the brother or sister of a new baby, no longer getting desired attention. *Apis* picture may be confused with *Pulsatilla*: both are better in open air, whine, are jealous and weepy, but where *Apis* is worse for touch, *Pulsatilla* is better for it – craves it even! In a fever, *Apis* types are tearful for no apparent reason, restless and fearful, with a fear of death, and/or of being alone.

Physical complaints

Bites/stings

BITES burning; itching; red; stinging; swollen. **Better** for cold. **Worse** for heat. **Cause** insect bites.

Bites react badly, causing a large, shiny, swollen red lump which itches and/or burns and/or stings.

NB *Apis* can be used for anaphylactic shock, the severe allergic reaction which may occur not just from a bee or wasp sting but from certain foods, like nuts, or even penicillin. This is always an emergency as it can be fatal: give *Apis* while you wait for emergency help to arrive. Classic symptoms are swollen eyelids, lips and tongue, urticaria (itchy lumps) and difficulty in breathing.

Carpal Tunnel Syndrome

In pregnancy.

Tingling and numbness in fingers, usually with some swelling of wrist or fingers.

Cough

Worse when lying down.

Cystitis

DESIRE TO URINATE constant: frequent. PAINS burning; pressing; stinging. URINATION constant; frequent.

Only small amounts of urine passed. May be blood in urine (it will look red); if so, and if the symptoms agree, take *Apis* but seek professional help immediately.

Diarrhoea

PAINLESS. Anus may be sore after passing a stool.

Earache

PAINS stinging.
Worse for swallowing.

With typical *Apis* general symptoms (worse for heat, pains starting on right side, etc.) and SORE THROAT.

Eye inflammation

In BABIES. EYES burning; red; sore; stinging; stitching. EYELIDS swollen.
Worse for heat.

Whites of eyes are red with visible bright-red blood vessels. Lower lids may be more swollen than upper.

Fever

HEAT burning; dry. With CHILLINESS; SENSITIVE SKIN.
Better for uncovering.
Worse for heat; for being in stuffy room; for warm covers; afternoon; morning; for washing.

Feels hot; finds heat intolerable, has a high fever and feels sleepy. This type of fever accompanies most acute complaints that call for *Apis*. Kicks off covers, then shivers (with chills) but keeps covers off.

Headache

HEAD feels full; hot. PAIN stabbing; sudden.

Scalp feels tight and sore.

Hives

With FEVER (see opposite); SWEATING.
Worse at night.

Joint pain

PAIN burning; stinging. With SWELLING.

Joints are red, swollen and shiny.

Measles

SKIN RASH slow to appear. With EYE INFLAMMATION (see opposite); FEVER (see opposite).

With typical emotional state and general symptoms.

Mumps

With typical general symptoms and emotional state (see p. 173).

Nappy rash (Diaper rash)

SKIN red; shiny; hot; sore.
Better for uncovering.
Worse for heat; for touch.

Retention of urine

In babies. Without cause.

Half-hourly doses of *Apis* will encourage urination to re-establish if the baby is drinking normally.

Scarlet fever

See MEASLES.

Sore throat

MOUTH dry. PAIN burning.

Thirstless although mouth is very dry. Throat is as red as tongue.

ARGENTUM NITRICUM (Arg-n.)

Other name: silver nitrate

General symptoms

Complaints from mental strain. **Cravings** for sugar/ sweets. **Exhaustion** with trembling. **Face** sallow. **Pains** needle-like. **Palpitations. Taste** in mouth sour. **Tongue** red-tipped. **Trembling.**

Better for fresh air.
Worse for heat; after eating sugar/sweets.

These are warm people, generally worse for heat, who suffer in warm stuffy rooms and feel better for fresh air. They have a sweet tooth and crave sugar and sweets but these make them sick. Their exhaustion is often accompanied by extreme anxiety and trembling may follow a period of intense mental work where the brain feels worn out and the memory lapses.

Emotional state

Anxious anticipatory; general. **Confused. Desires** company. **Excitable** babies. **Fearful** of being alone; of public speaking. **Hurried** while speaking; while walking; while waiting. **Impulsive**. Weak memory. Feeling of **panic. Restless.**
Better for company.

Argentum nitricum types dread ordeals, trembling with nervous excitement and suffering from diarrhoea. Anxious and impulsive thoughts torment them. They become fidgety and walk hurriedly around to calm themselves; time seems to pass inexorably slowly. They hate to be kept waiting, and doubt their ability to succeed: their lack of confidence may be well founded in that their anxiety can prevent them from doing well. They are not happy alone and are better for company. 'Birth' nerves during pregnancy may be alleviated but choose carefully between remedies, including *Argentum*, that have anticipatory anxiety or fear of childbirth in their picture.

Physical complaints

Diarrhoea

STOOLS green; smelly; watery. With FLATULENCE (see opposite); VOMITING.
Worse immediately after drinking; at night; after eating sugar.
Cause anticipatory anxiety; excitement; sugar; after weaning.

Liquids pass straight through, coming out as green diarrhoea, like chopped spinach. There may be vomiting. Newly weaned infants may produce this picture; or someone on sugar binge; or someone with acute anxiety and/or panics.

Eye inflammation

IN BABIES. DISCHARGE purulent; smelly; yellow. EYELIDS glued together; red. EYES red; sensitive to light.
Better for cold; for cold compresses.

For newborn babies with sticky eyes. Eyelids and corners of eyes are red and inflamed.

Flatulence

ABDOMEN/STOMACH feels bloated; intolerant of tight clothing. WIND loud; obstructed.
Worse after eating.

Wind is difficult to expel. Noisy, explosive burps provide relief from bloating and pain.

Headache

Better for binding up head.

Indigestion

ABDOMEN/STOMACH feels bloated; painful. BELCHES loud, difficult; empty. With FLATULENCE (see above); NAUSEA.
Better for belching.
Worse after eating; eating sweet foods/sugar.

Usually worse for eating, although it may help. Abdomen is as tight as a drum.

Sore throat

THROAT irritated; raw. PAIN splinter-like. VOICE hoarse; lost.
Cause singing; talking.

ARNICA MONTANA (Arn.)
Other name: leopard's bane

General symptoms

Breath smelly. **Complaints from** accident/injury/ surgery. **Pains** sore, bruised; glands.
Worse for jarring movement; lying on injured part; touch.

Arnica promotes healing, controls bleeding, reduces swelling, prevents pus forming: is an essential ingredient in any first-aid kit, the first to consider after an accident, injury, or any other trauma where there is shock, such as surgery or childbirth. Those needing *Arnica* usually feel sore, bruised and do not want to be touched or jarred, so that when lying down, the bed may feel hard.

Emotional state

Aversion to being touched/examined. **Complaints from** shock. **Denial** of illness; of suffering. **Fearful**

generally; of being touched. **Forgetful** following injury.

Denies being ill when is (sometimes very) sick. May moan and complain about pains, but more usually denies suffering, especially after an injury accompanied by delayed shock. After being knocked down by a car, for example, may stand up, maintaining that nothing is the matter, while blood pours from gaping wound in head. This can be dangerous because of possibility of delayed concussion. Actual concussion may cause hopelessness and indifference and stupor. On coming round, forgets words while speaking and does not want anyone near.

Physical complaints

Abdominal pain

In pregnancy. PAIN sore, bruised.
Cause an active baby.

Afterpains

PAIN sore, bruised.
Worse when baby nurses.

Given in labour, especially towards end and directly afterwards, *Arnica* lessens afterpains.

Bleeding (vaginal) in pregnancy

With PAIN; sore, bruised.
Cause an injury, fall or accident.

Blood blisters

Cause blow or injury.

Broken bones

With SWELLING/BRUISING.

Move on to *Symphytum* once swelling has reduced.

Bruises

With SWELLING. Without discolouration.
Cause childbirth; injury; surgery.

Give before skin begins to discolour – if given soon enough, even if there is already some swelling, bruise will not materialise, healing from inside. Given after bruise has formed, *Arnica* speeds healing and quickly reduces swelling. For bruises to shins see *Ruta*.

Bruised soreness that often accompanies and nearly always follows childbirth is greatly alleviated by *Arnica*. If severe and persistent, try *Bellis perennis*.

Cough

Whooping. EYES bloodshot. PAIN IN CHEST sore, bruised; must hold chest to cough. With NOSE-BLEEDS (see p. 177).
Worse for crying.

Babies cry before coughing in anticipation of pain, which may set off cough.

Eye injuries

BRUISING to eyeball; to surrounding area.

Give *Arnica* before discolouration if possible, even if eye is swollen.

Gums bleeding

Cause tooth extraction.

Arnica controls bleeding and speeds healing, especially where there is bruised soreness.

Head injuries

Give *Arnica* as routine after a fall or bang to the head, whether or not there is concussion. For maximum effect, wait for egg to appear (before it discolours), give *Arnica*, and watch the lump disappear!

Inflammation of penis

In babies.

Injuries

CUTS/WOUNDS with bruising. PAIN sore, bruised.
Cause after dental treatment; surgery.

Give *Arnica* in any injury to soft tissues, i.e. muscles, where there is swelling and bruising.

Joint pain

PAIN sore, bruised.
Worse for touch.

Joints are sore, bruised and very sensitive to touch.

Labour

TOO LONG.

Pains are sore; abdomen feels bruised. *Arnica* helps the muscles to do their work and minimises physical stress and strain on soft tissues. Women needing *Arnica* may brush off support saying they're fine – when they plainly aren't.

Nosebleeds

Cause injury.

Phlebitis

Cause childbirth.

Legs feel sore and achy.

Retained placenta

After a LONG LABOUR.

Retention of urine

After childbirth. After a LONG LABOUR. With painful URGE TO URINATE. With INCONTINENCE/ INVOLUNTARY URINATION.

Shock

Cause surgery; childbirth; injury.

Shock is suppressed (see Emotional state, p. 175).

Skin complaints

In pregnancy. BROKEN VEINS.

Sprains

Of ANKLE; of FOOT; of WRIST; in FIRST STAGE. With BRUISING (see p. 176); SWELLING.

Use *Arnica* to reduce swelling, prevent bruising, and speed healing.

Strains

PAIN sore, bruised.
Cause childbirth; overexertion.

For strained muscles which feel bruised, sore and no better for moving about. (If pains are stiff and better for moving about, even temporarily, see *Rhus toxicodendron*.) Jet-lag can produce this feeling.

ARSENICUM ALBUM (Ars.)

Other name: arsenic

General symptoms

Anaemia. Catches colds easily. Discharges burning; smelly; watery. **Dislikes** food in general; sight of food. **Dryness** generally. **Face** pale. **Likes** hot food/drinks. **Lips** cracked; dry; licks. **Mouth** burn-ing; dry. **Pains** burning. **Palpitations. Restless. Sweat** absent during fever; clammy; profuse; sour; cold. **Taste** in mouth bitter. **Thirsty** for large quantities or frequent small quantities; sips. **Tongue** red-edged or red-tipped.

Better for heat; for hot drinks; for warmth of bed; for lying down.

Worse for change of temperature; for cold; for damp; for exertion; after midnight; on waking; for wet weather; at 3 a.m.

Arsenicum types are extremely sensitive to cold *and* need fresh air so love to live in a house with the heating turned right up and windows open. When ill they typically look pale and anxious and quickly become weak and exhausted, sometimes to the point of collapse in an acute complaint, and often out of proportion to the severity of the illness. Tiredness often comes on suddenly, especially after physical exertion, even a short walk. They are generally better for lying down although many symptoms are worse for this, which causes general restlessness.

The pains are characteristically burning and, except for headaches, are better for heat (a useful, unusual symptom) and for warm drinks, food or compresses. Cold drinks and food aggravate, especially in gastric symptoms.

Emotional state

Angry. Anxious generally; on waking; at night (children); after midnight; during a fever; about others; when alone; at 3 a.m. **Complaints from** anger with anxiety. **Critical. Depressed. Desires** to be carried; company. **Despair** of getting well. **Expression** haggard; sickly; suffering. **Fearful** generally; of being alone; of death; at night (children). **Forgetful. Guilt. Irritable. Restless** babies; in bed; with anxiety. **Tidy.**

Arsenicum characters are more restless and anxious than virtually any other remedy type. If their anxiety goes unchecked it may turn to guilt, and self-criticism. When ill they become frightened of being alone for fear of death and want desperately to be looked after. They are demanding, difficult patients, who find fault and make a fuss. Obsessively tidy, they may clear up for visitors or the doctor in spite of being too weak to get out of bed to make a cup of tea! In labour women may become extremely anxious, dictatorial (bossy), fearful and irritable. Babies in need of *Arsenicum* may want to be carried around, but briskly, rather than gently (like *Pulsatilla*).

Physical complaints

Breathless

In pregnancy.

Worse for walking uphill; when lying down; at night in bed; for exertion.

Burns

PAIN burning. With BLISTERS.
Better for heat.

Carpal Tunnel Syndrome

In pregnancy.

Tingling and numbness in fingers.

Common cold

EYES burning; dry. EYELIDS puffy; red. NASAL CATARRH burning; profuse; watery. SINUSES blocked, painful. With frequent SNEEZING.
Worse during evening; on right side.
Cause getting chilled when overheated.

An acute cold with violent symptoms; may move on to the chest (see COUGH). Burning nasal discharge makes the area under the nostrils red and sore. Discharge may be blood-streaked. Lips may become so badly cracked they bleed.

Cough

Dry at night; exhausting; hacking; loose; tormenting. BREATHING difficult; fast; wheezing. LARYNX tickling. MUCUS copious; frothy; tastes salty. With SWEATING.
Better for hot drinks.
Worse for cold; for cold drinks; fresh air; during evening; for lying down; after midnight; at night; during fever.

Cough may be loose or dry but is more likely to be dry at night. Has to be propped up with lots of pillows even though wants to lie down. May wake up coughing around 1 or 2 a.m.

Cystitis

DESIRE TO URINATE ineffectual. PAIN burning. URINATION with unfinished feeling.
Better for heat; for sitting in hot bath.

Diarrhoea

Burning PAIN after passing stools. STOOLS smelly; watery. With EXHAUSTION (see below); SWEATING; ICY-COLD HANDS AND FEET; NAUSEA.
Worse for cold; after drinking; after eating fruit and any cold food; after midnight.
Cause food poisoning; ice-cream; fruit.

May be accompanied by intense exhaustion and nausea, which is aggravated by the sight, smell or even thought of food.

Exhaustion

EXTREME; PARALYTIC; SUDDEN. With FAINT FEELING; FEVER (see below); RESTLESSNESS.
Worse in morning; for movement; for passing stool.
Cause food poisoning; pain.

Comes on suddenly, especially after diarrhoea, and is worse for the slightest exertion. Is accompanied, unusually, by restlessness.

Eye inflammation

In BABIES. EYELIDS burning. EYES bloodshot; burning; gritty; sensitive to light.

Fever

HEAT burning; dry; dry at night; alternating with chills. With ANXIETY; DELIRIUM; EXHAUSTION (see above).
Worse in morning; at night; after midnight.

Feverishness or feeling hot alternates with feeling chilly, causing sweating. Head and face may feel hot to touch while body feels cold; or body may be hot to touch while chilled inside. At other times feels hot inside as though blood is burning in veins. With the characteristic *Arsenicum* thirst for sips.

Flatulence

ABDOMEN/STOMACH bloated. WIND smelly.

Flu

With symptoms of COMMON COLD (see opposite); FEVER (see above); RESTLESSNESS.
Cause change of temperature.

Cold and fever symptoms are accompanied by *Arsenicum* general symptoms.

Food poisoning

With DIARRHOEA (see above); NAUSEA; VOMITING (see below).

Cause rotten meat.

Nausea is intense – cannot bear sight, smell or thought of food.

Gastric flu

See FLU (p. 178) with DIARRHOEA.

Headache

PAIN burning; throbbing; in forehead; recurring at regular intervals.
Better for fresh air.
Worse for heat.

Wants to lie down with head high on lots of pillows. Pains may start at bridge of nose and spread to whole head. Feels like being wrapped in a duvet from neck down while sitting next to open window because unlike other *Arsenicum* pains, the headache benefits from fresh air and cold in general (or a cold compress).

Incontinence

In PREGNANCY. After CHILDBIRTH. DAY AND NIGHT.

With the emotional state and general symptoms.

Indigestion

Burning PAINS. With HEARTBURN.
Better for hot drinks.

Warm milk may be particularly soothing. Pains may be accompanied by HEADACHE (see above).

Insomnia

DREAMS anxious; nightmares. Restless SLEEP.
Worse after midnight.
Cause anxiety; overactive mind; shock.

In spite of complete exhaustion, anxiety prevents sleep. When sleep finally comes it is full of frightening dreams, of danger and dead people.

Measles

With *Arsenicum* general symptoms and emotional state.

Mumps

With *Arsenicum* general symptoms and emotional state.

Nausea

DEATHLY.
In PREGNANCY. With VOMITING (see below).

Retention of urine (after labour)

No desire to pass urine. With INVOLUNTARY URINATION.

For women who find it difficult to urinate after childbirth.

Piles

INTERNAL. BLEEDING. BURNING.
Better for bathing in warm water.

Sore throat

Burning PAINS. ULCERS in throat.
Better for hot drinks.
Worse for cold drinks; for swallowing.

Vomiting

VOMIT bile; food; smelly; watery. VOMITING easy; frequent; violent. With DIARRHOEA (see above); FAINTNESS after vomiting; SWEATING while vomiting.
Worse after eating/drinking; for movement.
Cause ice-cream; rotten meat.

Acute vomiting (and diarrhoea) of severe food poisoning. Everything is vomited immediately, even the smallest quantity of water (unlike *Phosphorus*, where vomiting occurs after a few minutes). Eventually there is nothing left in stomach and foul-smelling bile may be vomited.

ASARUM EUROPUM (Asar.)

Other name: European snake root

General symptoms

Senses hyperacute.
Better for bathing; cold drinks/food; fresh air; lying down; rest.
Worse for cold, dry weather; wet weather; heat; stuffy rooms; hot food/drinks; alcohol; movement.

Emotional state

Dull/sluggish. **Sensitive** to pain during pregnancy; oversensitive to noise. **Slow**.

The *Asarum* state is truly dreadful and unhappily common in pregnancy when some women become super-sensitive. Great sluggishness is accompanied by acute sensitivity to noise: ticking clock or dripping tap may drive to distraction and aggravate nausea.

Physical complaints

Nausea

CONSTANT. VIOLENT. In pregnancy. With RETCHING; VOMITING.
Worse for noise.

BARYTA CARBONICA (Bar-c.)

Other name: barium carbonate

General symptoms

Catches colds easily. Concentration poor. **Exhaustion** after eating. **Glands** swollen; sensitive. **Slowness** of babies to develop. **Sweat** one-sided. **Weight gain** poor in babies.
Worse for cold; for pressure; for getting feet wet.

Baryta carbonica types are sensitive to cold and need to wrap up warmly due to a tendency to catch colds and coughs, which usually come with swollen glands.

Young benefit most from this remedy. *Baryta carbonica* babies are slow, look 'old' and have big bellies with disproportionately skinny arms and legs.

Emotional state

Anxious during fever. **Dislikes** company (strangers). **Fearful** babies; of strangers. **Indecisive. Jumpy. Lack of self-confidence. Play** – doesn't want to. **Shy. Sluggish** babies.

Baryta carbonica types are serious, shy and nervous of strangers; although they can be cheerful and jokey, they hate to be teased.

Physical complaints

Blocked tear duct

In babies.

Common cold

GLANDS swollen. NOSE dry. With COUGH.
Worse at night.

Feels the cold and catches colds easily and often. These may be winter colds in babies who have developed catarrh from the first cold or damp weather of winter which remains until right through till warmth of late spring.

Mumps

With *Baryta carbonica* general symptoms and emotional state.

Sore throat

THROAT inflamed; raw. Roaring noises in EARS on swallowing. PAIN burning. TONSILS swollen. With INCREASED SALIVA.
Better for swallowing liquids.
Worse at night; for swallowing saliva; for swallowing food.

Can only swallow liquids; gags and chokes when swallowing food. Mucus drips down into the throat and saliva increases.

BELLADONNA (Bell.)

Other name: deadly nightshade

General symptoms

Complaints from cold, dry wind; getting head wet. **Eyes** shining. **Face** red; with toothache red in spots; dark red. **Glands** swollen; sensitive. **Sudden onset. Pains** come on suddenly; appear and disappear suddenly; in glands; shooting; throbbing. **Pupils** dilated. **Shock. Sweat** absent during fever; on covered parts. **Symptoms** right-sided. **Thirsty. Tongue** red or white-coated; strawberry.
Better for lying down.
Worse for jarring movement; for touch; for cold wind; at 3 p.m.; getting head wet.

A *Belladonna* illness – be it sore throat, earache or sunstroke – comes on suddenly and strongly, as does *Aconite*, and disappears as rapidly. A cold may start if head is chilled, especially if hair is wet (after swim or haircut). Generally, symptoms are worse at 3 p.m., although 3 a.m. may also be a bad time. Lying in quiet, darkened room helps, although some symptoms are better for standing. Eyes sparkle or shine, and pupils are usually dilated. Tongue may be red, coated with white dots, or have white coating. Face is flushed, and burns. With a fever blood vessels in neck may throb visibly.

Think of *Belladonna* where a part of the body becomes inflamed or infected, reddens and throbs painfully, radiating heat. Violent, throbbing pains are intensified by moving or being moved or touched, or jarred (for example, during a car journey).

Emotional state

Angry. Anxious. Aversion to being touched/

examined. **Biting**. **Confused**. **Delirious**. **Excit-able**. **Expression** fierce. **Hitting**. **Rage** with desire to bite or hit. **Restless**. **Screaming** with pain. **Sensitive** babies; to light; to noise. **Tantrums**. **Tearful** during a fever.

Belladonna suits happy, easy-going babies who become difficult and obstinate when ill, and are prone to tantrums where they may bite or hit those closest to them. Under stress anger surfaces more easily than fear. Someone needing *Belladonna* becomes agitated, excitable, restless and delirious with or without fever. Lies in bed moaning and jumps up from time to time; and becomes hypersensitive to light and noise. The delirium (with fevers) may be accompanied by hallucinations.

Belladonna is especially suited to women in labour having a first baby in their late thirties and forties. They rant, rage and quarrel with everybody, becoming uncontrollably angry with the pains.

Physical complaints
Backache

In pregnancy. **PAIN** dragging.

Bleeding (vaginal)

In pregnancy; after childbirth.

Sudden gushes of blood; flow of blood is dark red; with clots; with shooting pains that come and go suddenly.

Braxton Hicks contractions

In pregnancy.

Breast(feeding) problems

BREASTS engorged; hard; hot; inflamed; painful; with red streaks. **PAIN** throbbing. **MILK SUPPLY** overabundant.

When milk 'comes in', the breasts become red, hard, painful, and throb. Red streaks may radiate out from the nipples.

Chickenpox

With **FEVER**; **HEADACHE** (see p. 182).

With *Belladonna* general symptoms and emotional state.

Common cold

With **FEVER**; **HEADACHE**; **LOSS OF SMELL/TASTE**. **Cause** getting chilled; getting head wet.

Convulsions

In babies.
Cause teething.

With typical *Belladonna* general symptoms and emotional state. Some babies find teething difficult and can become ill with a fever and/or convulsions. Always seek professional help.

Cough

Barking; dry; exhausting; hard; hollow; in fits; irritating; racking; tickling; tormenting; violent. **BREATHING** fast. In **PREGNANCY**. **PAIN** sharp; in chest. With **HOARSE VOICE**.
Worse at night; for deep breathing.
Cause getting chilled.

Babies may cry before the cough anticipating pain.

Cramp

Worse during labour in hands or feet.

Dizziness

In pregnancy. With **HEADACHE**.
Worse getting up from bending down; stooping.

Earache

PAIN spreading down into neck; stitching; tearing; throbbing. With **FACE-ACHE**; **NOISES IN EAR**.
Worse on right side.

Pain is violent and causes great anguish.

Eye inflammation

EYES bloodshot; burning; dry; sensitive to light; watering. With symptoms of **COMMON COLD**.
Worse for light; for heat.

Fever

HEAT alternating with chills; burning; dry; at night; radiant. With **GRINDING OF TEETH**; **DELIRIUM**; **THIRSTLESS**. Without **SWEATING**.
Worse for light; for being uncovered; in afternoon; in evening; at night.

Radiates heat, especially from head, although limbs feel cold. Skin may be alternately dry and moist and if there is sweat it will be on covered parts of body.

Headache

PAIN in back of head; in eyes; in forehead; in temples; bursting; hammering; pulsating; throbbing; violent; starts and stops suddenly. In PREGNANCY.
Better for resting head; for lying in a darkened room; for pressure.
Worse for bending down; for cold; for heat; for light; for exposure to sun; for tying up hair; for walking.
Cause cold air; getting head wet (haircut); over-exposure to sun.

Injuries

CUTS/WOUNDS bleed freely.

Insomnia

SLEEP restless. With SLEEPINESS; GRINDING OF TEETH.

Moans in sleep; feels sleepy but is unable to sleep; has nightmares or dreams of falling.

Labour pains

SLOW or FALSE LABOUR. INEFFECTUAL: cervix doesn't soften. PAIN distressing; severe/violent; stops (or slows down); weak. With EXHAUSTION; CRAMPS in hands or legs; RED FACE.

Contractions are painful but ineffective.

Measles

ONSET sudden. SKIN RASH burns; hot; itches; red. With FEVER (see above); COUGH (see above); EYE INFLAMMATION (see p. 181).

With *Belladonna* general symptoms and emotional state.

Mumps

GLANDS painful; swollen; worse right side. ONSET sudden. With FEVER (see p. 181); HEADACHE (see above); SORE THROAT (see opposite).

The glands are painful to touch.

Roseola

See MEASLES (above) for symptoms.

Scarlet fever

See MEASLES (above) for symptoms.

Sore throat

THROAT constricted; irritated; raw. Swollen GLANDS. PAIN severe; stitching.
Worse on right side; for swallowing liquids.
Cause getting cold.

Neck is tender to touch, and talking is difficult. Constant desire to swallow despite extreme pain; pains may radiate from throat up into right ear on swallowing. Sips drinks with head bent forward.

Sunstroke

FEVER (see above). HEADACHE (see opposite).

Belladonna will cure sunstroke if *Glonoine* is indicated and fails (pictures are similar and difficult to differentiate).

Teething

PAINFUL IN BABIES. CHEEKS hot and red; swollen. SLEEP restless.

With severe pain and typical *Belladonna* restlessness.

BELLIS PERENNIS (Bell-p.)

Other name: garden daisy

General symptoms

Complaints from getting chilled when overheated; accident/injury; surgery.

A small but important remedy for the first-aider. For any illness that follows a plunge into cold water while hot (or overheated), i.e. sudden chilling either externally by bathing in cold water, or internally from cold drinks or ice-cream on a hot day. Also useful after an accident or surgery to aid recovery.

Physical complaints

Abdominal pain

In pregnancy. PAINS sudden. UTERUS feels sore. With STIFFNESS IN LOWER ABDOMEN.
Cause uterine ligaments stretching.

Pains are common towards end of pregnancy as these ligaments are stretched by expanding uterus.

Bruises

With BUMPS AND LUMPS. PAIN sore, bruised. MUSCLES sore, bruised.
Cause childbirth; injury; over-exertion; surgery.

Sometimes a bump or lump remains after bruising has disappeared, following a blow, knock or accident, or after a period of over-exertion, even if injury occurred a long time ago. *Bellis* is useful where *Arnica* has cleared bruising but a lump remains. It is deeper-acting than *Arnica* and relieves bruised soreness after childbirth where *Arnica* has not helped. Also useful for injuries to the breast, if *Conium* helps but a lump remains.

Groin pains

SUDDEN. In PREGNANCY. LEGS weak.

Pain, caused by a trapped nerve during the last few months of pregnancy, especially after the baby's head engages, comes on suddenly while walking and may last for only a few minutes. Groin pains are relatively common and can be severe enough to make walking impossible until they have passed. *Bellis perennis* will help them pass quickly and prevent recurrence.

Insomnia

SLEEPLESSNESS after 3 a.m.

Falls asleep easily and sleeps well before 3 a.m., but after this time cannot get back to sleep.

Joint pain

Cause getting chilled after being very hot.

BORAX VENETA (Bor.)

Other name: sodium biborate

General symptoms

Better for fresh air.
Worse for cold; for riding in a car.

Good for nervous babies who may have difficulty teething, becoming sensitive and prone to colds.

Emotional state

Anxious children; at night; of downward motion. **Clingy. Dislikes** strangers. **Expression** anxious. **Fearful** generally; of downward movement; of sudden noises (sneezing, etc.). **Irritable** before stools. **Jumpy. Screaming** in babies during sleep. **Tearful** babies at night.

Borax babies hate downward motion and scream on being rocked or put down in their cots. If asleep when you place them in their cots they wake immediately. They do not like to be thrown up (and then

down) in the air as do many babies. They are nervous, easily startled by sudden noises such as sneezing or the hoover being turned on. They may wake screaming from the slightest noise or scream suddenly during sleep and wake up screaming for no apparent reason, as if from a nightmare, and are particularly irritable leading up to passing a stool, and change dramatically to being cheerful directly afterwards.

Physical complaints

Breast(feeding) problems

BREASTS painful during feeding; aching after feeding.

Pain in breast opposite to one baby is feeding on. Afterwards when breasts are empty, breasts ache.

Diarrhoea

Painless. STOOLS with mucus.

In teething infants; may also accompany THRUSH.

Dizziness

Cause downward motion.

Hiccups

In babies.

Borax works in nervous babies who hiccup after feeds.

Thrush (genital)/Yeast infection

DISCHARGE like egg white; burning; white.
Worse between menstrual periods.

Thrush (oral)

In BABIES. THRUSH of mouth; of tongue. MOUTH bleeds easily; hot; dry. With EXCESS SALIVA.
Worse for breastfeeding; for touch.

Infant cries with pain while feeding or refuses breast altogether. The baby's mouth feels hot to the mother's nipple.

Travel sickness

With NAUSEA; VOMITING.
Worse for downward movement.

BRYONIA ALBA (Bry.)

Other name: white bryony

General symptoms

Complaints from change of weather from cold to warm; getting chilled; weaning. **Dizziness**. **Dryness** generally. **Face** dark red. **Likes** cold drinks; hot food. **Lips** dry. **Mouth** dry with thirst. **Onset of complaint** slow. **Pains** sore, bruised; stitching. **Sweat** absent during fever. **Taste** in mouth bitter. **Thirsty** for large quantities; at infrequent intervals. **Tongue** coated brown; dirty white.
Better for lying still; for firm pressure.
Worse for slightest movement; at 9 p.m.; for flatulent food (beans, cabbage, etc.).

Bryonia illness develops slowly over days, like *Gelsemium*. Acute complaints, such as flu, fevers and coughs, are often accompanied by headaches, a general dryness (mouth, lips, tongue, chest, eyes, etc.), and great thirst for large quantities (drinks are gulped straight down). Pains are 'stitching', and especially bad in evening around 9 p.m. although symptoms may also be bad on waking in the morning. The slightest movement aggravates the pains; the head, for example, aches even from rolling eyeballs. Firm pressure, lying on back and/or applying pressure to painful areas helps, as does lying on side that hurts. *Bryonia* types like fresh air and are generally worse in hot stuffy rooms (that is, from being overheated), although better for being kept warm and covered, especially if very ill.

Emotional state

Angry. **Anxious**. **Capricious**. **Desires** to be carried. **Irritable**. **Morose**. **Sluggish**.

Bryonia types are nicknamed 'the bear' because of their irritability. They are especially bad when disturbed. They may lie loglike, pretending to be asleep to avoid having to respond. They resent intrusion, wanting to be left alone when ill, and are touchy, not wanting to be questioned, examined or interfered with in any way. Babies want to be carried though not moved about too much. They are capricious and reject things – toys, food, etc. – they have just asked for.

Physical complaints

Abdominal pain

In pregnancy. With STIFFNESS in lower abdomen.

Towards end of pregnancy when muscles and ligaments are stretched and vulnerable to strain, great stiffness is felt in lower abdomen.

Backache

PAIN in LOWER BACK; stitching.
Worse for coughing; for slightest movement.

Breast(feeding) problems

BREASTS engorged; hard; hot; inflamed; pale; painful. MILK SUPPLY overabundant.
Worse for slightest movement.

Breasts look pale. Any movement is painful and the inflammation (mastitis) may be accompanied by fever and depression.

Breast pain

In pregnancy. With MASTITIS.

Broken bones

PAIN stitching.
Worse for slightest movement.

Bryonia may be given after a fracture where *Arnica* and *Symphytum* have been given and there is still tremendous pain.

Common cold

With HEADACHE; SNEEZING.

Nose may feel stuffed up after the watery discharge ceases; the cold quickly settles on the chest.

Cough

Dry; in fits; irritating; racking; vomiting; disturbs sleep. BREATHING fast. In PREGNANCY. PAIN IN CHEST stitching; holds chest with hands. PAIN IN STOMACH from coughing. With HEADACHE (see below).
Better for fresh air; for lying on painful side.
Worse for deep breathing; for slightest movement of chest; in right lung.

Accompanied by little or no expectoration. Eating or drinking may make the cough worse, because of the movement involved.

Diarrhoea

Worse after getting up; during morning; for movement.

Cause hot weather; excess of fruit.

Dizziness

Worse for slightest motion; walking.

Exhaustion

Extreme.
Worse for slightest exertion.
Cause breastfeeding.

Eye inflammation

EYES dry; sore.
Worse for moving the eyes.

Fever

HEAT burning; dry; alternating with chills; ONE-SIDED; WITHOUT SWEATING.
Better for complete rest.
Worse in autumn; around 9 p.m.

Feels hot internally and externally; the right side of body is hotter than the left. Chills may be present during day and in evening after lying down in bed.

Flu

With *Bryonia* general symptoms and emotional state.

Gastric flu

BILIOUSNESS. TASTE bitter.
PAIN aching; in stomach. With symptoms of FEVER (see above).
Better for belching.
Worse for coughing; after eating bread; for movement; for waking; in evening; lying down in bed.

All food and drink (except water) taste bitter. There is a sensation of a stone lying in the stomach, and the pains may be better for belching.

Headache

PAIN behind eyeballs, in forehead; bursting; violent.
Better for cold compresses; for pressure.
Worse for coughing; after getting up.
Cause breastfeeding; change of weather; cold, damp weather; ironing; overexposure to sun.

These headaches last all day.

Heartburn

In pregnancy. With INDIGESTION.

Hernia in babies

UMBILICAL.

Joint pain

PAINS stitching. With SWELLING.
Better for pressure; for rest.
Worse for cold; for slightest movement.

Joints look either pale or red, and are better for pressure – or resting on the painful parts. Tight bandaging helps.

Measles

ONSET slow. SKIN RASH slow to appear. With COUGH; FEVER; HEADACHE (see opposite).

With characteristic *Bryonia* dryness and dislike of movement.

Mumps

With *Bryonia* general and emotional/mental symptoms.

Phlebitis

PAINS in legs after childbirth.
Better for rest.
Worse for movement.

Sore throat

PAIN stitching. VOICE hoarse. With symptoms of FEVER (see opposite).
Worse for swallowing.

Varicose veins

Of vulva.
Worse during pregnancy.

Vomiting

VOMIT tastes bitter; watery.
Worse for movement; for coughing.

CALCAREA CARBONICA (Calc-c.)

Other name: oystershell

General symptoms

Anaemia. **Catches colds easily. Clumsy. Complaints from** getting wet; sprains. **Likes** boiled eggs;

strange things in pregnancy (chalk, coal etc.). **Discharges** thick. **Dislikes** coffee; meat; tobacco. **Face** pale. **Glands** swollen; painless. **Oedema** (swelling) of ankles/feet; of hands/fingers. **Pains** cramping. **Palpitations**. **Sense of smell** lost. **Slowness** of children to teethe/to walk. **Sweat** on head; sour; profuse; from slightest physical exertion; from mental exertion. **Symptoms** right-sided. **Taste** in mouth bad; sour. **Teeth** crumbling, decaying. **Tongue** white-coated. **Weight gain** easy, in babies.

Better for being constipated; for heat; for lying down.
Worse for cold; for damp; for draughts; for exertion; for fresh air; after drinking milk; for tight clothes.

Those needing this remedy tend to be sluggish, move slowly and look white and pasty and feel 'spineless' – adults have limp handshake and may slump in their chairs. Exertion leaves them weak and breathless; and they feel better for lying down. Babies are slow to walk and produce teeth and their fontanelles are slow to close. They have large heads and bellies.

Those who need this remedy are chilly and worse for cold and damp but may overheat easily and be subject to hot flushes. Their feet and hands are cold and often clammy, even in bed; they hate draughts or fresh air and may catch cold easily after swimming or getting wet. Warmth relieves their symptoms.

They sweat on their heads and at the back of the neck – especially while asleep – so profusely their sheets may be wet. Sweat and discharges smell sour.

Metabolism is slow and everything turns to fat. Milk turns sour in the stomach, causing nausea. The one unusual symptom is that they feel generally better for constipation.

Emotional state

Anxious about health; children, at night; during evening. **Confused. Depressed. Despair** of getting well. **Fearful** generally; children, at night; of death; in evening. **Melancholic. Slow. Sluggish. Stubborn** children. **Tearful** babies.
Worse for thinking.

Anxious, sluggish types, who find concentration difficult when ill. Babies are happy and content when well but may seem lethargic at times and more difficult to handle if teething or unwell as their stubborn side comes out more strongly.

Physical complaints
Backache

PAIN aching; in LOWER BACK; feels sprained.
Worse for damp; on getting up from sitting.

Cause lifting.

Back feels weak; cannot easily sit straight and soon slumps in a chair.

Braxton Hicks contractions

In pregnancy.

Breast(feeding) problems

MILK SUPPLY overabundant.

Breasts may be large and uncomfortable.

Breathless

In pregnancy.
Worse for walking uphill/upstairs; for exertion.

Broken bones

BONES slow to mend.

If a fracture fails to heal well after *Symphytum, Calcarea carbonica* or *Calcarea phosphorica* may be given (as a tonic, see p. 188) until it has healed. Use the general symptoms and emotional state to choose between them.

Carpal Tunnel Syndrome

In pregnancy.

With tingling and numbness in fingers and swelling of wrists/fingers.

Common cold

NASAL CATARRH dry; smelly; yellow. NOSE blocked. With LOSS OF SMELL; PAINLESS HOARSENESS.
Worse during the morning.

Constipation

STOOLS hard at first; large; pale; sour-smelling.
Better generally for being constipated.

Initial large, hard stool (which may be clay-like, or like a lump of chalk) may be followed by diarrhoea (see below).

Cough

Dry at night; loose during morning. In PREGNANCY. MUCUS copious; smelly; yellow; tough; tastes sour/sweet. With symptoms of FEVER.

Worse for playing piano; morning; evening in bed; at night; during fever.

Coughs up mucus with difficulty. Babies are prone to coughs when teething. The cough continues after the teeth come through.

Cradle cap

Sour-smelling, thick scales/crusts on the scalps of sweaty-headed babies.

Cramp

In calf; hand; sole of feet; toe.
Worse at night; during pregnancy; for stretching leg in bed.

Cramps come on when stretching limbs on waking up in bed, during the night or first thing in the morning.

Diarrhoea

In TEETHING BABIES. STOOLS containing undigested food; sour; watery.
Worse after drinking milk.
Cause drinking milk; teething.

Diarrhoea follows a formed stool, is full of undigested food and smells sour.

Dizziness

With HEADACHE (see opposite).
Worse for moving/turning head quickly.
Cause high places.

Sensitive to heights, becoming dizzy and headachy.

Earache

PAINS throbbing. With NOISES IN EAR.

With typical *Calcarea carbonica* general and emotional symptoms.

Exhaustion

With BREATHLESSNESS. DIZZINESS.
Worse for mental exertion; for slightest physical exertion; for walking; for walking upstairs.
Cause breastfeeding.

Eye inflammation

In BABIES. DISCHARGE purulent. EYES sensitive to light; watering. EYELIDS glued together; gritty. With symptoms of COMMON COLD.

Inflammation accompanies a cold; eyes may ooze a smelly discharge.

Flatulence

ABDOMEN/STOMACH feels bloated; intolerant of tight clothing.

Hair loss

After CHILDBIRTH.

Headache

PAINS burning; bursting; maddening.
Better for lying down.
Worse for light; for noise; on right side of head.
Cause cold, damp weather; getting wet.

Pains are worst at back of the head and spread up to the top. They are often worse while reading and for any jarring upward movement. Feels better for lying down with eyes closed.

Hernia in babies

UMBILICAL.

Hoarseness

PAINLESS.
Worse in morning.

Indigestion

ABDOMEN/STOMACH feels bloated; hard. BELCHES sour. PAIN pressing. With FLATULENCE; HEARTBURN during pregnancy.

Insomnia

Anxious DREAMS.
Worse before midnight.
Cause overactive mind; worry.

Sleepless from worry with persistently anxious thoughts. Anxious dreams may be interspersed with pleasant ones.

Joint pain

PAIN cramping.

Worse for wet weather; cold.
Cause wet weather.

When *Rhus toxicodendron* has worked well but has stopped having any effect, *Calcarea carbonica* often helps if typical general symptoms and emotional state are present.

Lochia

Lasts too long; intermittent; milky appearance.

Milk supply low

Breasts are full and may be sore but aren't producing much milk. With *Calcarea carbonica* general symptoms and emotional state.

Nausea

Worse for milk.

Sore throat

THROAT dry.
Cause change of weather.

Sprains

Of ankle; hand; wrist.
Worse for lifting.
Cause lifting heavy weights.

A useful remedy for clumsy people who stumble frequently while walking and sprain their ankles easily. Also for sprains from lifting heavy weights that do not clear up with *Rhus toxicodendron* and/or *Ruta graveolens*.

Teething

PAINFUL in babies. SLOW. DIFFICULT. With DIARRHOEA (see above).

Babies may make a chewing motion in their sleep and grind their teeth – or gums! Their teeth take forever to arrive.

Varicose veins

In pregnancy. Of the VULVA.

Vomiting

VOMIT curdled milk; sour.

CALCAREA FLUORICA (Calc-f.)
Other name: calcium fluoride

As with other *Calcarea* salts, those needing this remedy are generally worse for cold, damp weather. It is useful as a tonic for any tissues that have become worn out, flabby and lax. During pregnancy, *Calcarea fluorica* may be helpful if skin is dry and out of condition, or for varicose veins. Postnatally, repeated short courses are beneficial for mild prolapse with no other symptoms. Short courses of *Calcarea fluorica* can be repeated (say, once a month) if it helps during pregnancy or after childbirth.

Physical complaints
Backache

PAINS IN LOWER BACK.
Better for continued movement.
Worse on beginning to move.

If *Rhus toxicodendron* was indicated and only partially relieves pain, or if it fails, *Calcarea fluorica* usually helps.

Common cold

NASAL CATARRH dry. SNEEZING with difficulty.
Better for sneezing.

For stuffy head colds with dry catarrh.

Skin complaints

In pregnancy. STRETCH MARKS; DRYNESS.

CALCAREA PHOSPHORICA (Calc-p.)
Other name: calcium phosphate

General symptoms

Catches colds easily. Complaints from loss of body fluids. **Face** pale. **Slowness of babies** to learn/to teethe. **Thin. Weight gain** poor in babies.
Worse for cold; for damp; for draughts; for fresh air; for wet weather.

Calcarea phosphorica is useful as a tonic for worn-out nervous systems. Vital in the growth and maintenance of healthy cells, nourishes blood cells, bones, teeth and all connective tissue and therefore may be indicated in slow developers. Food is poorly assimilated which may cause anaemia, slow growth, and tooth decay, and fontanelles which close slowly. A wonderful tonic for children who have had a growth spurt and become pale and exhausted. Adults and children who are weak and tired while convalescing from illness will likewise benefit. The typical *Calcarea phosphorica* type is thin with long, dark eyelashes and dark hair. Sensitive to draughts, cold and damp, they have cold extremities.

Emotional state

Anxious. Discontented. Irritable children. **Restless. Screaming** in sleep. **Sighing. Slow. Sluggish. Worse** for mental exertion.

Calcarea phosphorica types (adults and babies) are discontented, complaining, grumbling and sighing when talking. They have no 'go', are sluggish *and* restless, not knowing what they want. Babies may be slow in their general development.

Physical complaints
Anaemia

With EXHAUSTION.
Cause acute illness.

For the convalescent stage of an illness, or post-childbirth, where regaining strength is proving difficult.

Breast pain

In pregnancy.

Broken bones

SLOW TO MEND.

For fractures taking longer than expected to heal. It may be given routinely after *Symphytum* has dealt with the pain of the fracture, as it will speed up the healing.

Cough

MUCUS yellow.
Worse when teething.

Useful for obstinate coughs (or whooping cough) which tend to be worse in cold-weather months, or precipitated by teething.

Cramp

In CALF.
Worse for walking.

Diarrhoea

In breastfeeding babies.

Exhaustion

With HEAVINESS in limbs. With WEAK LEGS.
Cause breastfeeding; pregnancy.

Headache

Cause mental exertion; overwork; anaemia.
Worse for cold wind, but cold bathing may help.

Insomnia

WAKING difficult; late.
Worse before midnight. Mornings are awful, waking is difficult.

Joint pain

In hips, in pregnancy.
Worse for cold, wet weather.

Foot joints may also be affected. Feet are always cold and there is a cramping and aching numbness.

Teething

PAINFUL in babies. SLOW. DIFFICULT. GREEN STOOLS.

Helpful for teeth that are slow in cutting through the gums. Teething children may develop diarrhoea, colds and coughs. Teeth are inclined to decay easily and prematurely. *Calcarea phosphorica* ensures better assimilation of calcium and encourages healthy dentine formation.

CALCAREA SULPHURICA (Calc-s.)

Other name: calcium sulphate

General symptoms

Abscesses discharging pus. **Discharges**, blood-streaked.
Worse for heat; for milk; for physical exertion; in stuffy rooms.

This remedy helps with abscesses or longstanding catarrh. Those needing it are prone to thick, lumpy, yellow or bloody discharges, and generally worse for warmth and overheating, unlike other *Calcarea* remedies, which are chilly, and unlike *Hepar sulphuris*, another important remedy for abscesses and catarrhs, which is also chilly. They like to be uncovered, if feverish, and are usually better for some fresh air, though they dislike draughts.

Emotional state

Anxious during evening. **Depressed. Irritable. Sluggish/dull. Tearful.**

Physical complaints

Abscess

DISCHARGING PUS; of GLANDS.

Speeds healing of discharging abscesses, i.e., those that have burst or broken and are discharging a thick, yellow, lumpy and possibly bloody matter.

Common cold

NASAL CATARRH blood-streaked; smelly; thick, yellow. With HEADACHE; LOSS OF SMELL. **Worse** after drinking milk.

For postnasal catarrh (where mucus drips down back of throat) or catarrh that is one-sided.

Cough

COUGH dry. MUCUS copious; lumpy; yellow.

Croup

Cough occurs only ON WAKING.

In croup, where *Hepar sulphuris* is indicated but fails, *Calcarea sulphurica* cures, especially if the baby is warm and wants to be uncovered and/or if croupy cough is only there on waking.

Earache

DISCHARGE blood-streaked; smelly; thick.

Eye inflammation

DISCHARGE thick; yellow.

Especially indicated if both nose and eyes are discharging thick yellow mucus.

Injuries

CUTS/WOUNDS SLOW TO HEAL; suppurating.

Where a wound has become inflamed and started to discharge thick yellow pus. (*Hepar sulphuris* is for the stage before this.)

CALENDULA OFFICINALIS (Calen.)
Other name: marigold

Physical complaints
Injuries

WOUNDS/CUTS LACERATED; suppurating. Painful out of proportion to injury.

Calendula is a great healer of wounds and cuts, both externally as an ointment (see External Materia Medica) and internally in potentised form (which helps wounds heal even more quickly). Use *Calendula* in straightforward injuries where the skin is broken but there are no other noteworthy symptoms. It works well if pains are stronger than the severity of injury warrants. Useful after childbirth to speed the healing of an episiotomy or tear – you can alternate with *Arnica* or *Bellis perennis* or any other remedy that is needed.

CANTHARIS VESICATORIA (Canth.)
Other name: Spanish fly

Physical complaints
Burns

Scalds; sunburn; second degree; with blisters. PAIN burning.
Better for cold compress.

Cystitis

DESIRE TO URINATE constant; frequent; ineffectual; urgent. PAINS before, during and after urination; burning; cutting. URINATION frequent. URINE hot; red; scanty.
Worse for cold drinks; before, during and after urination.

Pains come on suddenly and are violent and spasmodic. Despite a constant desire to pass water, bladder never feels empty. Although complaints are often aggravated by cold drinks, there may be a burning thirst. *Cantharis* is sometimes confused with *Apis* and *Arsenicum* because all suffer from severe burning pains and restlessness.

CARBO ANIMALIS (Carb-a.)

Other name: leather charcoal

General symptoms

Pains burning. **Sweat** exhausting; profuse; smelly.

This is a small remedy which has few general indications. The sweating is worse at night, or during/after eating.

Emotional state

Depressed. Desires to be alone. Dislikes company. **Uncommunicative.**

A remedy for anyone debilitated by illness.

Physical complaints

Exhaustion

Worse for walking; during a menstrual period.
Cause breastfeeding; after an acute illness; lifting; sweating.

The typical *Carbo animalis* sweat accompanies this exhaustion, which occurs in people recovering from an illness and also in nursing mothers. They may weep during meals because they feel too tired even to eat. Walking across a room seems too much. They may also have painful, lumpy breasts which hurt while the baby feeds.

Flatulence

ABDOMEN bloated.
Cause abdominal surgery.

Carbo animalis will provide some relief where the abdomen is bloated with wind that is difficult to pass after an abdominal operation such as appendicectomy, Caesarean or laparoscopy.

Strains

Strains muscles easily – of the wrist especially but also the back – from lifting even small weights; the strained muscle is worse for the slightest exertion.

CARBO VEGETABILIS (Carb-v.)

Other name: wood charcoal

General symptoms

Anaemia. Breath smelly. **Complaints from** measles; loss of body fluids. **Discharges** smelly. **Face** pale;
sallow or blue. **Feels faint** on getting up; on waking. **Sweat** cold; profuse. **Taste** bitter.
Better for fanning; for fresh air.
Worse for exertion; after eating rich/fatty foods; for humidity.

These are sluggish types with low vitality who want to lie down and sleep. The slightest exertion exhausts them; they have to force themselves to get going. They feel worse for lying down in spite of being too weak to do otherwise. Mornings and evenings are the worst times of day.

People recovering from an acute illness or chest infection often benefit from this remedy, as do children who have not fully recovered from a serious illness such as whooping cough or measles.

This remedy also deals with acute indigestion, in which case the emotional and general symptoms may not be present.

Emotional state

Anxious during the evening; in bed. **Confused. Indifferent** to everything. **Irritable. Sluggish.**

A remedy for inactive folk who find it difficult to rouse themselves. They may become indifferent to the point that they do not care if they live or die but suffer from anxiety in the late afternoon through to the evening, which intensifies when they go to bed and shut their eyes.

Physical complaints

Breathing difficulties

In newborn babies.

Breathless

In PREGNANCY.
Better for burping.
Worse when walking uphill/upstairs; lying down.

Common cold

NOSE blocked. SNEEZING frequent; with difficulty. With HOARSENESS; ITCHING THROAT.

Tickling in the throat may be acute; may not be able to sneeze at times in spite of wanting to.

Cough

Racking; in fits; suffocative; violent; whooping. BREATHING fast; wheezing. MUCUS green. VOICE HOARSE. With RETCHING.
Worse at night; evening; before midnight.

Coughing fits are often accompanied by the characteristic cold perspiration.

Exhaustion

BREATH cold. BREATHLESSNESS.
Better for being fanned.
Cause carbon monoxide poisoning; food poisoning; accident/injury; acute illness; loss of body fluids (diarrhoea, vomiting), breastfeeding; surgery.

Carbo vegetabilis is useful for extreme weakness – 'collapse' may be a more accurate label – commonly occurring after an accident or operation, severe vomiting, or during convalescence from a serious illness. The breath and sweat are cold, the skin feels cold to the touch but there is a feeling of heat internally and a desire for fresh, cool air. The face may be deathly pale or even blue, with bluish lips; the head feels heavy. I do not suggest that you treat anyone seriously ill without help, but if you are the only person available and this remedy fits the case, give it while you wait for help to arrive. *Carbo vegetabilis* may also be indicated to treat forms of poisoning: food; North Sea gas, or car exhaust fumes that may come on after sitting in a traffic jam on a hot, windless day for a long period.

Flatulence

ABDOMEN/STOMACH feels bloated; rumbling. WIND smelly. With DIARRHOEA.
Better for passing wind.
Cause abdominal surgery.

Abdomen is bloated below the navel as with *Lycopodium* flatulence.

Food poisoning

With FLATULENCE (see above).
Cause rotten fish/meat.

Hair loss

Cause acute illness; childbirth.

Headache

PAINS in back of head; heavy; pressing.

Head feels heavy, like lead.

Indigestion

ABDOMEN/STOMACH feels bloated. BELCHES empty; sour. PAINS burning; cramping. With FLATULENCE (see above); NAUSEA.

Better for belching; for passing wind.
Worse after eating rich/fatty food.

Carbo vegetabilis digestion is easily upset. The stomach feels full, becoming so bloated after eating that the skin is stretched as tight as a drum. Tight clothes feel uncomfortable. The nausea is worse in the mornings. Burping may relieve the bloatedness for a while but it builds up again quite quickly.

Mumps

GLANDS swollen/painful. PAINS spread to breasts, ovaries.

With typical *Carbo vegetabilis* pale face and cold sweat.

Nosebleeds

BLOOD dark.
Worse at night.

Good for weakened state after an acute illness such as measles, which results in night-time nosebleeds for no other apparent reason.

Spots

In babies (pimples). With FLATULENCE.

Varicose veins

In pregnancy. Of LEG/THIGH; of VULVA.

CASTOR EQUI (Cast.)
Other name: horn (horse's)

Physical complaints
Breast(feeding) problems

Sore/cracked NIPPLES.

This small remedy has few uses other than the treatment of sore, cracked nipples. Effective for women who are otherwise well with no other symptoms. Breasts may be engorged and the skin itchy; nipples are sore, cracked and very tender, quickly becoming raw if left untreated.

CAULOPHYLLUM (Caul.)
Other name: blue cohosh

Caulophyllum's major use is for establishing effective contractions in labour. Some homeopathic books advise pregnant women to take *Caulophyllum* during the last weeks or months before delivery to prepare them for an easy labour. Think carefully before doing this as some women have had short but violent labours after taking it or protracted ones (see Provings, p. 5). If this is not your first baby and you have a history of easy labours, do not take it. If it is your first baby and you are worried about the birth consult a homeopath, who will advise you properly on this remedy and any others that you might need.

Physical complaints

Bleeding (vaginal) in pregnancy

FLOW scanty. With bearing down PAIN; PAIN in back; weakness and trembling.

Braxton Hicks contractions

In pregnancy.

With no other symptoms.

Joint pain

PAIN in the small joints; flying around; irregular.

Pains occur in finger and hand joints and move around frequently.

Labour pains

LABOUR: late; slow. LABOUR PAINS: distressing; ineffectual (cervix doesn't soften); irregular; last a short time; stop (or slow down) from exhaustion; weak. With THIRST (during contractions); EXHAUSTION; TREMBLING. With IRRITABILITY.

Labour pains may appear in the groin, bladder and legs, and fly from one place to another. Cervix is rigid and does not dilate. Feels chilly, with trembling or shivering, even when covered up. Contractions are short and very painful. The only marked emotional state to look for is irritability (not anger) with the exhaustion and trembling.

CAUSTICUM (Caust.)

Other name: potassium hydrate

General symptoms

Appetite lost in pregnancy. **Blister** on tip of tongue; painful. **Clumsy** trips easily while walking. **Complaints from** change of weather to dry; getting wet. **Discharges** watery. **Dislikes** sweets/sweet things. **Exhaustion** during evening. **Eyelids** heavy. **Likes** smoked foods. **Loss of libido.**

Restless during evening. **Tongue** red stripe down centre (white edges).
Better for cold drinks; for heat; for warmth of bed.
Worse for changes in weather; for coffee; for cold; for draughts; during the evening; for fresh air; for walking; for getting wet.

These are chilly people badly affected by getting wet, draughts, changes in the weather and especially by clear, dry, cold weather. Mild, wet weather makes them feel better, especially their 'rheumatics' and their 'chests'; when everyone else is complaining about the damp they will be enjoying some relief from their pains. Evening weakness is overwhelming. Blisters often accompany a cough or sore throat. Women may lose their appetite when pregnant and develop a dislike of anything sweet.

Emotional state

Absent-minded. Anxious. Complaints from grief. **Concentration** poor. **Depressed. Fearful** children – at night; during evening. **Forgetful. Irritable. Memory** weak. **Sympathetic. Tearful** at least little thing.

These are sensitive, anxious souls who suffer when those close to them are hurt either emotionally or physically, and react against injustice in any shape or form. Pessimistic by nature, they may become gloomy and full of anxious forebodings when ill, despairing of getting well. Irritability sets in, and then depression. They cry easily, over a sad news item in the paper or on television. After the loss of someone close (even a favourite pet), they sink into a negative state, becoming irritable and then depressed. A woman may lose her sex drive during pregnancy and/or find that it takes a long time to return after the birth. Babies cry easily, are frightened of the dark and of going to bed on their own.

Physical complaints

Breast(feeding) problems

Cracked/sore NIPPLES.

May have difficulty in establishing a good milk supply because of exhaustion and anxiety.

Burns

BURNS third degree. PAINS burning. With BLISTERS.

For serious, third-degree burns, chemical burns, or scalds, with the characteristic *Causticum* pains. These *must* receive expert attention. You may prescribe *Causticum* on the way to hospital to provide some relief. *Causticum* may also help the soreness at the site of old burns.

Constipation

DESIRE TO PASS STOOL ineffectual. PAIN stitching.

Stool may be soft despite constipation. May have to stand up to pass a stool.

Cough

Constant; distressing; exhausting; hollow; racking; rattling; tormenting; violent; woken by cough at night. In PREGNANCY. MUCUS difficult to cough up; must swallow what comes up. PAINS raw in chest. With VOICE HOARSE.
Better for sips of cold water.
Worse for breathing in cold air; getting warm in bed; bending head forward; lying down.

Hoarseness with this cough is worse in the mornings. Coughing up mucus is difficult as it comes up to the throat and slips back again. Small sips of water are about the only thing that eases the cough and stops it, albeit temporarily.

Cramp

In FEET; in TOES; in SOLES OF FEET.
Worse at night.

Cystitis

DESIRE TO URINATE frequent, ineffectual. PAINS burning; during urination. URINATION difficult; frequent; involuntary; slow to start; with unfinished feeling.
Worse while urinating.

Feels the urge to urinate frequently but finds it difficult or impossible to pass water. May do so involuntarily when coughing, sneezing or blowing the nose.

Incontinence

In PREGNANCY.
Worse for coughing/sneezing/laughing or walking.
Cause becoming chilled.

Involuntary urination (stress incontinence) or leaking, either in pregnancy or after birth.

Indigestion

ABDOMEN/STOMACH feels full. BELCHES empty; tasting of food just eaten. PAINS cramping; pressing.

Joint pain

PAINS in back; in joints; in neck; burning; gnawing; pressing; stitching; tearing. With STIFFNESS.
Better for heat; for warmth of bed.
Worse for dry cold; getting up from sitting.

Pains cease on getting warm in bed to begin again on getting up in the morning. Restless at night.

Restless legs

In PREGNANCY.
Worse in the evening.

Retention of urine (after labour)

With frequent, painful, urgent desire to urinate.

Wants to pee but can't – and it hurts; or passes a little perhaps involuntarily.

Sore throat

CONSTANT THROAT burning; dry; raw. CHOKING sensation; constant DESIRE TO SWALLOW.
Worse for talking.

Swallowing is difficult as the throat feels too narrow. Cannot expectorate. Hoarseness remains after the sore throat has healed.

CHAMOMILLA (Cham.)

Other name: German chamomile

General symptoms

Complaints from coffee; teething. **Face** red; one-sided – in spots; with toothache (teething). **Likes** cold drinks. **Pains** unbearable. **Sweat** clammy; hot; better for uncovering.
Better for uncovering.
Worse during the evening; for fresh air; for coffee; for wind.

Especially suited to teething babies, women in labour, and anyone who has been in a highly emotional state (especially angry) for a long time, becoming over-sensitive, mentally or physically, as a result. Its keynote is unbearable pain. There may be sweating with the pains, especially on the scalp and face, along with a high fever. May feel better for sweating. Feels hot and doesn't like it, kicks off the bedclothes or sticks burning soles of feet out of bed. Is sensitive to wind and being chilled by cold, damp air.

Emotional state

Angry babies; women during labour; violently angry. **Complaints from** anger. **Depressed. Desires** to be carried; to be alone. **Dislikes/aversion** to company; being spoken to; being looked at; being touched. **Excitable. Hitting. Impatient. Irritable** babies; when teething; women in labour. **Quarrelsome** women during labour. **Restless** babies – better for being carried. **Screaming** with pain. **Sensitive** to pain. **Tearful** babies.

Is angry and excitable, tolerates nothing and nobody. Incredibly sensitive to pain and enraged by it. Snaps and snarls, demands relief from pain, but nothing helps. *Chamomilla* people say, 'I can't bear the pain any longer.'

Babies become spiteful, hitting parents. They whine, scream and cannot be comforted. They ask for things which they may immediately hurl across the room (drinks, toys, etc.). Babies insist on being carried and cry loudly when held still or put down. Even after being carried for a short time they may start to cry. The parents of a *Chamomilla* baby may soon reach the limits of their endurance and talk of adoption!

Physical complaints

Afterpains

PAIN unbearable.
Worse when the baby nurses.

Pains distressing, accompanied by frantic ill temper.

Braxton Hicks contractions

In pregnancy.

Colic

ABDOMEN/STOMACH feels bloated. **PAIN** unbearable. **Cause** anger.

Baby cries out while passing a stool. May have diarrhoea with green stools.

Cough

Dry during sleep; irritating; tickling. **MUCUS** (in adults) tastes bitter.
Worse at night.

Cough often worse at night; does not wake a sleeping baby.

Diarrhoea

STOOLS green; hot; smelling of rotten eggs; **PAINFUL**. In **TEETHING** and **BREASTFEEDING** babies.

Earache

PAINS aching; pressing; stitching; tearing; unbearable.
Worse for wind; bending down.

Effects of drugs taken during or after labour

IRRITABLE; and **SLEEPLESS**.
Cause morphine or pethidine.

Fever

HEAT burning; **ONE-SIDED**. With **THIRST**; **SHIVERING**.
Worse mid-morning.
Cause anger.

Face and breath are hot while body is chilly and cold. Face may sweat after eating.

Flatulence

ABDOMEN/STOMACH bloated.

Insomnia

With **SLEEPINESS**. **DREAMS VIVID** during pregnancy.

Results from pain, anger or stimulants (coffee, etc.), or too much chamomile tea even in babies.

Joint pain

PAINS violent. With **NUMBNESS**.

Driven out of bed by pain, helped by walking about.

Labour

LABOUR PAINS in the back; distressing; ineffectual (cervix doesn't soften); severe; stopping (or slowing down); unbearable. With **EXHAUSTION**.

Says she can't bear the pain and wants to die. Isn't anxious like *Aconite*, but angry and impatient as the cervix may be slow to dilate.

Teething

CHEEKS hot and red; pale and cold; red spot on one cheek. **PAINS** unbearable; cries out in sleep. With **DIFFICULTY TEETHING, RESTLESS SLEEP; DIARRHOEA; GREEN STOOLS; COUGH**.
Worse for heat of bed; warm food/drinks; for pressure; for warmth of bed.

May have at the same time one hot, red cheek or a red

patch on one cheek, and one pale, cold cheek. Babies don't want to chew on anything, as pressure aggravates their sore gums.

Vomiting

Easy. VOMIT bile.
Cause anger.

CHELIDONIUM MAJUS (Chel.)

Other name: celandine

Physical complaints

Jaundice

In newborn babies.

The main remedy for jaundice in little babies, it helps the liver adjust to life outside the uterus. If the baby is well in all other respects then give a short course of *Chelidonium*. If other symptoms are present, choose between other remedies that also have jaundice in their picture.

CHINA OFFICINALIS (Chin.)

Other name: cinchona officinalis

General symptoms

Anaemia. Appetite lost. **Complaints from** loss of body fluids. **Dislikes** bread; butter; food in general – in pregnancy; fruit; rich, fatty food; meat. **Eyes** sunken. **Face** pasty. **Likes** cold drinks; spicy foods; sweets. **Pains** sore, bruised. **Sweat** cold; on covered parts of the body, profuse; on single parts of the body; increased by slightest exertion. **Taste** bitter.
Better for firm pressure.
Worse for cold; for fresh air; for light touch; for movement; at night.

The *China* picture often emerges in someone anaemic, weak and depleted following a condition with a prolonged, exhausting discharge or loss of body fluids, such as diarrhoea, vomiting, perspiring, breastfeeding; or from prolonged mental or physical strain. The anaemia is temporary, but causes facial pallor and dark blue rings around the eyes. If indicated, *China* speeds up convalescence dramatically.

Lack of appetite is a curious symptom but one mouthful leads to it returning with a vengeance. The skin feels sore over the whole body, is aggravated by light touch but soothed by hard pressure. They are persistently chilly, worse for cold weather and sensitive to draughts and fresh air. Symptoms may recur at regular intervals or be worse, say, every other day. They sweat in their sleep, sleep restlessly and with difficulty and feel sluggish on waking.

Emotional state

Anxious. Apathetic. Aversion to being touched/ examined. **Depressed** generally; during pregnancy. **Despondent. Fearful** of animals; of dogs. **Irritable** children – in the mornings. **Screaming** – on waking. **Sensitive** generally; to noise. **Stubborn** children.

Apart from physical tiredness, feels emotionally weary. May formerly have been lively and active, both mentally and physically, but acute illness or stress causing the tiredness leads to complete debility, apathy, depression or despondency.

Babies are sensitive, dislike being examined, are irritable and mischievous, especially in the mornings, and lack vitality when unwell.

Physical complaints

Diarrhoea

In pregnancy. PAINLESSS. STOOLS containing undigested food. With INDIGESTION (see p. 197).
Worse after eating; during the afternoon; on alternate days; at night.
Cause acute illness; eating fruit; hot weather; weaning.

The digestion is slowed down. Newly weaned babies do not take well to solids.

Exhaustion

NERVOUS. Profuse SWEATING.
Cause loss of body fluids (diarrhoea, vomiting); breastfeeding.

Weakness characteristic during convalescence after heavy loss of body fluids (see General symptoms). May feel faint and have ringing in the ears as well as profuse sweating, especially on exertion and during sleep.

Flatulence

ABDOMEN/STOMACH feels bloated; obstructed (WIND difficult to expel); rumbling.
Cause eating fruit; abdominal surgery.

Abdomen distended (bloated) above the navel, with trapped wind, causes much discomfort and pain.

Headache

NERVOUS. PAIN sore, bruised; pressing; throbbing. SCALP sensitive.
Better for firm pressure.
Cause mental strain.

May feel as if the brain is beating against the skull. Pain relieved by hard pressure although scalp may be so sensitive that even individual hair follicles feel sore.

Indigestion

ABDOMEN/STOMACH feels bloated. BELCHES bitter; tasting of food eaten; ineffectual, incomplete; sour. FLATULENCE obstructed. PAIN pressing.
Worse after drinking; after eating; after eating fruit; after belching.
Cause abdominal operation.

Digestion is slow; feels as if all food turns to gas; much like *Carbo vegetabilis*, but in *China* burping relieves neither the discomfort nor the bloating. Abdomen is swollen tight like a drum, and it seems as if the wind is blocked. It may follow an operation to the abdomen. Fruit ferments in the stomach, turning to wind.

Jaundice

In newborn babies.

If your baby has *China* general or emotional symptoms then give it instead of *Chelidonium*.

Vomiting

VOMIT food; sour. VOMITING frequent.
Worse after eating.

CIMICIFUGA (Cimi.)

Other name: black cohosh

General symptoms

Complaints from childbirth. **Pains** sore, bruised. **Trembling.**
Worse for cold.

This remedy is useful in pregnancy. These are chilly types and with the exception of the headaches, their symptoms are worse for cold. Physical symptoms may alternate with depression. May be needed for post-natal complaints, with a *Cimicifuga* emotional state.

Emotional state

Depressed. Depressed/fearful and sensitive during pregnancy. **Depressed/screaming/sensitive** to noise during labour. **Fearful of death. Restless. Sensitive. Sighing.**

Useful for women who have bouts of gloominess or depression, as if a black cloud has settled over them, which can be common during pregnancy or after childbirth. May be afraid of death (like *Aconite*), and scared of losing her reason. During the gloomy phase, sits silently or sighs. When dejection lifts, may become excitable and talkative, jumping from one subject to another.

Physical complaints

Abdominal pain

In pregnancy. PAIN flying about abdomen.

Distressing shooting pains may occur during the later months of pregnancy.

Afterpains

PAIN unbearable.
Worse in the groin.

Headache

PAIN in back of head; top of head; pressing out; pressing up.
Better for fresh air.

Pain radiates from the back to the top of head, which feels as if it may fly off; it may start in the forehead and extend to the back of the head. Pain is severe and better for cool, fresh air.

Joint pain

In PREGNANCY.
Worse for cold.

Sore, bruised pains in joints and heaviness in lower back may also occur in pregnancy. They may alternate with feeling depressed.

Labour

LATE with FEAR OF BIRTH. LABOUR PAINS: in the back; in the hips; flying around the abdomen; ineffectual (cervix doesn't soften); stopping (or slowing down); weak. With CRAMP IN HIPS and/or SHIVERING/TREMBLING; feels FAINT.

Pains fly from one side of the abdomen to the other; whole body feels sore, bruised and sensitive to touch.

Retained placenta

With the SHAKES.

With exhaustion, trembling and shaking (or shivering).

CINA

Other name: European wormseed

General symptoms

Expression sickly. **Eyes** sunken. **Face** pale. **Likes** cold drinks. **Nose**: baby picks constantly.
Worse at night; for pressure.

Cina's general picture occurs most commonly in babies and may be an indication for worms but is useful for other complaints too, if whole picture fits. Despite being pale and sickly looking, has hot red cheeks.

Emotional state

Angry babies. **Anxious** – babies at night. **Aversion** to being touched/examined; being hugged; being looked at. **Capricious. Desires** to be carried. **Hitting. Irritable. Moaning/complaining. Restless** – better for being carried. **Screaming** on waking. **Stubborn. Tearful.**

These are angry, touchy and stubborn types. *Cina* babies dislike being looked at, touched, examined or interfered with in any way; may demand to be carried or rocked but are not better for it and kick and scream when picked up and cuddled (rather like *Antimonium crudum* and *Chamomilla*). Asks for things and rejects or throws them away.

Physical complaints

Convulsions

In BABIES.
Cause worms; teething.

Seek professional advice immediately.

Cough

In fits; suffocative. With RETCHING.
Worse after getting up.

Body stiffens before a coughing fit, and there is gur-

gling in the throat after coughing. May be almost constant (involuntary) swallowing with the cough.

Fever

THIRSTLESS. With HUNGER.
Worse at night.

The fever may recur daily at the same time.

Restless sleep

BODY twitching. LIMBS jerking. With GRINDING OF TEETH.

Babies scream out at night, and lie on their backs kicking their legs.

Worms

ANUS itches. APPETITE changeable; lost; ravenous. NOSE itches. With symptoms of FEVER (see above).

For worms in a baby who rubs and picks its nose continually; grinds the teeth while asleep; has an enormous appetite and asks for food soon after a meal, or wants to eat nothing but sweet things, and is generally irritable.

COCCULUS INDICUS (Cocc.)

Other name: India berry

General symptoms

Aversion to fresh air. **Dislikes** food in general; with hunger. **Hot flushes. Sweat** on single parts of the body; cold. **Taste** metallic. **Trembling** from emotion.
Better for lying down in bed.
Worse for exertion; for loss of sleep; for movement; for touch; for walking in the fresh air.

A remedy for complete exhaustion, usually from lack of sleep or irregular sleeping from working night shifts, looking after sick patients through the night, or nursing babies, etc. Trembles with tiredness and feels much worse for fresh air and physical exertion. Feels generally numb and as if specific parts of the body have gone to sleep. Wants to lie quietly in bed and sleep, but this is difficult because the habit of sleeping is lost. Is in a dreadful vicious circle of exhaustion.

Emotional state

Anxious. Complaints from anger; grief. **Confused.**

Dazed to others. **Forgetful. Introspective. Memory** weak. **Mild. Time** seems to pass too fast. **Uncommunicative.**

Emotional state results from stress, especially sleep deprivation, in normally easy-going characters. Grief (loss of a loved one, for example) or anger may also be part of the picture. Become introspective, uncommunicative and closed off from the world. Become trembly if confronted with difficult emotional situations. Time passes quickly, especially at night when they try to sleep but can't.

Physical complaints
Dizziness

In PREGNANCY. HAS TO LIE DOWN. With NAUSEA.
Worse for getting up from lying down.

Exhaustion

PARALYTIC. With DIZZINESS; NERVOUSNESS; NUMBNESS; STIFFNESS; TREMBLING; VERTIGO.
Worse for walking in fresh air.
Cause loss of sleep; irregular sleep; nursing the sick; nervous exhaustion.

Useful to combat exhaustion after working or caring for a baby through the night. Legs tremble while walking and hands while eating and when lifting them up high. Limbs may 'go to sleep' easily; back and neck feel weak and stiff. Needs to lie down and feels worse for sitting up.

Headache

PAIN in back of head; in forehead; at nape of neck. With NAUSEA (see below).
Cause irregular sleep; loss of sleep.

Head may feel empty, sore and bruised. Headaches from nervous strain, overwork or travel sickness.

Insomnia

DREAMS anxious; nightmares. Restless SLEEP.
Cause anxiety.

Nausea

ABDOMEN/STOMACH feels empty. APPETITE lost. BELCHES. TASTE metallic. With FAINTNESS.
Worse during the afternoon; after eating; after drinking; for movement; for sitting up in bed; for smell and sight of food; for travelling.

Nosebleeds

In PREGNANCY.

Thrush (genital)/Yeast

In PREGNANCY. DISCHARGE profuse; thin; watery.

Travel sickness

With DIARRHOEA; DIZZINESS; FAINT FEELING; HEADACHE (see opposite); NAUSEA (see opposite); VOMITING.
Better for lying down.
Worse for fresh air; after eating; after drinking; for movement; for sitting up.

Getting up causes dizziness and nausea; needs to lie down to prevent vomiting.

COCCUS CACTI (Cocc-c.)
Other name: cochineal

Physical complaints
Cough

Choking; in fits; irritating; violent; whooping; racking. Tickling in LARYNX. MUCUS copious after each coughing fit; sticky. THROAT dry.
Better for fresh air.
Worse in a stuffy room; around 11.30 p.m.

One of the main whooping-cough remedies. Mucus drips down back of throat, irritating larynx, causing hawking which in turn leads to coughing fits that end in retching and vomiting of mucus. Mucus hangs in strings from the mouth.

COFFEA CRUDA (Coff.)
Other name: coffee

General symptoms

Senses acute. Sensitive to pain; to noise.
Worse for fresh air; at night; for touch.

Coffea affects the nerves: look for overexcitement and oversensitivity. All senses, touch, sight, hearing, smell and taste, become acute.

Both coffee as a drink and *Coffea* can counteract the effect of some homeopathic remedies. See p. 21 for guidance.

Emotional state

Cheerful. Complaints from excitement; joy. **Despair. Euphoric. Excitable. Exhilarated. Fearful** of painful death – during labour. **Joking** during labour. **Lively. Moaning. Restless. Screaming** with pain. **Tearful** during labour.

A remedy for excessive euphoria, but also where the slightest pain induces despair: makes a fuss over minor aches and pains. During labour may be excitable and restless then despairing, fearing death, chattiness turning to moaning (wailing) and crying. May be sensitive to noise.

Physical complaints

Headache

NERVOUS. PAIN one-sided.
Worse for noise.

May be worse in the fresh air and may feel as if a nail is being driven into the brain.

Insomnia

With DREAMS, VIVID.
Worse during pregnancy.
Cause cramp, during pregnancy; overactive mind; over-excitement.

Sleeps lightly, waking at every sound; unable to sleep because of excitement, ideas and plans. Sleeplessness from good news!

Labour

LABOUR PAINS in back; distressing; ineffectual (cervix doesn't dilate); irregular; severe; stopping (or slowing down). With TALKATIVENESS.

Toothache

In NERVOUS PEOPLE. PAINS shooting/spasmodic.
Better for cold water.
Worse for hot food and drinks; heat.

Pain in the tooth is eased by holding cold water (especially ice-cold water) in the mouth, but returns as soon as the water warms up.

COLCHICUM AUTUMNALE (Colch.)

Other name: meadow saffron

General symptoms

Exhaustion. Sense of smell acute. **Sweat** sour. **Thirstless.**
Better for sitting.
Worse in the autumn; for cold; for damp; for movement; at night; for the sight of food; for touch.

These types are sensitive to cold and damp and their symptoms are worse at night. Movement of any sort, including walking, aggravates their pains and the only comfortable position is sitting. A keynote of the remedy is the heightened sense of smell; if unwell, cooking smells exacerbate symptoms and/or induce faintness. Sensitivity to smell is at its worst with egg, which induces nausea and/or vomiting.

Emotional state

Complaints from anger. **Memory** weak.

A small remedy with few strongly marked emotional characteristics. May be absent-minded and forgetful; sensitive to anger and conflict. Symptoms – diarrhoea, nausea or painful joints – are worse after, say, an argument.

Physical complaints

Diarrhoea

STOOLS jelly-like; with mucus; watery. PAIN on passing stools.
Cause damp weather.

Diarrhoea may accompany joint complaints that are worse in damp weather of autumn.

Flatulence

ABDOMEN/STOMACH feels bloated. WIND obstructed (difficult to expel).

Joint pain

PAIN in hands and feet; acute; tearing. With SWELLING.
Better for warmth.
Worse for cold, wet weather; for movement; for warm weather.

'Rheumatism' affects the small joints of the hands and feet, which may be better for being wrapped up and kept warm and are worse for touch. Toe joints become especially sensitive: accidental stubbing is agonisingly painful. Severe, tearing pains may be accompanied by general weakness.

Nausea

ABDOMEN/STOMACH feels bloated. APPETITE lost. With FAINTNESS; VOMITING (see below).
Worse after eating; for smell and sight of food.

Intense loathing at the sight, smell or thought of food, and nausea exacerbated particularly by the smell of eggs and fish. May be dry retching. The nausea is much worse than the vomiting.

Vomiting

PAIN burning; sore, bruised. With RETCHING after vomiting.
Worse for smell of eggs.

Stomach is distended and may feel cold.

COLOCYNTHIS (Coloc.)

Other name: bitter cucumber

Emotional state

Complaints from anger; humiliation; indignation. **Restless.**

Physical symptoms may develop from feeling angry or humiliated; pain causes intense anguish, restlessness and irritability.

Physical complaints

Colic

In BABIES. ABDOMEN/STOMACH feels bloated. PAINS cutting; griping; tearing; violent; in waves. With DIARRHOEA (see above); NAUSEA; VOMITING. **Dislikes** food in general; smell of food.
Better for bending double; for pressure; for passing a stool.
Worse after drinking; for cold drinks when overheated; before a stool; after eating fruit.
Cause anger; eating fruit; excitement; vexation.

Pains are so severe as to cause vomiting. A young baby commonly pulls its legs up to its abdomen and screams. Older sufferers double up with the pain and press hard on the affected area (they may dig their fists into the abdomen or bend over the back of a chair, twisting and turning to find relief). Eating, especially fruit, will aggravate the pain.

Cramp

In THIGH; LEG; CALF.

Diarrhoea

STOOLS green; pasty. With COLIC (see opposite).
Worse after eating fruit; after eating.
Cause anger; eating fruit.

Headache

PAIN on left side of face; spreads up to ear; tearing.
Worse for touch.
Cause excitement; vexation.

Sciatica

PAINS tearing.
Worse on right side of body.

Pains are usually worse for movement, pressure and touch and although they may be better for warmth are often worse for the warmth of bed at night.

CONIUM MACULATUM (Con.)

Other name: common hemlock

General symptoms

Complaints from accident/injury. **Dizziness. Palpitations** in pregnancy. **Sweat** during sleep; hot; at night; on closing eyes.
Worse on lying down.
Better for sitting down.

Those needing this remedy feel better when sitting letting the limbs hang (not cross-legged). Sweating may be profuse and occurs strangely on closing the eyes as well as during sleep.

Emotional state

Anxious. Apathetic. Depressed during pregnancy. **Memory** weak. **Sensitive** to noise. **Slow.**

Easily startled by noise, and sensitive to light, these are melancholic types whose brains seize up after a period of mental strain. Unable to read, they may sit looking vacant, feeling anxious and not wanting to work.

Physical complaints

Breast(feeding) problems

BREAST LUMPS worse in right breast.

Cough

Dry; irritating; tickling; violent; must sit up as soon as cough starts. EXPECTORATION difficult; must swallow what comes up.

Worse lying down in bed; in the evening; for deep breathing; during fever.

Cough caused by dry, tickling spot in larynx, brought on by lying down (day or night). Sits up to cough, then lies down to rest. Exhausting cough, often accompanied by a fever.

Dizziness

With TURNING SENSATION. With HEADACHE.
Worse for moving or turning the head quickly; for lying down.

Feels as if turning in a circle; cannot watch moving objects. Better when quite still with eyes closed.

Exhaustion

With TREMBLING; NUMBNESS.
Better for fresh air.
Worse for slightest exertion; after stool; for walking.

Injuries

To GLANDS, breasts. To HEAD. Stony hard lumps, sensitive, swollen, cold, inflamed.

Injured parts become lumpy and painful and feel stony hard. Tingling with stitching pains, after a bang or bruise.

Insomnia

In PREGNANCY. SLEEPLESS before midnight. With NIGHTMARES.
Cause movements of baby (in PREGNANCY).

Nausea

In PREGNANCY. With RETCHING and VOMITING.

CUPRUM METALLICUM (Cupr.)

Other name: copper

General symptoms

Extremities cold. **Face** blue; pale. **Lips** blue. **Pains** cramping. **Taste** sweet.
Better for cold drinks.
Worse for touch; for vomiting.

Cramp is an important part of the *Cuprum* picture; muscles feel knotted up. Tiredness is from mental exhaustion or sometimes loss of sleep; headaches and cramp may follow a period of heavy work. Looks pale and drawn.

Emotional state

Restless at night in bed.

This remedy does not have a strong 'character'; its general symptoms and physical complaints will lead you to prescribe it.

Physical complaints
Afterpains

With CRAMP IN FINGERS AND/OR TOES.

Especially useful for women who have had three or more children.

Colic

PAIN cramping; violent. With NAUSEA; VOMITING. Abdomen sore, bruised, tender and hot.

Convulsions

Cause teething in babies; vexation.

Accompanied by blue lips, cold hands and feet (see COUGH).

Cough

In long fits at irregular intervals; uninterrupted; suffocative; violent; whooping. BREATHING difficult; fast.
Better for sips of cold water (like *Causticum*).

Cold air may aggravate; mouth may taste metallic. During coughing fit, baby is breathless, becomes stiff, and a convulsion with fingers and toes twitching may follow. Between coughing fits, breathing is hurried and panting. A very serious cough, frightening for parents: professional help should always be sought immediately. Meanwhile, *Cuprum* will give relief and other medication may be avoided.

Cramp

In CALF; FOOT; LEG.
Cause childbirth (see LABOUR, p. 203).

Exhaustion

With HEADACHE between the eyes.
Cause loss of sleep.
Worse for mental exhaustion.

Labour

LABOUR PAINS with CRAMP in hand or leg, finger or toe. With vomiting.

CYPRIPEDIUM (Cypr.)

Other name: yellow lady's slipper

Physical complaints
Insomnia

In RESTLESS BABIES who wake to play at night.
Cause nervous exhaustion.

Overstimulation may cause chronic sleeplessness. Wakes in the middle of the night, is wide awake and plays happily for an hour or more. Nip this in the bud before it gets completely out of hand – the baby may sleep only a few hours every night, becoming hyperactive and unmanageable.

DIOSCOREA (Dios.)

Other name: wild yam

Physical complaints
Colic

In BABIES. ABDOMEN/STOMACH rumbling; windy. PAIN cramping; cutting; griping; around the navel; twisting.
Better for bending back; for stretching out.
Worse for bending forward; during the morning.

An infant arches back and screams (opposite of *Colocynthis* picture with its drawing up of legs). Has a rumbly, windy abdomen, does not want to lie down but is better for being held upright.

DROSERA ROTUNDIFOLIA (Dros.)

Other name: sundew

Physical complaints
Cough

Barking; deep; dry at night; in violent fits; hacking; irritating; suffocative; tormenting. BREATHING difficult; fast. LARYNX tickling. PAIN IN CHEST holds chest with hands to cough. With NOSE-BLEEDS; BLUE FACE; VOICE HOARSE; RETCHING; VOMITING of mucus.
Better for pressure.
Worse after midnight; after drinking; for lying down; for warmth of bed; for talking.
Cause after measles.

Typical severe cough of whooping cough often starts with tickling at back of throat, usually accompanied in its acute phase by retching and vomiting and sometimes nosebleeds. Breathing either speeds up during coughing or is difficult (coughing fits so violent that it is often impossible to breathe and cough at the same time so face becomes bluish). Coughing attacks follow each other rapidly, especially at night, and will often be set off as soon as the head touches the pillow. Cough is painful and chest becomes sore and bruised from coughing; holds chest with both hands when coughs as pressure helps to ease the pain. Voice becomes hoarse from coughing.

Sore throat

In BABIES. ABDOMEN/STOMACH rumbling, windy. PAIN.
Worse for swallowing.

Larynx sore and inflamed with an irritating feeling of dust in it. Voice becomes deep and husky.

DULCAMARA (Dulc.)

Other name: woody nightshade

General symptoms

Catches colds easily. **Complaints from** change of weather to damp; weaning.
Better for movement; for walking.
Worse for wet weather; for cold; for damp; for lying down; at night; for sitting still.

Lacking 'vital heat', these types are sensitive to cold and damp. They have a tendency to catch colds, especially in the winter. An unusual symptom is the strong need to urinate (or pass a stool) after becoming chilled or spending time in a cold place. A baby may develop rashes after weaning on to solid foods.

Emotional state

There are few strong emotional symptoms for this remedy; but they may be depressed, irritably impatient or quarrelsome.

Physical complaints
Backache

In LOWER BACK. PAIN aching; sore, bruised. With LAMENESS.
Better for movement; for walking.
Worse for wet weather.
Cause change of weather; damp weather; getting cold; getting wet.

Lower back aches as if from long stooping.

Breast(feeding) problems

MILK SUPPLY low in chilly women.

Common cold

NOSE blocked.

Nasal discharge may be thick and yellow but nose more likely to be blocked. Often better for keeping the head warm; may sit with head under a blanket or a scarf pulled up over the nose. Winter colds clear once summer warmth is established and return with cold weather the following autumn.

Cough

Rattling.
Cause damp weather.

Cough may develop from a sore throat. Has to cough for a long time before expelling mucus.

Cystitis

URINATION involuntary (incontinence).
Cause getting cold and wet.

Give after *Aconite* (if it hasn't helped), where cystitis developed after getting cold and wet, and where there are as yet no remarkable symptoms.

Diarrhoea

In TEETHING BABIES. PAINFUL. STOOLS yellow; watery.
Worse after eating cold food; at night.
Cause getting cold; getting damp; teething.

Pains are generally worse before the stool and may be accompanied by nausea.

Eye inflammation

Cause wet weather.

Often accompanies a common cold.

Flu

Cause cold, damp weather.

Hives

RASH lumpy.
Worse for heat; after scratching.
Cause getting cold.

Rash burns after scratching and, although brought on by getting cold, is worse for warmth, for example after exercise.

Joint pain

Better for movement.
Worse for sitting; at night.
Cause damp; getting cold.
Pains in joints come on after staying in a damp house, or sleeping in a damp bed.

Snuffles

In newborn babies. With EYE INFLAMMATION or COMMON COLD (see opposite).

EUPATORIUM PERFOLIATUM (Eup-p.)
Other name: agueweed

General symptoms

Pain sore; bruised; in bones. **Sweat** scanty. **Thirsty** for cold drinks; unquenchable.

Eupatorium resembles *Bryonia*: both have similar flu symptoms, but *Eupatorium* has terrible pains in the bones and great restlessness whereas *Bryonia* prefers to be completely still. *Eupatorium* symptoms may be better while sweating, except the headache.

Emotional state

Depressed.

Feels sad and depressed during flu, and lies about moaning during the fever.

Physical complaints
Fever

Sleepy, yawns and falls asleep all the time. With characteristic thirst and scanty sweat.

Flu

EYEBALLS ACHING. EYELIDS RED. PAIN in bones; bones feel broken. SKIN SORE. With SHIVERING; CHILLS in back; HEADACHE (see below); NASAL CATARRH; SNEEZING.
Better for sweating.

An awful flu with intense aching pains in the scalp, bones of arms, legs and lower back (sometimes the hips as well). The skin all over the body, even the scalp, feels dry and sore.

Gastric flu

With FEVER; NAUSEA; RETCHING; VOMITING of bile; of food.
Better after chills; during fever.

Very thirsty before vomiting.

Headache

PAIN in back of head; sore, bruised; throbbing. With FEVER (see p. 204).
Worse for sweating.

EUPHRASIA (Euphr.)

Other name: eyebright

Physical complaints

Common cold

NASAL CATARRH bland; watery. With COUGH (see below); EYE INFLAMMATION.

Nasal discharge irritates and the watering eyes do not. Throat may also be sore; if it is, it will burn (the opposite of *Allium cepa*).

Cough

DAYTIME only. MUCUS copious.
Better for lying down.
Worse during the morning.

Hawks up a mouthful of mucus at a time and clears throat frequently.

Eye inflammation

DISCHARGE burning; watery. EYES sensitive to light; watery. EYELIDS burning; red; swollen. With COMMON COLD.
Worse for coughing; for light; for wind.
Cause common cold.

Eyes stream on coughing and are sensitive to light.

Eye injuries

With EYE INFLAMMATION (see opposite).

Measles

With COMMON COLD (see opposite); COUGH (see opposite); EYE INFLAMMATION (see opposite).

Fever not usually very high. Does not necessarily feel very ill.

FERRUM METALLICUM (Ferr-m.)

Other name: iron

General symptoms

Appetite lost, alternating with hunger. **Face** pale; pasty; flushes easily; red with pain. **Gums** pale. **Oedema** (swelling) of feet/ankles; of hands/fingers. **Sweat** clammy; cold; profuse; worse for lying down and for slightest physical exertion.
Better for walking slowly.
Worse on beginning to move; at night; for lying down.

Becomes easily exhausted and breathless, and the typically pale face becomes flushed, not only with exertion but when excited, and when in pain or with a fever. Benefits from gentle exercise, which helps generally and relieves many symptoms.
    Not very hungry and appetite comes in bursts; experiences fullness after eating very little. Digestive disorders are marked and peculiar: has an intolerance of eggs; suffers from diarrhoea while eating (it actually comes on when they begin to eat, a symptom peculiar to *Ferrum metallicum*). Experiences periodic vomiting around midnight.

Emotional state

Depressed. Irritable. Moody. Restless in bed.

Anaemic, nervous, irritable and worn out. If stuck in bed feeling ill, will forever be getting out of bed to wander around aimlessly.

Physical complaints

Anaemia

In PREGNANCY. LIPS pale. With EXHAUSTION (see p. 206).
Cause loss of blood.

With characteristically pale face that flushes easily.

Backache

In LOWER BACK.
Better for walking slowly.
Worse on beginning to move.

Breathless

In PREGNANCY.
Better for gentle exercise; for a stroll.

Cough

In fits.
Better for walking slowly.
Worse after getting up; for movement.

Diarrhoea

TEETHING. PAINLESS. STOOLS containing undigested food; passed with wind. With BELCHING; FLATULENCE.
Worse after drinking water; for movement; at night; while eating.
Cause teething.

After eating burps taste of food recently consumed. Passes wind *with* the diarrhoea.

Dizziness

With NAUSEA.
Worse for getting up from bending down/lying down/sitting.

Exhaustion

With DESIRE TO LIE DOWN.
Better for walking slowly in the fresh air.
Worse for exercise.
Cause anaemia; sweating.

A mental as well as physical exhaustion. Person doesn't want to work.

Fever

Better for uncovering.

Has the typical pale face which flushes easily.

Headache

PAIN in forehead; hammering; throbbing. With THIRSTLESSNESS.

Better for firm pressure; for lying down.
Worse for moving head.

Headaches last 2–3 days at a time and are very draining. Has to lie down, and refuses drinks; face is alternately hot and flushed or pale and drained.

Joint pain

PAINS in shoulder; in upper arm; stitching; tearing.
Better for gentle movement.
Worse on beginning to move; for lifting arm up; for bending arm backwards.

Nosebleeds

In babies.

Sciatica

Better for gentle movement; for walking slowly.

Varicose veins

Of LEG/THIGH; of FOOT. PAINFUL; SWOLLEN.
Worse during pregnancy.

Often accompanied by anaemia and tiredness.

Vomiting

Sudden; of food.
Worse after eating eggs; after midnight; at night.

Food either comes up suddenly while eating or lies in the stomach all day, coming up around midnight.

GELSEMIUM SEMPERVIRENS (Gels.)

Other name: yellow jasmine

General symptoms

Exhaustion paralytic. **Eyelids** heavy. **Feeling of heaviness. Onset of complaint** slow. **Sweat** absent during fever. **Thirstless. Trembling**.
Better for sweating; for urination.
Worse for physical exertion.

Intensely weary types: body feels heavy (arms and legs feel as if weighted down with lead); becomes trembly with exhaustion and consequently worse for any additional physical exertion, only feeling better temporarily after urination.

Acute *Gelsemium* complaints (for example, flu) come on gradually, taking days to develop, coming on when the weather changes to warm after the cold of winter, for those who spend their lives in overheated houses. *Bryonia* is similar, but is thirsty and keeps still because of pain, whereas *Gelsemium* is thirstless and cannot move for heaviness and weariness.

Emotional state

Anxious babies. **Apathetic** during labour. **Clingy. Complaints from** receiving bad news; excitement. **Depressed** but cannot cry. **Desires** to be alone. **Despairing** during labour. **Dislikes** company. **Excitable** during pregnancy. **Fearful** of falling; of public speaking; in a crowd; of death. **Sluggish.**

These are dull, sluggish types who want to be left alone, to be quiet. *Gelsemium* is a favourite remedy for those paralysed with fear, mentally and physically, before an important event; not the active fear of *Argentum nitricum* or *Lycopodium*, more an acute anxiety. Tremble, stutter and cannot collect their thoughts. May even look, as well as feel, stupid. Like *Natrum muriaticum* and *Ignatia* find it difficult to cry if depressed, typically after receiving a piece of bad news. Likewise over-excitement causes illness, either emotional or physical.

Physical complaints

Braxton Hicks contractions

In pregnancy.

Diarrhoea

Cause anticipatory anxiety; bad/exciting news; fright/ shock.

Dizziness

In pregnancy.

Fever

Heat burning. With SHIVERING. WITHOUT SWEATING.
Better for sweating; for urinating.
Worse during the afternoon.

Waves of heat alternate with chills running up and down the back; although the teeth may chatter, doesn't feel cold. Chills begin in hands and feet and move up the body. May be breathing faster than normal.

Flu

EYEBALLS aching. PAIN in muscles. With EXHAUSTION (see General symptoms); HEAVINESS; NUMBNESS; SHIVERING/CHILLS in back.

Better for sweating; for urinating.
Worse for exertion; for walking.

A flu that may come on in mild, damp weather or from getting chilled. Tongue feels thick and heavy and speech is slurred. Back aches from the lower back up and over the head. Arms and legs ache and feel extremely heavy and tired. Extremely chilly, and cannot get warm.

Headache

FEET cold. HEAD feels heavy. PAIN in back of head; spreading to forehead; aching; sore, bruised. PUPILS dilated. URINATION FREQUENT. VISION blurred.
Better for urinating.
Worse for movement; for moving head.

Head feels so heavy that it needs support, of hands or a pillow; also feels constricted, as if a band or hoop were encircling it. Has difficulty opening the eyes or keeping them open as the lids feel so heavy. Urine is copious and colourless. Thirstless and feels better for urinating.

Labour

LABOUR LATE with anticipatory anxiety. LABOUR PAINS in back; distressing; false; ineffectual (cervix doesn't soften); weak. With TREMBLING.

A valuable remedy for backache in labour when baby is 'posterior'. Becomes apathetic, despairing and thirstless.

Measles

ONSET slow. With FEVER (see opposite); HEADACHE (see above).

With typical *Gelsemium* heaviness, drowsiness and lack of thirst.

GLONOINE (Glon.)

Other name: nitro-glycerine

General symptoms

Complaints from sunstroke. **Face** red.
Better for cold applications.
Worse for jarring movement; for heat; for exposure to sun.

The principal use of this remedy is for headaches after too much sun. Heat in any form aggravates, as does any jarring movement like walking.

Emotional state

Confused. **Forgetful**. **Time** passes slowly. **Uncommunicative**.

Unwilling to talk or answer questions. Appears dull and confused; familiar surroundings feel strange.

Physical complaints
Headache

EYES red. FACE red. PAIN bursting; hammering; throbbing; violent. With FAINTNESS; HOT FLUSHES.
Better for cold compresses; for pressure; at sunset.
Worse for heat; for jarring movement; at sunrise; during summer; for mental exertion; for walking.
Cause overexposure to sun.

Headache increases when exposed to the sun and is better for being pressed firmly with the hands. Feels faint and flushed and as if the head will burst. Ice pack may ease the pain.

Sunstroke

With HEADACHE (see above).

HAMAMELIS VIRGINICA (Ham.)
Other name: witch hazel

General symptoms

Pains sore, bruised.
Worse for touch.

A small remedy whose use for acute complaints is limited to nosebleeds, varicose veins and piles, but useful, taken as a tonic, for these symptoms. Pains are commonly worse for touch. No marked emotional/mental symptoms.

Physical complaints
Nosebleed

BLOOD dark; thin.
Worse during the morning.

Phlebitis

After labour. With prickling pains in veins/legs.

Piles

LARGE; BLEEDING. PAIN sore, bruised.
Cause childbirth; pregnancy.

These piles occur towards the end of pregnancy, and after childbirth (because of the pressure of the baby). Once *Arnica* has been given as a routine prescription for the bleeding, if soreness persists and a bigger remedy not indicated, *Hamamelis* will help. It is essential to seek professional help for both varicose veins and piles if the symptoms do not clear easily.

Varicose veins

Of LEGS/THIGHS; of VULVA. PAINFUL; SWOLLEN. PAIN stinging.
Worse for touch; after childbirth; during pregnancy.

Hard knotty varicose veins; sore, bruised and sensitive to touch.

HEPAR SULPHURIS CALCAREUM (Hep-s.)
Other name: calcium sulphide

General symptoms

Catches colds easily. **Complaints from** cold wind. **Likes** sour foods. **Pains** needle-like. **Sweat** cold; profuse; sour.
Better for warmth of bed; for heat; for wrapping up.
Worse for getting cold; for cold dry weather; for fresh air; for lying on painful side; at night; for pressure; for touch; for uncovering; for cold wind.

One of the chilliest remedies in the Materia Medica, these types hate the cold, especially dry cold, and because they lack internal warmth they catch colds more easily than others who are more resilient. Are so sensitive to cold when sick that if a part of the body – hand or foot – escapes the bedclothes feel worse and start to cough or sneeze. Highly sensitive to pain, may weep or even faint in anticipation of it. They do not want to be touched when sick.

Symptoms usually worse at night and may develop when asleep: may cough more in the night, for example. Only really better for lying in bed, well wrapped up, with the windows well shut and the heating on.

Emotional state

Violently **angry. Impulsive. Irritable. Play** – doesn't want to. **Sensitive** generally; to rudeness. **Hurried** generally; eating; speaking.

Over-sensitivity is the special feature that runs through this remedy. Morose, difficult individuals, they are easily offended and prone to fits of anger. When sick they are extremely difficult, and often obstructive in giving information while demanding angrily to be cured. They are also impulsive and speedy, like *Argentum nitricum*.

Physical complaints

Abscesses

Of GLANDS; of ROOTS OF TEETH; of BREASTS.

A major abscess remedy but generally only useful before the abscess has opened and started to discharge. Indicated at the swollen, painful stage, especially if this is accompanied by splinter-like pains and a great sensitivity to touch.

Common cold

NASAL CATARRH drips down back of throat; smelly; yellow. SNEEZING on uncovering.
Worse for uncovering.

Bones of the nose may feel sore and sense of smell may be lost. Sneezing brought on by draughts.

Constipation

STOOL soft.

Constipation may accompany any of the acute symptoms, such as cough or earache. Stool is passed with difficulty.

Cough

Barking; dry during the evening/night; loose during the morning; hacking; irritating; suffocative; violent. MUCUS copious; sticky; thick; tough; yellow. With HOARSE VOICE; RETCHING; SWEATING; VOMITING.
Worse for cold dry air; for being uncovered; on single parts of body; for uncovering hands; evening in bed; before midnight.
Cause exposure to cold dry wind.

A bad cough with irritation in the larynx; chest becomes sore from coughing. The simple act of going to bed may also set off the cough (as soon as eyes are closed cough starts up again).

Croup

RECURRENT. With symptoms of COUGH (see above).

Many of the general symptoms and cough symptoms are present in the croup. *Hepar* croup is usually worse in the early morning (if it is worse in the evening it is more likely to be *Aconite*); slightest breath of cold air causes coughing, as does uncovering. Chokes,

wheezes and rattles, but bringing up mucus is difficult.

Diarrhoea

PAINLESS.

Rumbling in the abdomen accompanies this diarrhoea.

Earache

DISCHARGE smelly. PAINS stitching.
Better for wrapping up warmly.
Worse for cold.

Fever

HEAT alternating with chills.
Better for heat.
Worse for being uncovered.

Slightest exertion can bring on coughing and sweating, which is cold, sour-smelling and profuse. Sweating provides no relief.

Inflammation of navel

In newborn babies.

If it doesn't help within 48 hours give *Silica*.

Injuries

CUTS/WOUNDS with inflammation; SLOW TO HEAL; PAINFUL. PAIN sore; splinter-like.

For cuts, including episiotomy, and injuries where the skin is broken and healing taking longer than expected. Redness (inflammation) develops around the site of the injury which is generally sensitive to touch.

Joint pain

In fingers; hip; shoulder; sore, bruised; pulling; tearing.
Better for heat.
Worse for cold.
Cause getting cold.

Sore throat

PAIN spreading up to ear; raw; splinter-like. TONSILS swollen.
Better for hot drinks; for warm compresses.
Worse for breathing in cold air; for coughing; for swallowing; for turning the head; for cold drinks; in winter.
Cause getting cold; exposure to wind.

Throat feels as if there were a splinter or a fish bone stuck in it and the pains radiate up to the ear on swallowing, turning the head and sometimes even when yawning. Tonsils are swollen and ulcerated and the neck is sensitive to pressure/touch and better for being wrapped up warmly.

HYPERICUM PERFOLIATUM (Hyp.)
Other name: St John's wort

General symptoms

Complaints from accident/injuries to nerves/coccyx.
Pains shooting.
Worse for cold; for pressure.

The first remedy to think of when a nerve-rich part of the body is injured, that is, fingers, toes, spine (especially the coccyx), eyes, lips, and so on. Intense pains, usually tearing, severe and sensitive to touch, shoot along the course of wounded nerves towards the trunk or up the spine. Give *Arnica* first to prevent swelling and bruising and follow with *Hypericum*, repeated every few minutes if the pain is excruciating. Use external remedies to clean dirty wounds.

Emotional state

Shock from injury.

Has no major emotional symptoms apart from the shock.

Physical complaints
Afterpains

With HEADACHE.
Cause forceps delivery.

PAINS may be bad in hips and lower back.

Backache

PAINS in COCCYX; in LOWER BACK; sore, bruised; shooting; tearing.
Cause childbirth; forceps delivery; epidural; injury to coccyx; injury to spine.

Useful for any trauma to spinal nerves, which might occur during childbirth, or after an injury to the coccyx causing lasting pain and soreness.

Bites/stings

BITES inflamed. PAIN shooting; tearing up nerve pathways.
Cause animal bites; insect bites.

Inflamed, exceptionally painful bites on nerve-rich parts.

Injuries

CUTS/WOUNDS to nerve-rich parts; crushed; punctured; lacerated; slow to heal. PAINS shooting.
Cause accident; dentistry; splinter; surgery.

Wounds are inflamed and very painful. The pain is often more severe than the injury seems to warrant, because the nerves are injured (squashing a finger in a car door, stepping on a nail, tearing off a finger- or toenail, cutting the lips, or a splinter in the hand). If the pains are severe and shoot up the body, *Hypericum* is the correct first-aid remedy. Also useful after any type of surgery where nerves are cut and painful or feel frayed or sore, for example, in teeth (root canals); gums (after dental work and/or extraction); abdominal surgery (appendicectomy, Caesarean).

IGNATIA AMARA (Ign.)
Other name: St Ignatius's bean

General symptoms

Aversion to fresh air. **Dislikes** fruit; milk; tobacco. **Sweat** hot; on single parts of body. **Symptoms** contradictory.
Better after eating; for heat.
Worse after drinking coffee; for tobacco.

They experience contradictory symptoms, such as an empty feeling in the stomach that is not relieved by eating, or a sore throat that is worse when not swallowing. They are generally sensitive to coffee which brings on shakiness, and tobacco, which results in headaches. They feel worse for fresh air, which quickly chills them, and better for warmth.

Emotional state

Anxious during pregnancy; after shock. **Broody. Complaints from** anger; anger with anxiety; death of a child; disappointed love; fright; grief; humiliation; reprimands; shock; suppression of emotions. **Conscientious. Depressed** from suppressed grief; during pregnancy. **Desires** to be alone. **Despair. Disappointment. Dislikes** consolation; contradiction. **Guilt. Idealistic. Indeci-**

sive. **Introspective. Involuntary** weeping. **Moody. Quarrelsome. Resentful. Sensitive** generally; to pain. **Sentimental. Sighing. Tearful** cries on own; during pregnancy.

The *Ignatia* character is formed largely by the suppression of emotions, rather than any general physical characteristics. *Ignatia* complaints come on typically after emotional upset, be it grief (a loss or bereavement), or shock, or anger where anxiety is also present, or from being told off, punished or contradicted. They suffer inwardly, becoming introspective and moody.

They experience great highs and lows: the highs are when everything is OK – only the sighing may give the game away – and the lows are rarely seen because of their innate secretiveness. They torment themselves with recollections of the offence or (emotional) injury they have received. Also for emotional shock, when feelings have been suppressed and 'hysterical' symptoms developed as a result. They become nervous and excitable.

Physical complaints

Bleeding (vaginal) in pregnancy

Cause grief; emotional shock.

Cough

Dry; irritating; racking; short; violent. PAIN IN CHEST stitching. With THROAT tickling.
Worse for coughing; during the evening in bed.

Feels as if a feather or dust is in the pit of the throat. Suppressing cough helps – the more the coughing, the worse it becomes (this contradictory symptom should guide you straight to this remedy). May be useful in croup or whooping cough if the symptoms fit.

Fever

THIRST with chills.
Better for uncovering.
Worse during the afternoon; on front of body; for warm covers.

Thirsty during the chilly stage rather than when hot and feverish – an *Ignatia* contradictory symptom.

Headache

PAIN in forehead: stabbing; violent.
Worse in a smoky room.

Nervous headaches that start gradually and stop sud-

denly, or start and stop suddenly. Feels as though a nail were being driven into the side(s) of the head. Often set off by emotional upsets.

Indigestion

ABDOMEN/STOMACH feels empty. BELCHES sour.
Better for belching.
Cause grief.

Insomnia

In pregnancy.
Cause shock.

Piles

INTERNAL. PAINS shooting.
Better for walking.
Worse after childbirth; after passing stool.

Shock

Cause emotional trauma.

Like *Phosphoric acid*, shock needing *Ignatia* will have been sparked off by some emotional shock or loss.

Sore throat

PAIN stitching. With LUMP SENSATION in throat; CHOKING SENSATION.
Better for swallowing.
Worse when not swallowing; evenings.

The sore throat is worse when not swallowing (a contradictory symptom). Liquids may be more difficult to swallow than solids. There is often a sensation of a lump in the throat – often associated with suppressed desire to cry or express some upset.

IPECACUANHA (Ip.)

General symptoms

Dislikes food in general; smell of food. **Face** red, one-sided; blue during cough. **Nausea** persistent; violent. **Sweat** hot or cold.
Worse at night.

Violent and persistent nausea accompanies virtually all complaints (headache, diarrhoea, labour pains, whooping cough, haemorrhage, etc.). Looks deathly, with a drawn, bluish face and dark-ringed eyes; may be covered with a hot or cold sweat. May feel chilly externally and hot inside. Complaints recur periodically, at regular or intermittent intervals.

Emotional state

Anxious during a fever. **Capricious. Complaints from** anger; vexation.

The *Ipecacuanha* baby is capricious, pleased by nothing; screams or howls with frustration if thwarted. When ill, is anxious and generally difficult to look after. Complaints come on after getting angry or frustrated.

Physical complaints

Bleeding

After childbirth (haemorrhage). FLOW OF BLOOD bright red. With severe NAUSEA.

Colic

PAINS aching; cramping; griping.
Worse for movement.

Often accompanies the *Ipecacuanha* nausea and vomiting.

Cough

Choking; dry; in fits; irritating; rattling; tormenting; vomiting; whooping. BREATHING difficult; fast; wheezing. MUCUS bloody; difficult to cough up. With NAUSEA (see opposite); NOSEBLEEDS; RETCHING; BLUE FACE.
Worse during a fever.

May complain of irritation in the larynx or air passages. Nosebleed produces bright red blood. Babies go stiff during coughing fits and have difficulty breathing (catching their breath).

Diarrhoea

In BABIES. STOOLS grass green.

Fever

With ANXIETY. CHILLINESS worse for heat; better for fresh air.

Flu

CHILLS. PAINS in bones; in back; in legs; aching; sore, bruised.

Feels weary, as if has carried a heavy load; bones may feel torn to pieces. Chills are worse in a warm room and better for fresh air. Nausea may well be present.

Gastric flu

See FLU (opposite).

Headache

PAINS sore, bruised. With VOMITING (see below).

Labour

LABOUR PAINS. With constant NAUSEA.

Nausea

BELCHES empty. With PALLID FACE; RETCHING; copious SALIVA.
Worse after eating; for movement; for smell of food; for tobacco.

Feels nauseous but finds vomiting difficult and the nausea will persist even if able to vomit. The tongue is usually clean.

Vomiting

VOMIT bile; food; green. With HEADACHE.
Worse after eating; after bending down; for coughing.

JABORANDI (Jab.)

Other name: Pilocarpus pinnatifolius

Physical complaints

Mumps

With FACE RED. GLANDS swollen. PAINS spread to breasts, ovaries. Copious SALIVA. Profuse SWEATING.

Sweat starts on the face and spreads over the body. Saliva is like egg white, and although it runs freely the mouth feels dry. The jaw is stiff and the tonsils are often swollen. Given early enough, *Jaborandi* prevents involvement of other glands (breasts, ovaries, testicles). The sweaty stage is accompanied by an acute thirst, followed by prostration and drowsiness and a general feeling of dryness. *Mercurius solubilis* presents a similar picture with its salivation and sweating but the smelly breath and sweat is less marked with *Jaborandi*.

KALI BICHROMICUM (Kali-b.)

Other name: potassium bichromate

General symptoms

Discharges stringy/sticky; thick. **Pains** appear and disappear suddenly; in a spot; wandering. **Tongue** white-coated.

Worse in morning on waking; at night; for getting cold; after eating; in summer.

Smallish remedy, useful for colds and sinusitis. These are chilly individuals who are worse for cold, whose symptoms come on after getting cold. Become chilly when ill, yet feel worse in the summer's heat. The pains can usually be located with a fingertip and may wander about the body.

Physical complaints

Burns

DEEP. SLOW TO HEAL.

Common cold

NASAL CATARRH crusty; dry; hard crusts; smelly; thick; green; yellow; yellow-green; sticky; stringy. PAINFUL SINUSES with DRY THROAT.

Catarrh forms sticky crusts in nostrils, which are difficult to remove, leaving raw, sore patches, and then re-form. Catarrh drips down back of throat, accumulates overnight, and is difficult to hawk out in morning; or may block nose entirely and be impossible to blow out.

Cough

COUGH croupy. MUCUS ropy; sticky; tough; thick; difficult to cough up. PAIN IN CHEST sore, bruised. With VOICE HOARSE.

Worse after eating; on waking in the morning.

Pain in the chest spreads from front to back, and air passages are irritated and aggravate the cough. Ropy mucus tends to be coughed up only in the morning.

Croup

With COUGH symptoms (see above).

Earache

DISCHARGE thick; yellow; smelly. PAIN stitching.
Worse on left side.

Headache

PAIN recurring at regular intervals; in sinuses.

Usually comes on at the same time each day and although initially pain is in a small localised spot, it may extend to the whole head, especially if sinus congestion is severe.

Joint pain

PAIN alternating with indigestion; alternating with cough; in one spot; sore, bruised; wandering.

Unlikely to suffer joint pain and common cold symptoms at the same time.

KALI CARBONICUM (Kali-c.)

Other name: potassium carbonate

General symptoms

Anaemia. Catches colds easily. **Dislikes** bread. **Exhaustion. Hot flushes. Pains** stitching. **Sweat** on single parts of the body; after eating; after the slightest physical exertion; profuse.

Better for warmth of bed.

Worse for becoming cold; for cold, dry weather; for draughts; for lying on side; around 2–4 a.m.; for getting overheated; at night; for touch; for uncovering.

This picture may be hard to spot. These types are extremely weak, wary and often anaemic. They sweat easily and, being chilly, they catch cold easily. They are sensitive to draughts but dislike being overheated as this produces hot flushes. They feel generally better for warmth. Pain is characteristically sharp, stitching, and worst between 2 and 4 a.m. They look puffy, especially around eyes and upper lids. Symptoms are worse for lying on the affected part.

Emotional state

Angry. Anxious children; during labour. **Desires** company; to be carried. **Dictatorial** (bossy) during labour. **Dislikes/aversion** to being touched; being alone. **Expression** haggard; suffering. **Fearful** of being alone during labour. **Irritable** during labour. **Jumpy. Sensitive** to noise. **Sluggish. Touchy.**

These are touchy individuals who are anxious, irritable and sluggish all at the same time. They do not want to be alone and yet they are not the welcoming type! They are highly strung, being easily startled both by noises and by unexpected touch, either while awake or asleep. They often talk and moan in their sleep.

Physical complaints

Afterpains

PAIN stitching; shooting down into buttocks/hips/legs.

Backache

In LOWER BACK. PAIN dragging; sore, bruised; stitching.
Better for pressure.
Worse around 3 a.m.; before menstrual period; after long sitting; for walking.
Causes pregnancy; childbirth.

May occur after injury, and pain, which is much worse in the early hours of the morning, may drive the sufferer out of bed.

Bleeding (vaginal) in pregnancy

With PAIN IN BACK spreading down into buttocks and thighs.

Constipation

In PREGNANCY. Large, hard STOOL. PAIN before a stool, with unfinished feeling.

Cough

BREATHING wheezing. COUGH dry; hard; irritating; loose; racking; vomiting; violent; disturbs sleep. PAIN IN CHEST cutting; stitching. With NAUSEA; VOMITING.
Worse for deep breathing; for becoming cold; during fever; during evening; for heat; for lying down; in morning; at night; for talking; around 3 a.m.
Cause getting chilled.

Has to sit up and lean forward to cough (typically rests elbows on knees) to get some relief. Chest pain with a cough (chest infection) is often right-sided and cutting, knife-like or stitching, with a feeling of irritation throughout respiratory tract. Coughs in those who are worn out.

Faintness

In PREGNANCY. HAS TO LIE DOWN.

Fever

SWEATING profuse; after slightest exertion.
Better in bed; for heat.
Worse after eating.

Headache

PAIN above eyes; in forehead; shooting; tearing.
Worse for cold; on left side of head.
Cause eye strain.

Indigestion

ABDOMEN/STOMACH feels bloated; full. PAIN sore, bruised.
Better for belching.
Worse after eating.

Feels bloated after eating: everything turns to gas.

Insomnia

DREAMS anxious; nightmares.
Worse before midnight; around 1–2 a.m.

Feels drowsy in the evening but is unable to get to sleep, or alternatively falls asleep easily, has awful and/or anxious dreams and wakes in the early morning, unable to get back to sleep again.

Joint pain

ARMS feel weak. RESTLESS LEGS. PAIN in arms/hip/legs/shoulder; sore, bruised; stitching; tearing.
Better for movement; for walking.
Worse around 2–3 a.m.; for lying on painful part.

Jerks on going to sleep. Hands and feet feel cold and numb and legs fall asleep easily.

Labour

PAIN in back, buttocks or thighs; distressing; ineffectual (cervix doesn't dilate); stops (or slows down); weak. With CHILLINESS (after a contraction); EXHAUSTION.
Better for hard pressure.

Piles

LARGE, protruding when passing a stool or coughing.
Worse for touch.
Cause childbirth.

KALI MURIATICUM (Kali-m.)
Other name: potassium chloride

General symptoms
Discharges white. **Tongue** white-coated.

This is a small remedy whose keynote is whiteness – and this is found everywhere: tongue, mouth, and all discharges. Consider it for any cold that has moved beyond the first stage and settled in but has not turned into a more serious infection (with yellow/green discharges).

Physical complaints

Common cold

NASAL CATARRH white. With DEAFNESS AFTER A COLD.

It is for stuffy head colds with thick white mucus and swollen glands.

Cough

Barking; hard; short.

Earache

With NOISES IN THE EAR. GLANDS swollen. **Worse** for swallowing.

Ears crackle and pop on blowing the nose or swallowing.

Indigestion

With DIARRHOEA; STOOLS pale. **Worse** after eating starchy food.

Sore throat

TONSILS swollen; white.

Thrush (oral)

In BREASTFEEDING BABIES. TONGUE/GUMS coated white.

KALI PHOSPHORICUM (Kali-p.)

Other name: potassium phosphate

General symptoms

Anaemia. **Exhaustion** caused by flu; nervous. **Sweating** when tired; profuse; after the slightest physical exertion.
Better for heat; for rest.
Worse for cold; for exercise; for excitement; for mental exertion; for worry.

Kali phosphoricum is a nerve nutrient found in tissues and fluids of brain and nerve cells, indicated in cases of nervous exhaustion where anaemia, nervous headaches and/or insomnia are present. Especially useful for exhaustion following a bad case of flu and also in convalescent stage of acute illness where there is muscular weakness. Sensitive to cold, cold in general, they feel much better for warmth.

Emotional state

Anxious babies – at night. **Complaints from** mental strain; overwork. **Depressed. Fearful** babies – at night. **Forgetful. Jumpy. Screaming** on waking. **Sensitive** babies.

For exhaustion with frayed nerves, following a heavy work or study period. The memory becomes unreliable. With resultant anxiety and the mind exhausted and sluggish. Sensitivity to noise and light is often present; may startle easily.

Physical complaints

Backache

Pain in SPINE; sore, bruised.
Better for movement.

Headache

NERVOUS. PAIN one-sided.
Cause mental exertion; overwork.

Indigestion

NERVOUS. ABDOMEN/STOMACH feels empty.
Cause nervous exhaustion; overwork.

Nervous, empty feeling in the stomach is only temporarily relieved by eating. Accompanies nervous exhaustion.

Insomnia

With EMPTY FEELING in pit of stomach.
Cause anxiety; excitement; mental strain; nervous exhaustion.

Sleeplessness following a period of intense work or excitement. With no other symptoms to guide you to another remedy take *Kali phosphoricum* for simple insomnia at bedtime, every 5–10 minutes until sleep falls.

Labour pain

With EXHAUSTION.

Marvellous for simple exhaustion in labour with no

other symptoms (or too few to prescribe on). Take one between every contraction until energy levels rise.

KALI SULPHURICUM (Kali-s.)

Other name: potassium sulphate

General symptoms

Complaints from change of weather from cold to warm. **Discharges** thick; yellow. **Pains** wandering. **Tongue** yellow-coated.
Better for fresh air.
Worse for heat; for change of temperature.

Similar to *Pulsatilla*: its symptoms are aggravated by warmth and relieved by fresh air, especially a walk outside. Both remedies have thick yellow discharges and wandering pains. *Pulsatilla* has a very clear emotional state, especially in babies who are clingy, weepy and shy. *Kali sulphuricum* has similar physical symptoms without a strong emotional picture to prescribe on.

Emotional state

Angry. Anxious when indoors; when overheated. **Irritable.**

These types may be ratty and anxious, especially when stuck inside.

Physical complaints
Common cold

NASAL CATARRH profuse; thick, yellow.
Better for fresh air.
Worse in stuffy room.

If *Pulsatilla* is well indicated for a cold but either does not or only partly helps, *Kali sulphuricum* will finish the cure.

Cough

RATTLING; WHOOPING. MUCUS yellow; difficult to cough up; has to swallow what comes up.
Worse at night; in warm room.

Earache

DISCHARGE thin; yellow. With CRACKLING IN EARS when chewing.

Causes temporary deafness, especially in babies, because Eustachian tubes are blocked with mucus.

Headache

PAIN in forehead; in sides of head; stitching.
Better for fresh air.
Worse during evening; in warm room.

Joint pain

FEET cold. PAIN in hips; in legs; wandering.
Better for fresh air; for movement; for walking.
Worse for heat; in summer.

Although feet feel cold, the symptoms are worse for heat.

KREOSOTUM (Kreos.)

Other name: beechwood kreosote

Emotional state

Capricious. Desires to be carried. **Screaming** (babies).

Babies are obnoxious during teething (rather like *Chamomilla*). In women, marked burning and smelliness of discharges, rather than the emotional state, guide you to this remedy.

Physical complaints
Bleeding (vaginal) in pregnancy

In EARLY PREGNANCY. FLOW CLOTTED; dark; black; smelly.

Gums bleeding

Lochia

DARK (brown); LUMPY; SMELLY; BURNS. Returns, having almost stopped.

Nausea

In PREGNANCY. With VOMITING; COPIOUS SALIVA.

Teething

TEETH decay as soon as they come through. PAIN severe. With RESTLESS SLEEP.

Thrush (genital)

In PREGNANCY. DISCHARGE burning; milky; profuse; smelly; thin; watery. With ITCHING (vulva, vagina).

LAC CANINUM (Lac-c.)

Breast(feeding) problems

WEANING to dry up milk.

To help your milk dry up after weaning, or to decrease your supply if it is over-abundant and gushing everywhere.

LAC DEFLORATUM (Lac-d.)

Breast(feeding) problems

MILK SUPPLY LOW in women who are generally chilly and exhausted from loss of sleep.

LACHESIS (Lach.)

Other name: bushmaster snake

General symptoms

Breath smelly. **Lips** blue. **Nosebleeds. Palpitations. Sweat** from mental exertion; from pain. **Symptoms** left-sided or start on left and move to right.
Better for fresh air; while eating.
Worse for humidity; for heat; during the morning; for pressure; after sleep; for tight clothes; on walking.

Generally, *Lachesis* types are worse for heat (they suffer easily from hot flushes) and feel better for cold compresses and fresh air. Their tiredness, which is often accompanied by trembling and a faint feeling, is not helped by sleeping. They and their symptoms are worse on waking and they may even begin to dread falling asleep because of this. They suffer from left-sided complaints, which may then move across to the right side of the body.

Emotional state

Anxious on waking. **Aversion** to being touched/examined (babies); to company during pregnancy. **Cheerful. Complaints from** grief; mental strain. **Confused. Depressed** generally; in pregnancy; on waking. **Desires** to be alone. **Excitable. Exhilarated. Expression** sickly. **Jealous. Lively. Sensitive** to pain; to touch. **Shock** from injury. **Sluggish** on waking. **Talkative. Tearful** during pregnancy.

These are lively, excitable characters who are so talkative it is hard to get a word in edgeways. Ill-health often follows overwork or a personal loss which causes depression and anxiety (worse on waking) and mental exhaustion. Acutely sensitive to touch, they cannot tolerate the slightest pressure, especially around the neck.

Physical complaints

Bites/stings

Better for cold.
Worse for heat.
Cause insects/animals.

Area around the bite looks bluish.

Carpal Tunnel Syndrome

In pregnancy.
With tingling and numbness in the fingers.

Cough

CHOKING on falling into deep sleep; dry; hacking; suffocative; violent; from tickling in larynx.
Worse for touch; at night.

The larynx is irritated as if a crumb were lodged in it; sets off desire to cough, as does having neck touched. Wakes with a choking cough immediately after falling into a deep sleep.

Croup

With symptoms of COUGH (see above); LUMP SENSATION in throat.
Worse after sleep; on waking.

The voice is hoarse and the air passages feel irritated.

Earache

PAINS on left side. With SORE THROAT (see p. 218).
Worse for swallowing; for exposure to wind.

Exhaustion

Worse during morning after getting up; for heat of sun; for slightest exertion; for walking; for mental exertion.
Cause mental exertion.

Hair loss

Cause pregnancy.

Headache

Head feels heavy; hot. PAIN in forehead; spreading to back of head; in temples and top of head; bursting; pressing; throbbing; violent.

Better after eating.
Worse on left side of head; for lying down; on waking; for pressure; for walking.
Cause over-exposure to sun.

Headaches begin on the left side of head and may move to the right. Dreads going to sleep, knowing pain will be awful on waking.

Injuries

CUTS/WOUNDS bleed freely; slow to heal. SCARS become red.

Skin around wound looks dark or bluish and blood is dark.

Mumps

GLANDS swollen/painful. With SORE THROAT.
Worse on left side.

The neck and glands are especially sensitive to touch; swallowing is painful and difficult.

Piles

PAINFUL. In pregnancy. BLEEDING; BLUISH; EXTERNAL; LARGE.

Scarlet fever

RASH looks bluish.

With typical *Lachesis* general and emotional/mental symptoms.

Sore throat

PAIN spreading up to ears; splinter-like. With CHOKING SENSATION; LUMP SENSATION in throat.
Better for swallowing solids.
Worse for heat; on the left side; for pressure; for touch; for swallowing liquids or saliva.

Throat is very painful; feels better for swallowing hard foods, such as toast, because hard pressure eases the pain. Swallowing saliva or drinks, especially warm ones, hurts. There's a sense of constriction around the neck; cannot bear to be touched there; a constant desire to swallow to dislodge the 'lump'. Hawking may relieve this feeling.

LEDUM PALUSTRE (Led.)
Other name: wild rosemary

General symptoms

Pains wandering.
Better for cold bathing.
Worse for heat; for movement; for touch; for walking.

Effective for acute rheumatic complaints of the joints. Injured or painful parts puff up, become numb and are sensitive to being touched; they may look mottled, bluish or pale. The painful part (injury or rheumatic joint) feels cold (internally and externally), but pains are relieved by cold compresses or being bathed in cold (even icy-cold) water. Pains are generally worse for movement and warmth.

Physical complaints

Bites/stings

Better for cold.
Worse for heat.
Cause insects/animals.

Ledum prevents sepsis: give it routinely after a bite by any animal, poisonous or not. Also for insect bites or stings unless another remedy is strongly indicated; use the appropriate external remedy as well.

Bruises/black eye

Cause injury.

If *Arnica* has been given but bruising comes out, i.e. you give *Arnica* a bit too late, give *Ledum*.

Eye injury

BRUISING and discolouration.
Better for cold compress.

Injuries

CUTS/WOUNDS lacerated; punctured; to palm of hand/sole of foot.
Better for cold compresses.
Worse for heat.
Cause splinter; nail; knife; needle.

If prescribed early, *Ledum* will prevent sepsis from developing in wounds where the skin is punctured by a sharp, pointed instrument. If a splinter is still in the wound, press gently around it to encourage bleeding and to expel it or give *Silica* (see p. 252).

Joint pain

Hot; icy-cold; stiff. PAIN in hands and feet; in right hip; in left shoulder.

Better after common cold; for being uncovered; after cold compresses; after cold bathing.

Worse for movement; for heat; for warmth of bed; at night.

Pains may start in the lower limbs, especially in the small joints, and move upwards, for example from feet to hands. Feels cold, but warmth of bed is unendurable.

LILLIUM TIGRINUM (Lil-t.)
Other name: tiger-lily

General symptoms

Worse at night; for heat.

These are hot people who feel worse (emotionally and physically) at night.

Emotional state

Apathetic about anything being done for them. **Depressed. Hurried**, doing several things at once. **Irritable. Restless**.

These types are always on the go. They are snappy, busy people who feel better for being occupied, nothing anyone else does for them has an effect.

Physical complaints
Palpitations

In pregnancy.

Piles

With dragging down sensation.
Worse for standing.
Cause childbirth.

Prolapse

With BEARING DOWN SENSATION.

Feels as if everything will fall out.

LYCOPODIUM (Lyc.)
Other name: club moss

General symptoms

Blisters on tip of tongue. **Discharges** yellow. **Expression** confused. **Face** pale; sickly. **Likes** sweets; chocolate. **Oedema** (swelling) of ankles/feet; of hands/fingers. **Pains** in glands. **Sweat** cold; profuse; clammy; smelly; sour; worse for slightest physical exertion; better for uncovering. **Symptoms** right-sided; start on right side and move to left. **Taste** sour.

Better for fresh air; for warmth of bed.

Worse around 4–8 p.m.; during afternoon; during evening; for pressure; in stuffy rooms; for tight clothes; for wind; for onions; for flatulent food (beans; cabbage, etc.).

They have trouble with food: either feeling full up and bloated after eating very little or having no appetite at all until they start eating, and then becoming ravenous. Sweet-cravers, often eating several bars of chocolate a day. They may feel sleepy after eating. They digest their food poorly and become bloated with gas, with acidity and sourness. Despite being chilly and worse for extremes of heat and cold, they feel generally better for fresh air. Babies may sleep well at night but cry all day.

Emotional state

Angry babies; from contradiction. **Anxious** generally; during labour; indoors; anticipatory. **Aversion** to being consoled; own babies. **Complaints from** humiliation; mental strain; suppressed anger. **Concentration** poor. **Depressed** on waking. **Desires** company; to be carried. **Despair. Dictatorial** during labour. **Dislikes** being contradicted; being alone; company. **Fearful** babies, of strangers; of public speaking. **Forgetful. Hitting. Indecisive. Irritable** babies – after a sleep; in the mornings; daytime (good all night and cross all day); when sick; on waking. **Moody. Rage. Resentful. Restless sleep** during labour. **Screaming** during sleep; on waking. **Lack of self-confidence. Sensitive. Shy. Sluggish** better for fresh air. **Tantrums. Tearful.**

Lycopodium individuals are anxious and worry about many things because they lack self-confidence. They dread taking on new things, but in anticipation of an event prepare meticulously and usually shine! Sensitive and shy; their rude and difficult behaviour is a front for their low self-confidence. They hate to be alone, but are not keen on company, either; their ideal is to know that there is someone else in the house – in another room! They are irritable intellectuals who find it difficult to express their feelings. They become forgetful and indecisive when tired, especially after mental strain.

Lycopodium babies are irritable and dictatorial; having tantrums if contradicted; kicking and screaming after a nap or on waking in the morning. They are generally difficult to live with.

Physical complaints
Backache

In LOWER BACK. With STIFFNESS.
Better for movement; for passing wind; for urinating.
Worse on beginning to move; while passing a stool; on getting up from sitting.
Cause lifting.

Lower back feels sore, often because of wind that cannot escape.

Carpal Tunnel Syndrome

In pregnancy.

Tingling and numbness in fingers, with or without swelling of wrist.

Common cold

NASAL CATARRH yellow. NOSE blocked; dry. SINUSES blocked. With HEADACHE (see below).
Worse on right side.

Nose and sinuses are blocked so sleeps with mouth open. Nursing infants cannot breathe; this is a major remedy to consider for new babies with the snuffles.

Constipation

In BABIES. In pregnancy. DESIRE TO PASS STOOL ineffectual. STOOLS hard; knotty. With FLATULENCE.

Cough

Constant; disturbs sleep; dry; irritating; painful. BREATHING difficult; fast. MUCUS green; yellow; white; copious; tastes salty.
Better for hot drinks.
Worse on going to sleep; at night; in evening in bed.

Overpowering tickling in larynx, as if being touched by a feather. It is worse in the evening on going to bed and can prevent sleep. A feeling of constriction or tightness in the chest can develop.

Cradle cap

In thin, gassy babies.

Cramp

In calf.
Worse at night.

Cystitis

DESIRE TO URINATE frequent; ineffectual. PAIN aching; cutting; pressing; stitching. URINATION frequent; slow (waits a long time for it to start).
Better after urination.

Passes only a few drops or a dribble of urine at a time. Child screams before urinating because of difficulty or pain.

Earache

With BLOCKED FEELING; PAIN TEARING. NOISES IN THE EAR.

Eye inflammation

DISCHARGE purulent. EYES sensitive to light; stitching; watering. EYELIDS glued together.

Fever

One-sided; on left side.
Worse in evening.

One-sided sweating, or feeling hot on one side of the body and cold on the other, is a common symptom.

Flatulence

ABDOMEN/STOMACH feels bloated; intolerant of tight clothing; rumbling.
Better for passing wind.
Worse after eating; before and after passing stools.

Bloated and uncomfortable below navel; has to loosen clothing around the waist.

Hair loss

Cause childbirth.

Headache

PAIN in forehead; in temples; pressing; throbbing.
Better for fresh air.
Worse for coughing; during menstrual period; for overheating; for warmth of bed; for wrapping up head.
Cause eye strain; mental strain.

Hernia in babies

INGUINAL on right side.

Indigestion

ABDOMEN/STOMACH feels empty; feels full very quickly. BELCHES acrid; empty; sour. PAINS in stomach; pressing; cramping. With HEARTBURN.
Better for belching.
Worse after eating; for onions; for tight clothing.

Insomnia

SLEEPLESS in daytime (babies).

Sleeps at night but is bad-tempered all day.

Joint pain

PAIN tearing.
Better for movement; for walking; for warmth of bed.
Worse on beginning to move; during a fever; for sitting down.

Rheumatic pains occur in joints, but knee and finger joints are especially sore and stiff. Pains often start on right and move to the left.

Labour

LATE – with anticipatory anxiety; too FAST.

Women in labour are anxious, restless and dictatorial.

Mouth ulcers

UNDER TONGUE.

Mumps

GLANDS swollen/painful. With FEVER (see above); SORE THROAT (see below); typical *Lycopodium* general and emotional/mental symptoms. SWELLING MOVES from right to left.

Nausea

In pregnancy. With VOMITING.

Piles

BLEEDING. EXTERNAL. ITCHING. With CONSTIPATION.

Snuffles

In newborn babies. With COMMON COLD.

Sore throat

THROAT dry; with lump sensation. PAIN raw; sore. TONSILS swollen.

Better for warm drinks.
Worse at night; on right side.

Throat sore and inflamed, and feels full of dust. Chokes while drinking though warm drinks soothe the pains.

Varicose veins

During pregnancy. Of LEG/THIGH; of VULVA. Painful.

MAGNESIA CARBONICA (Mag-c.)

Other name: carbonate of magnesia

General symptoms

Discharges sour. **Insomnia** after 3 a.m.; sleep unrefreshing. **Sweat** oily; sour. **Taste** in mouth sour. **Weight gain** poor in babies.
Better for fresh air.
Worse during evening; at night.

Puny, sickly babies, or individuals of any age worn out from too many cares and not enough good food. They snack for comfort on junk food and look 'unloved'. They are generally worse at night, when they cannot sleep; wake more tired than when they went to bed. A walk in fresh air helps a little. Nursing babies may refuse the breast; milk passes through undigested. Weaning children won't eat vegetables but want meat.

Emotional state

Anxious in bed. **Irritable** babies. **Screaming** on waking.

Babies are particularly irritable and anxious during a fever. Sleep is restless and disturbed.

Physical complaints

Diarrhoea

PAIN colicky; cramping. STOOLS frothy; green; slimy; sour-smelling.
Worse in morning; before passing a stool.

Milk is poorly tolerated, passes through undigested; nursing babies may even refuse the breast. Stools are like the scum of a frog pond.

Flatulence

ABDOMEN/STOMACH feels bloated. With RUMBLING before passing a stool.

Headache

PAIN recurs at regular intervals; spasmodic; shooting; tearing.
Better for pressure; for walking.
Worse for lying down.

May be obliged to walk about all night because pains return in force on stopping to rest.

Indigestion

ABDOMEN/STOMACH feels bloated; rumbling. **BELCHES** greasy; sour. With **HEARTBURN; NAUSEA.**
Worse after eating cabbage; after drinking milk.

MAGNESIA MURIATICUM (Mag-m.)

Other name: chloride of magnesium

General symptoms

Discharges sour.
Better for fresh air; for pressure.
Worse after drinking milk; at night; for swimming in sea.

For babies' colic or digestive upsets that are worse for milk or caused by drinking milk. Generally better for fresh air; pains are better for pressure. Sweat and stools smell sour.

Emotional state

Anxious. Restless in bed.

Feels rushed and hurried; must be doing something all the time. Though present during the day, anxiety is always worse in bed at night, causing insomnia.

Physical complaints
Colic

In **BABIES**; cramping; sore, bruised. With **CONSTIPATION** (see below); **DIARRHOEA** (see opposite); **INDIGESTION.**
Worse after drinking milk.
Cause milk; teething.

Common cold

Cause swimming in sea.

Constipation

STOOLS passed with difficulty; crumbling; small balls; knotty. With **STRAINING** ineffectual.

Cause drinking cow's milk.

Diarrhoea

STOOLS green. In **BABIES.**
Cause drinking milk.

Headache

PAIN in temples; spreading to eyes. With **BELCHING; THIRST.**
Worse for pressure; for wrapping up head.

Insomnia

SLEEP unrefreshing.

Restless and anxious in bed, especially on closing eyes; may be over-sensitive to noise then, and unable to get to sleep.

Teething

PAINFUL in babies. With **COLIC; GREEN STOOLS.**

MAGNESIA PHOSPHORICA (Mag-p.)

Other name: magnesium phosphate

General symptoms

Pains cramping.
Better for heat; for firm pressure.
Worse for cold; for swimming in cold water; for touch, light pressure; for being uncovered; for walking in fresh air.

Nicknamed the 'homeopathic aspirin' because of its success in easing minor aches and pains, such as headaches, earaches, teething pains or even neuralgic pains of the face. For greatest effect, the general symptoms (above) must be present.
Pains are greatly relieved by heat and pressure, and are much worse for cold.

NB This remedy is best given dissolved in warm water. Add 4 tablets to a glass of boiled and partially cooled water and stir vigorously. Sip frequently until the pains ease. Repeat as and when needed. Scald glass and spoon afterwards or the next person to use them may get an inadvertent dose of the remedy.

Physical complaints
Colic

PAIN cramping; drawing.
Better for warmth; bending double.

Cramp

In arm; finger; hand; wrist.
Better for heat.
Cause prolonged use of hands.

For writers, musicians, typists and others whose occupations involve prolonged use of fingers and hands.

Earache

PAIN spasmodic; shooting.
Better for heat; for firm pressure.
Worse for cold; for turning head.
Cause cold wind.

Comes on after a walk in cold wind.

Headache

PAIN on right side of head; spasmodic; shooting.
Better for heat; for firm pressure.
Worse for cold.
Cause getting chilled.

Often right-sided; may be accompanied by pains in the face that come and go throughout the day.

Hiccups

In babies; violent.
Worse after eating or drinking.

Labour pains

With CRAMP (see above) in hand or leg.

Sciatica

Better for heat.
Worse for cold.

Sciatica or any cramping, neuralgic pains in back. Pains often caused by cold, and are much better for hot applications and firm massage.

Teething

PAINFUL in babies.
Better for external heat.

Hot-water bottle (wrapped in towel) relieves the pains. *Magnesia phosphorica* in a bottle or cup can also help.

MERCURIUS CORROSIVUS (Merc-c.)

Other name: mercuric chloride

General symptoms

Breath smelly. **Exhaustion. Gums** pale; bleeding. **Likes** cold drinks. **Oedema** (swelling) ankles/feet; hands/fingers. **Sweat** cold. **Thirst** extreme. **Tongue** yellow-coated.
Worse for pressure.

This remedy has a similar sphere of action to *Mercurius solubilis* (below) but its general picture is stronger: has more pains and more burning and more thirst and is more violent, more active.

It does not have any marked emotional symptoms. The physical symptoms are nearly always accompanied by general feeling of **nervous exhaustion**, and, because of seriousness of the physical symptoms, there will also be some anxiety, irritability and/or depression.

Physical complaints

Cystitis

DESIRE TO URINATE constant; painful; frequent. PAIN burning. URINE dark; green; red; scanty. URINATION dribbling; frequent; difficult.
Worse during urination.

Severe cystitis where terrible pains are felt both in bladder and rectum. Little urine is passed in spite of constant, painful urge to urinate. Has to strain to pass urine which is also excruciatingly painful. Urine burns and may have blood in it. Seek professional help immediately.

Diarrhoea

PAIN severe. STOOLS bloody; frequent; green; slimy; smelly; yellow. STRAINING frequent; painful.
Worse before/during/after passing a stool.

Severe diarrhoea (dysentery) where there is constant, incessant, excruciatingly painful straining that is not relieved by passing a stool. May be accompanied by vomiting of bile which will eventually cause a bruised stomach. Seek professional help immediately.

Sore throat

GUMS bleeding; swollen. PAIN burning; raw. With SALIVA increased. ULCERS in throat.
Better for eating.
Worse for pressure; for swallowing liquids.

Choking sensation in the throat and an increase of

sticky saliva in the mouth, which create a constant desire to swallow. Breath is smelly and gums may be swollen and bleed easily.

MERCURIUS SOLUBILIS (Merc-s.)

Other name: ammonio-nitrate of mercury

General symptoms

Breath smelly. **Complaints from** getting chilled. **Discharges** burning; blood-streaked; smelly; yellow; watery. **Face** pasty. **Glands** swollen. **Likes** bread and butter; cold drinks. **Mouth** dry. **Mouth ulcers** on gums, on tongue. **Pains** in bones; pressing. **Saliva** increased; during sleep. **Sweat** cold; profuse; smelly; from pain. **Taste** mouth tastes bad; bitter; metallic. **Thirst** extreme. **Tongue** cracked; coated yellow.

Worse for heat and cold; for lying down; during evening; at night; for light touch.

All discharges – stools, urine, sweat, saliva, catarrh, etc. – smell strongly. They sweat profusely, without relief, especially at night. Symptoms are worse at night generally and especially if they become hot.

They are sensitive to extremes of temperature; disliking both heat and cold. They may feel chilly and want a hot-water bottle, then feel overheated so open the window, which chills them quickly, whereupon cycle begins again. A change of 2 degrees either way makes them feel worse. Resting in bed in a moderate temperature affords the greatest relief.

They have a burning thirst in spite of having a lot of saliva which they are constantly swallowing – it may dribble on to their pillows at night. They have a bitter, metallic taste in the mouth; and their flabby tongues take the imprint of their teeth so that they are indented around the edges.

They suffer with mouth ulcers; abscesses; colds; painful, swollen glands and pains in the teeth.

Emotional state

Confused. Depressed. Dictatorial. Discontented. Forgetful. Restless children.

These are nervous, anxious, restless types who find it difficult to stay still. They do slow down, both mentally and physically, when they become sick, appearing apathetic but always feel hurried inside. In this slowed-down state, their memories weaken, confusion sets in and they may have trouble thinking. They may feel depressed and weepy but crying alternates with laughter – they are restless even in their emotions!

Physical complaints

Abscesses

Of GLANDS; of ROOTS OF TEETH.

With *Merc-s.* general symptoms: increased saliva, foul taste and smelly breath.

Backache

In LOWER BACK. PAIN burning; shooting.
Worse for breathing; for coughing; on getting up from sitting; for sweating.

Breast(feeding) problems

BREAST ABSCESS painful.

Chickenpox

With *Merc-s.* general symptoms: worse at night, weak and smelly. Rash suppurates and is smelly.

Common cold

NASAL CATARRH bloody; burning; green; yellow; yellow-green; smelly; watery. Blocked, painful sinuses. With FEVER (see p. 225); HEADACHE (see p. 225); HOARSENESS; LOSS OF SMELL; frequent SNEEZING; SORE THROAT (see p. 225).
Worse for cold and for heat; at night.

Nasal discharge burns upper lip, nostrils may become ulcerated. Nose may bleed during sleep.

Cough

Racking; MUCUS green.
Worse during evening in bed; at night; for lying on right side.

Cystitis

DESIRE TO URINATE constant; ineffectual. PAIN burning; URINE dark; scanty. URINATION frequent.
Worse at beginning of urinating; when not urinating.

Pains are terrible and urinating is slow and difficult.

Diarrhoea

In BABIES. PAIN burning. STOOLS bloody; green; slimy; smelly; yellow. With SWEATING before/during/after stool; LOUD WIND.
Worse for cold; during the evening; at night after passing a stool.

Burning pains come on when passing a stool and remain for a time afterwards. Feels faint and weak (see EXHAUSTION). Desire to pass a stool may be worse *after* the stool has been passed.

Earache

DISCHARGE from ears blood-streaked; smelly. PAIN boring; burning; pressing; tearing. With BLOCKED FEELING in ears.
Worse at night; for warmth of bed; fresh air.

Eardrum may perforate; discharge will be smelly and blood-streaked.

Exhaustion

With HEAVINESS in limbs.
Worse after sweating; after passing a stool.
Cause sweating.

Accompanies a fever or an attack of diarrhoea; waves of tiredness with a feeling of heaviness come on after passing a stool or after a heavy bout of sweating. Trembles with exhaustion.

Eye inflammation

DISCHARGE purulent. EYES sensitive to light; watering. With symptoms of COMMON COLD (see p. 224).
Worse for heat of fire; warmth of bed.

Fever

HEAT alternating with chills. With SWEATING (see General symptoms).
Worse for fresh air; at night in bed.

Feels chilled in the fresh air, but overheated in a stuffy room. Fever may precede a common cold.

Headache

PAIN in forehead; burning; pressing; sore, bruised.
Worse at night; for bending down.
Cause common cold; rheumatism.

Feels as though there is a band around the forehead or the head is in a vice. With increased saliva as well as other *Merc-s.* general symptoms.

Heartburn

In pregnancy.
Worse at night.

Stomach feels empty and out of sorts with hiccups and burping.

Joint pain

PAIN burning; tearing.
Worse in bed; at night; for wet weather.

Rheumatic pains are severe and always worse at night in bed, when they drive the sufferer out of bed.

Mouth ulcers

On gums; on tongue. PAIN stinging; throbbing.

Major mouth-ulcer remedy, but take general symptoms into account – increase in saliva and flabby, indented tongue – as well as ulcers themselves.

Mumps

GLANDS hard; swollen/painful. With FEVER (see opposite); COPIOUS SALIVA; PROFUSE SWEATING.
Worse for blowing nose; at night; on right side.

Typical *Merc-s.* tongue and smelly breath also present. Bones in face may ache.

Scarlet fever

With *Merc-s.* general symptoms and emotional state.

Sore throat

PAIN spreading up to ears and neck; sore; stitching. TONSILS swollen; ulcerated.
Worse at night; on right side of body; for swallowing.

Very painful sore throats with ulcers on the tonsils and swollen glands. Pains shoot up into the ear or into the neck on swallowing.

Thrush (genital)/Yeast

DISCHARGE burning; greenish; smelly. With ITCHING.
Worse at night.

Thrush (oral)

In BABIES. With EXCESS SALIVA.

Characteristic smelly breath is usually present.

NATRUM CARBONICUM (Nat-c.)
Other name: sodium carbonate

General symptoms
Complaints from sunstroke. **Dislikes** milk. **Face**

pale. **Sweat** from slightest physical exertion; from pain. **Taste** in mouth metallic.

Better after eating; for massage.

Worse before eating; during stormy weather; for fresh air; mid-morning; for milk; for physical exertion; for sun.

These people have pale faces with blue circles around the eyes; eyelids may be puffy. They dislike exposure to the sun (especially the head); and are also averse to fresh air. Once run down, any exercise will aggravate their general condition. They are sensitive to thunderstorms; can sense them coming. They suffer from poor digestion, but feel better after eating, when they feel warmer. They dislike milk – this can cause diarrhoea. Babies, even breast-fed babies, have difficulty digesting milk.

Emotional state

Anxious. Cheerful. Complaints from mental strain. **Confused. Depressed. Fearful. Forgetful. Gloomy. Jumpy. Lively. Sensitive** generally; to music. **Shy. Sluggish.**

These people put on a brave face when really they feel miserable. They are sensitive generally; harbour emotional hurts inside, though without feeling bitter. They avoid conflict by appearing cheerful, but this masks feeling of being cut off, depressed and anxious with persistent sad thoughts. Listening to music increases their sense of melancholy. They are easily startled by noise.

They become mentally weakened by emotional pressure, can find it difficult to think. Complaints come on in this weak state, after mental strain (overwork) or when feeling sad and depressed.

Physical complaints

Common cold

NOSE blocked. NASAL CATARRH drips down back of throat; smelly; thick.

Wants to hawk up catarrh. May have a sour or metallic taste in the mouth.

Dizziness

Worse for mental exertion; in a stuffy room.

Exhaustion

WEAK LEGS. NERVOUS EXHAUSTION. With COLD EXTREMITIES; HEAVINESS in the limbs.

Worse for exposure to sun; for mental exertion; for slightest physical exertion.

Cause mental strain; over-exposure to sun.

Nervous exhaustion follows a period of overwork: feet and hands become cold and legs feel heavy and weak. Can also be caused by an overdose of sunshine (which need not be a great deal), these types become tired in hot weather, and thinking, sunshine or exertion make tiredness worse.

Headache

HEAD feels heavy. PAIN pressing. With SWEATING on forehead.

Worse after eating; for thinking.

Cause mental strain; mental exertion; summer; sunstroke.

Feels generally better after eating, but the headache itself may be worse. After too much study or mental strain, the brain feels worn out. May also be a hot-weather headache.

Indigestion

BELCHES sour. PAIN in stomach; sore, bruised. With NAUSEA.

Feels nauseous in a stuffy room and has trouble digesting food because nervous system is run down.

Insomnia

DREAMS, ANXIOUS. WAKING early.

Often cannot get back to sleep again.

NATRUM MURIATICUM (Nat-m.)

Other name: sodium chloride

General symptoms

Anaemia. Appetite lost in pregnancy. **Blisters** on tip of tongue. **Catches colds** easily. **Discharges** like egg white. **Dislikes** bread; food in general; the thought of food – in pregnancy; with hunger. **Dryness** generally. **Face** pasty. **Gums** bleeding. **Likes** salty things, especially in pregnancy. **Lips** cracked. **Mouth** dry; with thirst. **Palpitations** in pregnancy. **Oedema** (swelling) of ankles/feet; of hands/fingers. **Taste** in mouth bitter. **Thirst** extreme; for large quantities.

Better for lying down; after rest; after sweating.

Worse 10 a.m.; after eating; for exposure to sun; for heat; mid-morning; for physical exertion.

Dryness and extreme thirst are characteristic, especially with a fever. Lips dry up and become cracked; lower lip often has a centre crack. Hangnails are also common. Discharges are profuse and watery (often like egg white) or thick and white. They sweat a lot when ill and feel better for doing so.

People needing this remedy feel chilly in their bodies but dislike hot weather and feel worse for sun's heat or being in stuffy rooms. May have cold hands and feet in winter, but it doesn't bother them. An uncommon symptom that suggests this remedy is an inability to pass urine in the presence of others, such as in a public toilet.

Emotional state

Absent-minded. Angry. Aversion to consolation. **Complaints from** disappointed love; grief; humiliation; suppression of emotions. **Confused. Depressed** in pregnancy but cannot cry; from suppressed grief. **Desires** to be alone; in pregnancy. **Despair** during pregnancy. **Discontented. Introverted. Irritable**, worse for consolation. **Loss of libido. Resentful. Sensitive** generally. **Tearful** in pregnancy; with difficulty crying; cries on own. **Worse** for consolation.

Despite being emotional types, they may appear cool and prickly because of their difficulty expressing emotions. They close themselves off to avoid being hurt, suppress their grief, and so may appear quite hard. Their feelings can burst out uncontrollably under certain conditions, especially to a sensitive, sympathetic ear; they may cry in spite of themselves. In that state they hate to be consoled and feel worse for any comforting. They prefer to cry alone, it is rare to see them crying in public; this humiliates them.

When depressed they refuse all invitations, preferring to stay at home alone. If hurt (which is very easy!) they do not show it; they harbour hurts inside and become bitter. They are haunted by persistent, unpleasant thoughts, and dwell on things in the past. This can make them ill.

Babies are serious and dislike too much physical contact. They hate to be teased, and are also often slow to talk and walk.

Physical complaints
Backache

In **LOWER BACK. PAIN** aching; back feels as if broken; sore, bruised.
Better for lying on a hard surface.
Cause manual labour.

Back feels weak and tired after exertion or bending down for a long time (after gardening, for example).

Cold sores

SORES on lips; around mouth.
Cause sun; suppressed grief.

This is a major cold sore remedy, but it is a mistake to prescribe it on this symptom alone: the general symptoms and the emotional state are both important. A *Natrum muriaticum* type will often produce cold sores after a disappointment or a loss that wasn't expressed. The sores are usually found at the corners of the mouth.

Common cold

DISCHARGE FROM EYES watery. **NASAL CATARRH** drips down back of throat; profuse; white, watery alternating with blocked nose; like egg white. With **LOSS OF SMELL; LOSS OF TASTE.**

Sneezes a lot in the early stages of the cold.

Constipation

STOOLS crumbling; small balls; **STRAINING** ineffectual; feels unfinished.

Cough

Dry; hacking; irritating; tickling. **MUCUS** like egg white; transparent; white.
Worse during fever; evening in bed; from tickling in larynx.

Cough is set off by tickling in the larynx and air passages. Eyes water when coughing.

Diarrhoea

ABDOMEN/STOMACH feels bloated. **DIARRHOEA** during day only. **STOOLS** gushing; painless; smelly; watery.
Worse after eating starchy food.

May be pains before passing stool.

Dizziness

In **PREGNANCY.**
Worse for getting up from lying down; for tobacco; for walking.

Exhaustion

With **HEAVINESS.**
Worse during evening.
Cause loss of sleep (broken nights).

Energy may increase for a short while after eating, but feels tired and heavy, especially in the evening.

Eye inflammation

Gritty; sensitive to light; watering.

Fever

HEAT burning. With NAUSEA.
Better for uncovering.
Worse mid-morning; in the autumn.

Looks dazed and sleepy and falls asleep when hot. Feeling of burning heat may alternate with intense chilliness. Sweating helps. An extreme thirst for large quantities of liquids.

Hair loss

Cause childbirth.

Headache

EYES sore; watering. PAIN in forehead; in temples; hammering; pressing; splitting; throbbing.
Better for firm pressure.
Worse around 10 a.m. to 3 p.m.; after eating; for coughing; for emotions; for excitement; during a fever; on waking; for reading/writing; talking; thinking.

Trouble with vision, with flickering and zig-zags appearing before the eyes during the pains. Typical of migraines; always seek professional help.

Heartburn

In PREGNANCY. With INDIGESTION (see below). BELCHES sweetish; watery.

Incontinence

In PREGNANCY.
Worse for laughing; for coughing; for sneezing; for walking.

Involuntary urination, with leaking on exertion.

Indigestion

BELCHES incomplete, ineffectual; sour; tasting of food just eaten. MOUTH tastes bitter; salty. PAIN in stomach cramping; pressing. With violent HICCUPS.
Worse after eating starchy food.

After suppressing emotions the stomach becomes 'disordered', and stodgy foods are no longer easily digested. Burps after eating but with difficulty and this does not relieve the indigestion. May also have violent hiccups.

Insomnia

DREAMS anxious; vivid.
Cause grief.

Finds it difficult to get to sleep after a loss or disappointment; wakes in the night and cannot get back to sleep. May have anxious, vivid dreams.

Labour

PREMATURE. SLOW. LABOUR PAINS stopping or slowing down; weak. With EXHAUSTION.

During labour women become depressed, withdrawn and want to be alone – they don't ask for anything and become difficult to reach.

Piles

In PREGNANCY. BLEEDING. With CONSTIPATION (see p. 227).

Prickly heat

With typical general symptoms.

Retention of urine

Cause presence of strangers.

Can only pass urine when alone.

Sore throat

PAINS burning. THROAT dry; with LUMP SENSATION. VOICE HOARSE.

Can only swallow liquids; solids come back up, and person may choke (also when drinking). Hawks up egg-white mucus from back of throat.

Thrush (genital)/Yeast infection

DISCHARGE burning; like egg white. With ITCHING.

Thrush (oral)

GUMS/TONGUE white-coated.

With characteristic dry mouth and thirst.

NATRUM PHOSPHORICUM (Nat-p.)
Other name: sodium phosphate

General symptoms

Discharge sour. **Exhaustion**, nervous. **Tongue** yellow
at back.
Worse during the evening.

This picture is full of sourness: sour sweat, stools,
urine and so on. Yellow-coated tongue (usually base
only) accompanies nearly all symptoms. General
weakness, acidic digestion, weak ankles and cold
extremities (like *Natrum carbonicum*).

Emotional state
Apathetic. Indifferent.

These types are apathetic and dull, like *Phosphoric
acid*.

Physical complaints
Colic

VOMIT sour; acid; curdled milk. DIARRHOEA.

For simple colic with acidity (and sourness) when
there are no other guiding symptoms leading you to
another remedy. Babies may vomit curdled milk and
suffer from sour-smelling, green, watery diarrhoea.

Headache

FACE pale. PAINS in the forehead.
Cause mental exertion.

Indigestion

ABDOMEN/STOMACH feels bloated. BELCHES sour.
With HEARTBURN.
Acidity comes on two hours after eating. Heartburn
of pregnancy may be relieved if the characteristic
sourness is present.

NATRUM SULPHURICUM (Nat-s.)
Other name: sodium sulphate

General symptoms

Complaints from accident/injury to the head. **Hot
flushes. Likes** cold drinks. **Sweat** from pain. **Taste**
in mouth bad (in morning); bitter. **Tongue** green.
Better for fresh air.
Worse for damp; for humidity; for wet weather; for

lying down; during the morning; after eating
starchy food.

These types are sensitive to damp: cold and wet, or
hot and wet. Complaints may result from living in a
damp house. This remedy is most often needed for
complaints arising from head injury.

Emotional state
Depressed. Jumpy. Weary of life.

After a head injury they become sick and tired of life
(having been quite happy before) and over-sensitive
to noise.

Physical complaints
Backache

PAIN sore, bruised.
Cause injury to spine.

Colic

With INDIGESTION (see p. 230).

Cough

DAYTIME only. MUCUS green.
Worse for damp, wet weather.

Diarrhoea

ABDOMEN/STOMACH gurgling; rumbling. STOOLS
smelly; thin; watery. WIND loud; smelly; spluttering.
Better for passing wind.
Worse after getting up; during morning; after eating
fruit/starchy food.
Cause fruit.

Feels exhausted after the diarrhoea; or may want to
pass a stool but manages only to pass wind. May also
be sensitive to starchy foods (potatoes or bread) or
vegetables.

Flatulence

Loud; loud during stool; smelly. With DIARRHOEA.
ABDOMEN/STOMACH rumbling.
Better for passing wind.
Worse after breakfast.

An urge for a stool but only sputtering wind is
passed.

Headache

EYES sensitive to light.
Cause head injury.

Give after *Arnica* if pains remain after a head injury.

Head injuries

See HEADACHE (above).

If *Arnica* has been given for a head injury, and the swelling has subsided but pain remains, or there are other symptoms after a bang or fall, *Natrum sulphuricum* will clear these symptoms. Sometimes babies change character after a bad fall, from being cheerful and easy-going to distressed – don't mistake this for teething and give *Chamomilla*.

Indigestion

ABDOMEN/STOMACH feels bloated. BELCHES bitter; sour. With FLATULENCE after breakfast.
Better after passing a stool.
Worse after eating starchy food.

Cannot digest starchy food, such as potatoes, and the tongue may look greenish brown or dirty green.

Jaundice

In newborn babies.

If *Chelidonium* doesn't help, choose between *Natrum sulphuricum* and *Lycopodium*. Babies who had a long and difficult birth, especially with forceps, may need *Natrum sulphuricum* to help heal minor head injury from birth.

NITRICUM ACIDUM (Nit-ac.)

Other name: nitric acid

General symptoms

Anaemia. Breath smelly. **Discharges** like ammonia. **Dislikes** cheese. **Likes** fat/fatty foods. **Pains** in bones; flying around; needle-like; splinter-like; appear and disappear suddenly. **Sweat** on single parts of body; smelly; sour; worse for slightest physical exertion. **Tongue** cracked.
Better for lying down.
Worse for cold; for fresh air; at night; on waking; for loss of sleep; for touch; for jarring movement; for walking.

These are chilly types – worse for cold in any form. They are very sensitive to being touched or jarred. Their urine smells strong (like a horse's); sweat is also foul-smelling. They crave fatty, fried foods and fat on meat. They are always better for lying down.

Emotional state

Violently **angry. Anxious** about health. **Depressed. Fearful** of death. **Irritable. Sensitive** to noise; to pain. **Sluggish. Tantrums. Unforgiving.**

These types become anxious and depressed when ill – anxious about their health; believing they may have something serious wrong with them.

They may become sick because of harboured anger and their unforgiving streak which eats away like an acid. Their anger can explode volcanically. They overwork and become worn out and over-sensitive, especially to noise.

Physical complaints

Common cold

NASAL CATARRH bloody; burning; dirty yellow; thin; watery in the fresh air.
Worse for fresh air; at night.

Nose is blocked, feels sore and bruised and sensitive to touch. There may be ulcers in the nostrils.

Earache

CRACKLING IN EARS when chewing. PAIN splinter-like; throbbing. With symptoms of SORE THROAT (see p. 231).
Worse on right side, for swallowing.

Pains are usually splinter-like and hearing becomes acute – more sensitive than normal.

Exhaustion

NERVOUS.
Worse after passing stool; for walking.
Cause diarrhoea; loss of sleep (broken nights); nursing the sick.

Weakness results from loss of sleep or accompanies or follows an attack of diarrhoea.

Eye inflammation

In BABIES. EYES watering. EYELIDS swollen.

Flatulence

Smelly; obstructed (difficult to expel).

Hair loss

Cause childbirth.

Headache

HEAD feels constricted. PAIN spreading to eyes; in bones; recurring at regular intervals; pressing.
Worse for jarring movement; for movement; at night; for noise; for pressure; on waking; for walking.

Severe headache that is worse at night. Bones of face are sore, and the slightest pressure, even that of a hat, makes it worse. Pressing pains (as if the head were bandaged tightly) may come and go suddenly.

Insomnia

DREAMS anxious. SLEEP unrefreshing.
Worse after 2 a.m.

Wakes around 2 a.m. and is unable to get back to sleep.

Joint pain

PAIN in bones; in legs; splinter-like; stitching; tearing.
Worse at night.

Mouth ulcers

On edges of tongue; painful.

There is more saliva and the gums may bleed more easily. Breath is smelly.

Piles

PAIN burning; splinter-like. PILES bleeding; large.
Worse after a stool.

Pains may last for 1–2 hours, even after a soft stool.

Sore throat

PAIN burning; pressing; raw; splinter-like; stitching; spreading up to ears. TONSILS swollen/inflamed; ulcerated.
Worse for swallowing.

Pains are severe and extend to ear on swallowing. Swallowing is extremely difficult.

Thrush (genital)/Yeast infection

DISCHARGE burning; smelly; thin. With ITCHING.

NUX MOSCHATA (Nux-m.)

Other name: nutmeg

General symptoms

Thirstless.
Better for heat.
Worse for cold; for fresh air.

Emotional state

Apathetic. Dreamy. Sluggish. Stupor.

Physical complaints

Sleepy babies

Don't wake to feed, especially after the birth. This is for newborns who are difficult to wake up – even for a feed.

NUX VOMICA (Nux-v.)

Other name: poison nut

General symptoms

Catches colds easily. **Complaints from** getting chilled; cold, dry wind. **Dislikes** coffee; food in general, with hunger; meat; tobacco; water. **Likes** spicy food. **Pains** cramping. **Sense of smell** acute. **Sweat** hot; one-sided; smelly. **Symptoms** right-sided. **Taste** in mouth bitter; sour in morning.
Better for heat; for lying down; for sitting down; for hot drinks.
Worse after drinking coffee; after eating cold food; for tobacco; for cold, dry weather, cold wind, fresh air; for loss of sleep; during morning; in winter; for touch; for uncovering; for walking.

These are extremely chilly individuals who hate the cold, catch cold easily, especially if exposed to draughts or wind or after becoming chilled. If sick they become so sensitive to cold that the slightest draught upsets them; they want only to sit or lie down and keep warm, and this is what helps.

Nux vomica is useful for disturbances that follow over-indulgence in food, coffee or tobacco. Once sick, any further indulgence makes them worse, but they find it hard to stop.

Mornings are their worst time of day, especially after a disturbed night.

Emotional state

Angry violently; when has to answer questions.

Anxious about others. **Aversion** to consolation. **Complaints from** anger; anger with anxiety. **Concentration** poor. **Dwells on the past. Excitable. Hitting. Impatient. Impulsive. Irritable. Mischievous. Quarrelsome. Screaming. Sensitive** generally; to rudeness; to light; to music; to noise. **Spiteful. Stubborn. Tidy.**

Self-indulgent workaholics who overdo everything: work too hard, stay out too late, take no exercise, eat too much rich food, drink too much alcohol, become too wound up to sleep and then consume vast quantities of coffee to get going the next day. Then they find it difficult to concentrate, lose interest in their work, become nervy, highly sensitive and irritable.

Impulsive, quarrelsome, stroppy individuals who know what they want and want it now. They are critical, fussy and can be exacting, easily frustrated by limitations. They may be tidy but not fanatically so. They dislike contradiction, are irritable if questioned and if anger is suppressed they feel awful and get sick. Babies become irritable if chilled or tired or if they eat too much of the wrong sort of food.

Physical complaints

Abdominal pain

In pregnancy. With NAUSEA (morning sickness).

Afterpains

With DESIRE to pass a stool during the pains. Feels FAINT after the pains have passed.

Backache

In LOWER BACK. PAIN aching; dragging down; pressing; sore, bruised. In PREGNANCY.
Worse in bed; during morning; for movement.
Cause getting cold; childbirth.

Has to sit up to turn over in bed. Pain comes on after being chilled, and is often accompanied by the desire to pass a stool.

Colic

PAIN cramping; griping; pressing; sore, bruised.
Better for passing a stool; for hot drinks; for warmth of bed; for passing wind.
Worse after eating; for coughing; in morning; during a fever; for tight clothing.

Pains come on after over-indulging. May accompany nausea or indigestion (see p. 233). Also in babies whose breastfeeding mothers eat too much spicy food or drink too much coffee and tea (or Coca-Cola).

Common cold

EYES watering. NASAL CATARRH burning; watery. NOSE runs during day, blocked at night. With HEADACHE (see p. 233); frequent SNEEZING; SORE THROAT (see p. 234). With blocked, painful SINUSES.
Better for fresh air.
Worse after eating; after getting up; during morning.
Cause draughts.

May start with an irritated spot high up at the back of the nose/nostril. Breastfeeding babies whose blocked noses make feeding difficult will benefit, particularly if also sensitive to what their mothers eat.

Constipation

Alternates with DIARRHOEA. DESIRE TO PASS STOOL ineffectual; constant. In BABIES. In PREGNANCY. STOOLS hard; large. With UNFINISHED FEELING.
Cause bottle-feeding; over-eating; pregnancy; sedentary habits; weaning.

Wants to pass a stool but cannot, or passes only small amounts each time.

Cough

BREATHING difficult. COUGH distressing; dry; racking; suffocative; tickling; in violent fits. LARYNX raw. MUCUS tastes sour. With VOMITING when hawking up mucus.
Better for hot drinks.
Worse for becoming cold; for cold air; during early morning; on waking in the morning; for slightest movement of chest; after eating; during fever.

Cough is dry during the fever; it is also dry, and worse, after midnight until daybreak. May cough up sour-tasting mucus; tickling in the larynx excites the cough.

Cystitis

DESIRE TO URINATE frequent; ineffectual; urgent. PAIN burning; pressing. URINATION frequent; ineffectual. URINE burning; scanty.
Worse during urination.

Constant urge to urinate, and slight incontinence; then wants to pee but can't.

Dizziness

In PREGNANCY. With HEADACHE.
Worse for getting up from lying down or sitting; loss of sleep; stooping; tobacco; walking.

Earache

PAIN stitching. With ITCHING IN THE EAR.
Worse for swallowing.

Eustachian tubes itch making swallowing compulsive although it hurts. Hearing is acute.

Effects of drugs taken during or after labour

With IRRITABILITY and INSOMNIA (see opposite).

Helps to rid the body of drugs taken in labour (as a general clear-out).

Exhaustion

NERVOUS.
Worse on waking in the morning.
Cause loss of sleep (broken nights).

Fever

HEAT alternating with chills; dry; one-sided. With BACKACHE; extreme CHILLINESS; SHIVERING; SWEATING (see General symptoms).
Worse for fresh air; for draughts; for movement; for being uncovered; for slightest movement of bed-clothes.

Becomes chilled if a mere hand is poked out of bed. Fever may be on one side only; feels dry and hot externally and chilly internally. Limbs feel heavy and tired. Is usually thirsty.

Flatulence

ABDOMEN/STOMACH feels bloated; intolerant of tight clothing; rumbling.
Better for passing wind.
Worse for eating.

Flu

PAIN in bones; in joints; sore, bruised. With symptoms of COMMON COLD (see p. 232); EXTREME CHILLINESS; FEVER (see above).
Better for warm compresses; for warmth of bed.
Worse in bed; for cold; during the morning.

Similar to the common cold; feels extremely chilly and unable to get warm.

Gastric flu

See Flu (above).
With a disordered digestive system (see INDIGESTION, opposite).

Headache

HEAD feels heavy. PAIN in back of head; in forehead; pressing; sore, bruised; stupefying; tearing. With BILIOUSNESS; DIZZINESS.
Better for excitement; on getting up in morning; for pressure; for wrapping up head; during evening in bed.
Worse after eating; for cold; for moving eyes; for shaking head.
Cause cold wind; common cold; damp weather; loss of sleep; mental strain; over-eating.

Eyes often feel sore.

Heartburn

In PREGNANCY. With INDIGESTION (see below). With sour BELCHES.

Hernia (in babies)

INGUINAL. Left side.
Cause constipation.

Hiccups

In babies. VIOLENT.
Worse after eating or drinking.

Indigestion

ABDOMEN/STOMACH feels bloated; empty. BELCHES bitter; sour. PAIN in stomach; cramping; pressing; sore, bruised. With HEARTBURN. See also COLIC.
Better for hot drinks; for warmth of bed.
Worse after eating; for tight clothing.
Cause coffee; mental strain; over-eating; rich food.

Food lies like a knot in the stomach for 1–2 hours after eating, and stomach feels full, heavy and tender.

Insomnia

In PREGNANCY. With DREAMS, VIVID. WAKING early; late; around 3 a.m.
Cause cramps (in pregnancy); excitement; mental strain; overwork; overactive mind.

Sleepy on going to bed but cannot sleep, or gets to sleep but wakes in the early hours with anxious thoughts. May fall into deep sleep just before the alarm goes off, and so wakes tired and worn out.

Labour

PREMATURE. LABOUR PAINS in back; ineffectual (cervix doesn't soften); severe/violent; stopping (or slowing down). With CRAMPS in hands or legs. With EXHAUSTION; FAINT FEELING. With an URGE TO PASS A STOOL during contractions.

With the typical *Nux vomica* emotional state.

Nausea

CONSTANT. With COPIOUS SALIVA; INABILITY TO VOMIT; RETCHING; VOMITING.
Worse after eating; in morning; in bed; for sweating; for tobacco.
Cause pregnancy; travelling.

May feel faint with the nausea.

Piles

In PREGNANCY. BLEEDING; INTERNAL; ITCHING; LARGE. With CONSTIPATION (see p. 232).
Better for bathing in cold water.

Snuffles

Of newborn babies. With symptoms of COMMON COLD (see p. 232).

Sore throat

PAIN spreading up to ears; raw; stitching. With LUMP SENSATION in throat.
Worse for cold air; for swallowing; for uncovering.

Swallowing is difficult; the throat feels rough and pains radiate to the ears on swallowing. The rawness may have been caused by coughing.

Toothache

Better for external warmth; for wrapping up head; for heat; in winter.
Cause filling/extraction.

Lying on a hot-water bottle wrapped in a towel helps.

Travel sickness

FAINT-LIKE FEELING; HEADACHE; NAUSEA.
Better for lying down.
Worse for tobacco.

Vomiting

VOMIT bile; mucus; bitter; sour; smelly.

Worse for expectorating (hawking up mucus).
Cause anger; pregnancy.

Biliousness (with or without vomiting) occurs after over-eating or indulging in rich or unusual foods. Can feel like food poisoning; can occur when travelling.

OPIUM (Op.)
Other name: white poppy

General symptoms

Eyes glassy. **Face** dark red or blue. **Faintness** after excitement; after fright. **Pains** absent. **Pupils** contracted. **Shock** from injury. **Sweat** profuse; hot; on single parts of body; from fright.
Worse during sleep; on getting up; for warmth of bed.

This remedy is for a particular type of shock: those needing *Opium* appear glassy-eyed and stupefied, suffer from inertia, and feel faint, numb and/or trembly. There is an abnormal lack of pain, as if the senses have been blunted. The face is red and drawn, sunken and old-looking, possibly with a bluish tinge. Children are unable to urinate after shock.

In a fever *Opium* types feel worse for heat and sweating and will kick off the covers in bed. Generally, profuse sweating with scanty urination.

Emotional state

Apathetic and doesn't complain; during fever; during labour. **Complaints from** anger; reprimands; shock. **Confused. Depressed. Dreamy. Drowsy. Exhilarated. Expression** sleepy. **Fearful** during labour. **Indecisive. Indifferent** during a fever. **Lively. Senses** dull. **Stupor.**

In acute illness like fever or after a shock, *Opium* types become dull, confused and apathetic to the point of stupor. Before reaching this state of stupor, however, they may go through an exhilarated and delirious stage.

People in a state of fear after a bad fright or shock or an operation may look similar to *Aconite* (that is, enormously shocked) but are also in a dream-like state they cannot snap out of. *Opium* helps that 'spaced out' feeling after a general anaesthetic. The *Opium* individual recreates during waking hours the image or situation that caused the shock. *Arnica* types, on the other hand, are fine during the day but have bad dreams.

Physical complaints

Bleeding (vaginal) in pregnancy

At any time in pregnancy.
Cause fright.

Constipation

In BABIES. DESIRE TO PASS STOOL absent. STOOLS
black balls; hard; small balls; 'shy' (they recede).
With UNFINISHED FEELING.
Cause bottle-feeding; weaning.

There is no desire to pass a stool; no pain either. May
be acute after an operation; may alternate with
diarrhoea after sudden joy or a fright. Babies may
react badly to bottled milk or prepared baby foods
and become completely bunged up, going for weeks
without passing a stool.

Cough

BREATHING difficult; slow; snoring.
Worse during sleep; on falling asleep; on waking.

Breathing slows down during sleep and when the
fever is strong; it becomes irregular and laboured, like
a waking snoring.

Effects of drugs taken during or after labour

DROWSY, SLEEPY, SPACED OUT.
Cause general anaesthetic; morphine or pethidine.

May feel as though on another planet and can't quite
wake up.

Fever

HEAT burning; intense. With DEEP SLEEP; SWEATING
(see General symptoms).
Better for uncovering.
Worse during sleep; for sweating.

Overpowering sleepiness and yawning; falls asleep
and then breathes slowly and loudly as if snoring.
Heat comes on during sleep; sweating does not
relieve the symptoms. If woken, wants to uncover,
and is either delirious and excitable or stupefied and
semi-conscious.

Insomnia

With SLEEPINESS.

Sleeps lightly and restlessly and hears every sound.
Sleepy but cannot fall asleep; bed may feel hot.

Labour

PREMATURE caused by fright/shock. LABOUR PAINS
stopping or slowing down; weak. With EXHAUS-
TION. With red face.

Apathetic and fearful in labour.

Retention of urine

Cause childbirth; shock.

After a shock or fright is unable to pass urine.

PETROLEUM (Petr.)

Other name: coal oil

General symptoms

Dislikes meat; fatty, rich food. **Sweat** one-sided;
smelly.
Worse for fresh air; during morning; travelling (boat,
car, train, bus, etc.).

There is a general dislike of fresh air which also
aggravates the nausea of travel sickness or
pregnancy.

Emotional state

Confused in fresh air. **Forgetful. Irritable. Quarrelsome.**

These are irritable types who feel confused outside
(partly because it aggravates their physical
symptoms).

Physical complaints

Diarrhoea

DAYTIME ONLY. PAIN pressing. With ravenous
APPETITE.

The diarrhoea occurs only during daytime and is not
accompanied by loss of appetite.

Dizziness

With NAUSEA (see p. 236).
Worse for getting up from lying down/sitting.

Headache

PAIN in back of head; pressing. With HEAVINESS;
NAUSEA (see p. 236).

Usually comes on when travelling and accompanies
nausea.

Nappy rash (Diaper rash)

Skin red; itches; cracked – dry or weepy; bleeding.
Worse in the folds of the skin.

Nausea

With DIZZINESS (see p. 235).
Worse for fresh air.

Usually accompanied by dizziness and/or headache.

Thrush (genital)/Yeast infection

DISCHARGE like egg white; burning; copious.

Travel sickness

With HEADACHE (see p. 235); NAUSEA (see above);
　VOMITING.
Worse for fresh air.

One of the main travel-sickness remedies and is
indicated where fresh air aggravates. Opposite of
Tabacum.

PHOSPHORIC ACID (Pho-ac.)

General symptoms

Anaemia. Complaints from loss of body fluids. **Eyes**
glassy. **Face** pale. **Gums** bleeding. **Likes** fruit;
refreshing things. **Pains** in bones. **Sweat** clammy;
profuse. **Symptoms** one-sided. **Thirstless.**
Better after a good sleep.
Worse for cold; for sweating; during evening; during
morning; on one side of body.

This remedy benefits those who are weak and tired
from studying too much or from losing body fluids,
for example after diarrhoea, a heavy period, bleeding
or vomiting. It is also for those who are convalescing
from an acute illness. They look pale and sickly; with
dark rings around their eyes and sweat a lot. They
want refreshing food to eat, such as fruit and vegetables (to replace the liquid), but may not be thirsty
and often feel tired after eating. They are generally
worse for cold and better for a sleep, even a short
nap.

Emotional state

Anxious about others. **Apathetic. Brooding. Complaints from** disappointed love; excitement; fright;
grief; humiliation; shock. **Depressed. Disappointment. Dwells on past. Forgetful. Homesick.**

Indifferent during fever. **Irritable. Uncommunicative.**

Emotional trauma such as disappointment in love,
shock or homesickness results in mental apathy.
Phosphoric-acid types beome depressed, they do not
want to talk, think or answer and may even forget
words while they are speaking. They appear indifferent to everything and lack even the energy to cry.

Physical complaints

Cough

Dry; tickling; violent.

Diarrhoea

ABDOMEN/STOMACH rumbling. STOOLS profuse;
　thin; watery; white. Without WEAKNESS.
Worse after eating solid/dry food.
Cause summer; hot weather.

May pass an involuntary stool at the same time as
passing wind. There may be gurgling and cramping,
gripping pains, and a bloated, full feeling in the
abdomen, although it is usually painless. Exhaustion
does not accompany the diarrhoea but sets in once it
has stopped.

Exhaustion

NERVOUS; PARALYTIC.
Worse after eating; in morning on getting up; for
　slightest exertion; for walking.
Cause breastfeeding; loss of body fluids (diarrhoea,
　vomiting, etc.); flu.

Hair loss

Cause grief.

Headache

EYES smarting. HEAD feels heavy. PAIN top of head;
　back of head; nape of neck; one-sided; pressing.
Better for excitement.
Worse for getting up from lying down.
Cause eye strain; grief; mental exertion/strain,
　especially from studying.

Insomnia

SLEEP unrefreshing. WAKING frequent; SLEEPLESS
　after midnight.

Shock

Cause emotional trauma.

For shock caused by emotional trauma and accompanied by the typical emotional state.

PHOSPHORUS (Phos.)
Other name: white phosphorus

General symptoms

Anaemia. Bleeding occurs easily; bright red; profuse. **Complaints from** change of weather; getting chilled. **Discharges** blood-streaked. **Dislikes** fruit; hot food; water during pregnancy. **Face** red in spots. **Haemorrhages. Hair loss. Heavy feeling. Hot flushes. Likes** cold drinks; cold food; spicy food; ice-cream; milk; chocolate; salt. **Nosebleeds. Pains** in glands; burning. **Sweat** on single parts of body; worse for slightest physical exertion; clammy. **Taste** in mouth sour. **Thirst** unquenchable for ice-cold drinks; for water. **Tongue** red-coated.
Better after a good sleep; for cold drinks; for massage.
Worse for cold; before eating; for change of weather; during evening; during morning; for windy weather.

These types are usually tall and slim. They burn up food quickly and therefore need to eat often, are also thirsty and want cold or iced drinks (especially cold milk). Chilly individuals who are sensitive to changes in the weather, feel worse for getting cold, and hate wind. They bleed easily and copiously; suffering from heavy periods and nosebleeds of bright-red blood which is slow to coagulate. They are prone to anaemia and hair loss because of blood loss. Pains are usually burning pains, wherever they are. Mornings and evenings between dusk and midnight are their worst times of day.

Emotional state

Affectionate. Anxious about health. **Apathetic** indifferent to children or relatives. **Clingy. Desires** company. **Euphoric. Excitable. Fearful** generally; of being alone; of the dark; of death; during a thunderstorm. **Irritable. Jumpy. Sensitive** generally; infants to pain; to light. **Slow. Sympathetic. Uncommunicative.**

When healthy they are lively, affectionate and excitable – although may also have classic *Phosphorus* fears: they hate to be alone, especially in the dark at night when their vivid imaginations go to work; scared of thunderstorms. They are gregarious types, who feel things strongly, are sensitive, highly strung and easily startled.

When sick they become irritable, mentally sluggish (like *Phosphoric acid*), apathetic, and don't want to think, talk or work. Illness debilitates them; their energy may flare up in bursts, but is followed by a return to their exhausted state. They need sympathy when ill and, despite being fearful and irritable if tired or upset, they are easily comforted and reassured. They love massage, touch and affection.

Physical complaints
Backache

BETWEEN SHOULDER BLADES. In LOWER BACK; back feels broken; burning.
Better for rubbing/massage.
Worse on getting up from sitting.
Cause childbirth.

Bleeding

After childbirth. FLOW OF BLOOD is bright red.

Common cold

NASAL CATARRH blood-streaked; profuse; one-sided; dry. With SENSE OF TASTE/SMELL lost. HOARSENESS; SORE THROAT (see p. 238).

Nose runs profusely or is blocked and dry with no discharge.

Cough

BREATHING difficult; fast. COUGH dry at night; during fever; hacking; irritating; racking; tickling; tight; violent; from tickling in larynx; wakes person at night; must sit up at night. LARYNX raw. MUCUS tastes sweet; salty; transparent; white; yellow; green; copious; bloody. PAIN IN CHEST burning. With SWEATING. In PREGNANCY.
Better for heat.
Worse for change of temperature; for cold air; for fresh air; during fever; for lying on left side; during the morning after getting up; during the evening until midnight; reading aloud.

Chest feels weighted down and burning pains are worse for coughing. Air passages feel irritated and worse for cold air. Coughs up copious quantities of sputum, especially in the morning.

Croup

See COUGH (above).

Diarrhoea

STOOLS blood-streaked; frequent; PAINLESS; profuse; watery. With ICY-COLD HANDS AND FEET. In PREGNANCY.
Better after cold food.
Worse during morning; after getting chilled.

Abdomen may be bloated and gurgling, and stools are blood-streaked. Cold drinks may help.

Dizziness

HAS TO LIE DOWN.
Worse for getting up from lying down/sitting.

Effects of drugs taken during or after labour

DROWSY, SLEEPY, SPACED OUT. With VOMITING (see opposite).
Cause general anaesthetic.

Exhaustion

NERVOUS. PARALYTIC. With FEVER (see below).
Worse for slightest exertion; for walking.
Cause breastfeeding; diarrhoea; fever; sweating.

So tired during acute illness that cannot stay upright in bed but continually slides down.

Fever

Increased APPETITE. HEAT dry at night; burning; ONE-SIDED; worse on right side.
Worse in afternoon/evening/night.

Has an unquenchable thirst for cold drinks and a good appetite. May not appear as ill as fever indicates they might.

Gums bleeding

Cause tooth extraction.

Hair loss

Falls out IN HANDFULS.
Cause acute illness.

Headache

HUNGER before/during headache. PAIN in forehead; sides of head; burning; bursting; pressing; throbbing.
Better after sleep; for cold; for cold compresses; for fresh air; on getting up; for massage; for walking.
Worse for getting cold; for coughing; for daylight; for hot drinks; in stuffy room; for wrapping up head.
Cause imminent thunderstorm.

Nervous headache, the head feels heavy and the sense of smell is often acute, the eyes water in cold air.

Indigestion

PAIN in stomach burning; sore, bruised.
Worse after eating.

Injuries

CUTS/WOUNDS bleed freely; blood bright red; slow to clot.

Insomnia

Anxious DREAMS. With SLEEPINESS.

Sleeps on the right side cannot fall asleep when lying on the left side, especially with a chest infection or cough. Has anxious, vivid dreams.

Nausea

ABDOMEN/STOMACH feels empty. BELCHES sour.
Worse for putting hands in warm water; for hot drinks; for drinking water.

The empty feeling is not relieved by eating.

Nosebleed

Blood bright red; persistent. With SWEATING.
Worse for blowing nose.

Shock

With VOMITING (see below).
Cause surgery.

Sore throat

PAIN raw; sore. TONSILS swollen. VOICE hoarse.
Worse for breathing in; for coughing; during morning/evening; for pressure; for talking.

Sore throats often accompany a cold. Can hardly talk as the throat is so painfully hoarse.

Vomiting

Burning PAIN IN STOMACH. VOMIT bile; mucus; bitter; yellow; violent.
Worse after drinking/eating.

Vomits food and drink – even the smallest quantity – as soon as it becomes warm in the stomach (after a little while). May be burning pains in the stomach or a bruised soreness.

PHYTOLACCA DECANDRA (Phyt.)
Other name: poke-root

General symptoms

Breath smelly. **Pains** shoot upwards. **Tongue** red-tipped.

These types feel exhausted, stiff and worn out. Smelly breath and a red-tipped tongue accompany many of the complaints.

Physical complaints
Breastfeeding problems

BREASTS inflamed; lumpy. ABSCESSES. NIPPLES cracked/sore. PAIN while nursing.

This remedy is a specific for sore, cracked nipples where pain radiates from the nipple all over the body. Also useful for infections and abscesses where the breast is hard, nodular and lumpy; or if a lump in the breast becomes painful and an abscess threatens. It can take 12–24 hours to act (unlike the quick action of *Aconite* or *Belladonna*).

Mumps

GLANDS hard; painful; swollen. PAINS spread to breasts, ovaries. With COPIOUS SALIVA; PROFUSE SWEATING; SORE THROAT (see below).

Sore throat

THROAT dark red. TONSILS swollen.
Better for cold drinks.
Worse for hot drinks.

Swallowing is difficult and causes pains to shoot through both ears (in *Belladonna* sore throats the pains shoot up only to the right ear). The throat may also hurt on sticking out the tongue.

Teething

PAINFUL IN CHILDREN. With CRYING.
Better for biting gums together hard.

Teething babies will bite their teeth (or gums) together – on anything and everything!

PODOPHYLLUM (Podo.)
Other name: mandrake

Physical complaints
Diarrhoea

ABDOMEN/STOMACH gurgling; rumbling. STOOLS frequent; gushing; involuntary; painless; profuse; smelly; sudden. With EXHAUSTION after passing stool.
Worse after drinking water; immediately after drinking; after eating; for hot weather; mid-morning; around 4 a.m.; at night.

Diarrhoea may alternate with other symptoms such as a headache or even constipation. Dull aches or cramping pains may accompany much gurgling before a stool; the stools are usually painless and shoot out. They may be frothy, of a changeable colour and consistency, and are usually accompanied by loud wind. Feels drained, faint and weak after a stool. Teething babies sometimes produce this type of diarrhoea.

Flatulence

ABDOMEN/STOMACH gurgling before stool. WIND loud during stool.

PULSATILLA NIGRICANS (Puls.)
Other name: meadow anemone

General symptoms

Anaemia. Breath smelly. **Complaints from/after** measles; getting wet; getting feet wet; weaning. **Discharges** thick; yellow; bland. **Dislikes** bread; butter; food in general; fruit; tobacco; hot food/drinks; fatty, rich food; meat. **Faintness** in a warm room. **Glands** swollen. **Lips** dry. **Mouth** dry. **Oedema** (swelling) of ankles/feet; hands/fingers. **Pains** on parts lain on; wandering. **Sweat** smelly; single parts of body; one-sided; worse at night. **Symptoms** right-sided; changeable. **Taste** in mouth bad in morning. **Thirstless. Tongue** coated white/yellow.
Better for bathing; for fresh air; for movement; for pressure; for walking in fresh air; for crying.
Worse for getting cold; for exposure to sun; for rich fatty food; for getting feet wet; for heat; in stuffy rooms; at twilight; for wet weather; for wind.

These types have dry mouths and lips and an absence of thirst. They may be chilly, with cold hands and feet, but dislike heat and stuffy rooms, becoming quickly flushed. Always feel better in the fresh air, where their moods lift and their symptoms (especially coughs) disappear, returning only back in the warm. But they are sensitive to getting wet or being exposed to wet, windy weather, when they may start a cough or cold.

They hate rich, fatty food, which gives them indigestion and nausea. They may, however, have a craving for butter. Chests and joints are worse for rest and better for moving about, especially in fresh air; twilight is their worst time.

Also useful in pregnancy where anaemia in *Pulsatilla* type may result from an excess of ordinary iron pills, so stopping iron is essential (see *Ferrum metallicum*). Their physical symptoms may be hard to pin down, changing from one moment to the next, rather like their moods.

Emotional state

Affectionate. Angry (morose) babies. **Anxious** at night; indoors. **Capricious. Changeable. Clingy. Complaints from** fright; grief; shock. **Depressed** worse before menstrual period, during pregnancy, in stuffy room, in evening, from suppressed grief; better for fresh air. Desires to be carried (infants). **Disappointment. Excitable. Fearful** at twilight; in evening. **Gentle. Introspective. Irritable. Jealous. Lonely. Moody. Sensitive** babies. **Shy. Sluggish/dull. Tearful** during a fever; while breastfeeding, in pregnancy; better for fresh air. **Whiny.**

These types are gentle, yielding, mild; easily moved to laughter or tears; highly emotional and cry easily. They are clingy and dependent, particularly when sick, when they also become irritable and whiny and feel hard done by. Especially useful for babies as so many of them go through a *Pulsatilla* phase – weepy, clingy, whiny and wanting to be carried.

Pulsatillas are affectionate creatures who love animals and cannot bear to see them hurt. They too are easily hurt but may suppress it and become introspective, moody, even irritable. Depression (even post-natal) will be better for fresh air, and worse during the evening and in warm, stuffy rooms. A breastfeeding mother may weep while nursing. Generally, these types moan and weep during fever, and cry when talking about their illness. They crave sympathy which makes them feel better.

Physical complaints

Afterpains

With classic *Pulsatilla* general and emotional/mental symptoms: thirstless and weepy.

Backache

In LOWER BACK; in SMALL OF BACK. PAIN aching; dragging down; pressing. In pregnancy.
Better for gentle exercise; for walking slowly.
Worse on beginning to move; on getting up from sitting; before menstrual period.

Back feels weak and tired. Getting up after a long period of sitting or bending down is almost impossible. Back may feel sprained.

Bleeding (vaginal) in pregnancy

FLOW OF BLOOD stops and starts; changeable; with clots.

Breast(feeding) problems

MILK SUPPLY overabundant. PAIN IN BREAST when baby nurses.

Breathless

In PREGNANCY.
Better for fresh air.
Worse for exertion.

Breech baby

This can help to turn some babies in late pregnancy.

Chickenpox

With COUGH (see p. 241).

With a low fever and typical general symptoms and emotional state. Itching is worse for heat.

Common cold

NASAL CATARRH dirty yellow; green; yellow-green; bland (non-irritating); smelly; thick; dry alternating with profuse; watery in fresh air. With SENSE OF SMELL/TASTE lost. With SNEEZING in stuffy room. Blocked, painful SINUSES.
Better for fresh air.
Worse in a stuffy room.

Nose is watery in fresh air, blocked in evenings, in a warm room, though there will be much sneezing then too. Sense of taste is lost altogether or there is a bitter taste before and after eating.

Constipation

In PREGNANCY. STOOLS changeable.

Cough

Constant in evening; dry at night; during fever; loose in the morning; exhausting; irritating; racking; in fits; violent; disturbs sleep. MUCUS yellow; green; yellow-green; copious; sticky; difficult to cough up (must sit up). With NAUSEA (see p. 242); RETCHING. In PREGNANCY.

Better for fresh air; for sitting up.

Worse for getting hot; for physical exertion; for heat; for lying down; after meals; during the morning; at night/evening; in a stuffy room; getting warm in bed.

The cough disturbs sleep; breathing is loud and rattling. Sputum is characteristically thick, difficult to cough up, may taste unpleasant, and is worse in the morning on getting up.

Cystitis

DESIRE TO URINATE frequent; ineffectual; painful; urgent. Spasmodic PAIN. Frequent URINATION. URINE copious. In pregnancy.

Worse after urinating.

Cause getting cold and wet.

Hurries to pass urine to prevent it escaping, but once there the urine dribbles slowly.

Diarrhoea

In BABIES. In PREGNANCY. STOOLS changeable; greenish-yellow; slimy; watery.

Better for fresh air.

Worse after eating; after eating starchy or rich food; at night; for getting overheated; in stuffy room.

Cause rich food; fruit.

Dizziness

HAS TO LIE DOWN.

Worse for getting up from lying down; sitting; stooping; walking.

Earache

DISCHARGE smelly; thick; yellow; yellow-green. EAR (external) red; EAR (internal) feels blocked. PAIN aching; pressing; pressing outwards; stitching; tearing; throbbing. With DEAFNESS; ITCHING; NOISES in ear.

Worse at night.

Cause after common cold; after measles.

Exhaustion

NERVOUS.

Worse for heat of sun; in stuffy room; mental exertion; morning in bed.

Cause loss of sleep (broken nights).

Eye inflammation

In BABIES. DISCHARGE purulent; smelly; thick; yellow. EYES aching; burning; itching; watering. EYELIDS glued together; itching in evening. With symptoms of COMMON COLD (see p. 240).

Better for cold bathing; for fresh air; for cold.

Worse during evening; in warm room.

In the morning the eyes are sticky and the inner corners discharge. They ache and burn in a warm room, and water in cold air or wind and/or with a cough.

Faintness

In PREGNANCY.

May accompany mild anaemia.

Fever

HEAT burning; dry during the evening; ONE-SIDED. With CHILLINESS.

Better for uncovering.

Worse for heat; for washing; in the afternoon; in the evening; at night; in morning in bed; for warm covers; in stuffy room; for being uncovered.

Wants to be covered but gets overheated, kicks covers off and then gets cold. The fever (heat) may be on one side only and is often worse in early afternoon, followed by a chill around 4 p.m. Sweating may also be one-sided (usually the left) or localised. Sweats while asleep and wakes up chilled, then finds it difficult to get back to sleep.

Flatulence

ABDOMEN/STOMACH rumbling/gurgling. WIND smelly; obstructed (difficult to expel).

Better for passing wind.

Food poisoning

With DIARRHOEA (see opposite).

Cause rotten meat; rotten fish.

Headache

NERVOUS. PAIN in forehead; one-sided; pressing; sore, bruised; throbbing. In PREGNANCY.

Better for firm pressure; for fresh air; for lying with head high; for walking in fresh air.

Worse after eating; for bending down; for blowing nose; for hot drinks; for running; for standing; in a stuffy room; in heat.

Cause breastfeeding; excitement; ice-cream; running.

Pulsatilla types are prone to nervous headaches over the eyes, usually on one side; worse for movement and better for fresh air. Can be caused by too much sun or too much rich food.

Incontinence

In PREGNANCY.

Worse for coughing, laughing, sneezing, walking.

Indigestion

ABDOMEN/STOMACH feels empty. BELCHES bitter; empty; tasting of food just eaten. PAIN in stomach; pressing. With HEARTBURN. In PREGNANCY.

Worse at night; for rich, fatty food.

Cause rich, fatty food.

Abdomen/stomach gurgles and rumbles during the evening.

Insomnia

DREAMS anxious, vivid. SLEEP restless. With SLEEPINESS. WAKING from cold; frequent. In PREGNANCY.

Worse before midnight.

Cause overactive mind; repeating thoughts.

Pulsatilla insomniacs like to sleep on their backs, arms above their head, and feet poked out of bed. They sleep restlessly, with twitchy arms and legs, and have anxious dreams and nightmares.

Joint pain

PAIN in bones; in joints; pulling; sore, bruised; wandering.

Better for cold compresses; for fresh air; for gentle movement; for walking.

Worse after a common cold; on beginning to move; for heat; for warmth of bed; for wet weather.

Labour

LABOUR PAIN in back; false; ineffectual (cervix doesn't dilate); irregular; short (each contraction lasts a short time); stop or slow down; weak. With FAINT FEELING; EXHAUSTION (see p. 241); NAUSEA (see below); VOMITING.

With characteristic general symptoms and emotional state. Women are pathetic, depressed, clingy and weepy in labour.

Lochia

SCANTY, MILKY, RETURNS (having almost stopped).

Measles

With COUGH (see p. 241); COMMON COLD (see p. 240); EYE INFLAMMATION (see p. 241).

With characteristic weepiness and lack of thirst.

Mumps

GLANDS swollen/painful. PAINS spread to breasts, ovaries. In pregnancy. With VOMITING; FEVER (see p. 241).

With characteristic general and emotional mental symptoms.

Nausea

With VOMITING.

Better for cold drinks; fresh air.

Cause pregnancy.

Worse after drinking/eating; for coughing; during morning; for hot drinks; for rich food; ice-cream.

Phlebitis

With stinging pains in the veins/legs.

Piles

INTERNAL. After CHILDBIRTH.

Prolapse

With a sense of PRESSURE IN THE ABDOMEN and the SMALL OF THE BACK.

Retained placenta

With INEFFECTIVE, SPASMODIC CONTRACTIONS and the 'weeps'.

Roseola

See MEASLES (above) for symptoms.

Sciatica

Better for fresh air.
Worse in a warm room.

Snuffles

In newborn babies. With symptoms of COMMON COLD (see p. 240).

Sore throat

THROAT dry. LARYNX irritated; tickling. PAIN raw; scraping; stitching.
Worse for heat.

Larynx feels as though there is dust in it; feels rough, and raw from coughing. Chokes when swallowing solid food.

Styes

Worse on upper eyelids.

Teething

PAINFUL.
Better for cold water; fresh air.
Worse for heat of bed, warm food/drinks.

Thrush (genital)/Yeast infection

In pregnancy. DISCHARGE burning; cream-like; milky; thick.

Varicose veins

Of LEG/THIGH/FOOT. PAINFUL. PAIN stinging.
Worse during pregnancy.

Limbs lain on become numb and cold, indicating poor circulation.

Weaning

To dry up milk.

Breasts are sore and swollen after weaning in spite of having taken *Lac canninum*.

PYROGEN (Pyr.)

Other name: sepsin

General symptoms

Discharges (breath, pus, sweat) smelly. **Pain** in parts lain on; sore, bruised. **Pulse** rapid. **Thirsty**.

Better for movement.
Worse for cold; for cold, wet weather.

This is an important flu remedy, for those very severe flus with terrible pains and smelly discharges. The cold in any form aggravates.

A severe acute complaint such as blood poisoning always needs professional care. I have also given indications for emergency treatment of this complaint. If indicated it works quickly and may make antibiotics unnecessary.

Physical complaints

Blood poisoning

With fever (see below); extreme chilliness.
Worse for cold.
Cause childbirth; surgery; infected wounds.

Give *Pyrogen* every 5 minutes after calling for emergency help. A keynote for the use of *Pyrogen* is smelly discharges. The urine may be clear.

Fever

HEAT. With CHILLINESS internal; extreme; SWEATING; SHAKING.
Worse for being uncovered.

During a fever parts lain on feel sore and bruised (like *Arnica*). A low fever is usually accompanied by a fast pulse and is not a cause for immediate concern. If the fever is high and the pulse slow this may indicate acute blood poisoning. Always seek help if these symptoms occur. Feels extremely chilly and cannot get warm. May be anxious, unusually talkative and slightly delirious.

Flu

PAIN aching; in bones of legs. With FEVER (see above); extreme THIRST; SHIVERING; CHILLINESS in back.
Better for movement; for walking; for warmth of bed.
Worse during chilly stage; for sitting.

RHEUM (Rhe.)

Other name: palmated rhubarb

General symptoms

Discharges (stools, sweat, etc.) sour.

These are pale babies who have a hard time assimilating food when producing (or trying to produce) teeth. Sourness is the keynote of this remedy. The baby smells sour, despite frequent washing.

Emotional state

Capricious. **Irritable** with teething. **Play** babies don't want to. **Restless** with teething. **Screaming**. **Tearful** babies at night.

Rheum is for teething children who are colicky, irritable, difficult, peevish, restless and don't want to play. They may sleep very little and seem to survive remarkably well (you don't).

Physical complaints

Diarrhoea

In teething babies. STOOLS sour smelling; pasty. **Cause** teething.

Food is not assimilated well and colicky pains cause babies to cry and be restless at night.

Teething

PAINFUL in babies. With DIARRHOEA (see above).

RHODODENDRON (Rhod.)

Other name: Siberian rhododendron

General symptoms

Complaints from change of weather to stormy. **Better** for movement. **Worse** for cold; for cold, wet weather; for stormy weather; before a storm; for wind.

These types are extremely sensitive to the change in pressure that precedes a storm; their symptoms come on then or are generally worse. They are also sensitive to changes in the weather, particularly to cold, wet and windy weather, and are worse during the seasons of change – spring and autumn. Their symptoms may abate when the storm breaks.

Emotional state

Fearful during a thunderstorm.

May feel apprehensive, fearful or just 'unwell' before and, to some extent, during a storm.

Physical complaints

Backache

In LOWER BACK; in NECK. PAIN rheumatic; sore, bruised. **Better** for movement. **Worse** for wet weather.

Headache

PAIN tearing. **Better** for getting up; for walking; for walking in fresh air; for wrapping up head. **Worse** before/during thunderstorm; for damp weather.

The pains in the face and eyes are always worse before and during a storm.

Joint pain

PAIN in arms/legs/shoulders; drawing; tearing. **Better** for movement; for stretching out limb. **Worse** for change of weather; for sitting down; for stormy weather; for wet weather.

RHUS TOXICODENDRON (Rhus-t.)

Other name: poison ivy

General symptoms

Complaints from getting wet; change of weather to cold/damp; getting chilled. **Face** red. **Glands** swollen. **Likes** milk. **Lips** dry. **Oedema** (swelling) of ankles/feet; hands/fingers. **Pains** burning; pressing; shooting; sore, bruised. **Sweat** worse for lying down; uncovering; slightest physical exertion. **Taste** in mouth metallic. **Tongue** red-tipped. **Better** for changing position; for fresh air; for movement; for sweating; for warmth of bed; for hot drinks. **Worse** in the autumn; for change of weather; for cloudy weather; for cold; for cold/wet weather; for foggy weather; for cold drinks/food; for damp; for draughts; on beginning to move; for lying down; for uncovering; swimming in cold water.

Rhus-t pains are typically aching, sore and bruised with tearing or stitching pains that are worse on first moving after rest. These ease off after joint has been gently exercised by, for example, a little walk. But after a while tiredness sets in and the pains start up again, requiring rest followed by gentle exercise, and so the cycle continues. They find any position uncomfortable, are restless, and need to move around, seemingly constantly. Their pains cause them to get up at night, preventing sleep. Lying on a hard floor may help.

The tongue has a characteristic triangular red tip that may be sore and/or it may be coated.

These people feel better generally for sweating, especially during a fever, but getting chilled while sweating aggravates their condition and can produce a cough or cold. They are chilly people, hate the cold in any form: cold food or drink, swimming or washing in cold water, and cold and wet weather in any form. Even touching cold things, putting a hand out of bed into cold air, or eating ice-cream on a hot day can make them feel bad. They feel better for heat, for warm, dry compresses (heat packs) and for hot baths.

They are sensitive to the damp, especially of autumn, when they may suffer from joint pains or a bad flu.

Emotional state

Anxious indoors; in bed. **Confused. Depressed. Desires** to be carried (babies). **Irritable. Restless** generally; babies; in bed. **Tearful.**

Restlessness is the key, whether caused by physical pain or by nervousness. It can be seen during an acute illness with a fever where a person tosses and turns and has to get up. The anxiety is worse in bed at night because of having to be still then, especially after midnight when the mind dwells on unpleasant thoughts. Also they feel worse in other ways at night, being irritable and fearful. Their depression is not very deep, but it may be constant, and they may suddenly and involuntarily burst into tears without knowing why.

Physical complaints

Abdominal pain

In PREGNANCY. With STIFFNESS IN LOWER ABDOMEN; restlessness.
Worse as uterus expands (towards end of pregnancy).
Cause ligaments of uterus stretching.

Afterpains

Frequent. With RESTLESSNESS.
Better for moving about.

Backache

In LOWER BACK; in SMALL OF BACK; in NECK. PAIN aching; dragging down; sore, bruised; rheumatic. With STIFFNESS.
Better for lying on hard surface; for movement; for walking; for heat.
Worse on beginning to move; on getting up from sitting; for reaching up; for wet weather.
Cause damp weather; draughts; injury; lifting; pregnancy; sprain.

Back feels weak, lame and tired, and pains compel constant moving about in bed. Getting up after lengthy sitting down is difficult. Pain may result from

sitting in a draught, from lifting or a sprain, or it may be rheumaticky pain in damp, wet weather. It is always better for warmth, but aggravated by first movement.

Bleeding (vaginal) in pregnancy

FLOW clotted. With LABOUR-LIKE PAINS.
Cause over-exertion; strain.

Carpal Tunnel Syndrome

In pregnancy.

With tingling and numbness in fingers.

Chickenpox

SKIN RASH itches maddeningly.
Restlessness with the itching, and characteristic *Rhus-t.* red-tipped tongue.

Cough

Irritating; short; tickling.
Better for hot drinks.
Worse for becoming cold; for uncovering; on single parts of the body; for uncovering hands.
Cause swimming in cold water.

Cough is aggravated if part of body is uncovered and consequently becomes cold.

Diarrhoea

STOOLS mushy, watery.
Cause getting wet, getting feet wet.

Exhaustion

NERVOUS. With HEAVINESS; RESTLESSNESS.
Better for walking in fresh air.
Worse for slightest exertion; for sitting down; for walking in fresh air.

Slightest exertion is an effort but a gentle walk in the fresh air helps. With characteristic *Rhus-t.* restlessness.

Eye inflammation

EYES sensitive to light; sore; watering. EYELIDS glued together; itching; swollen.
Worse for moving eyes.
Cause cold, wet weather.

Eyelids are stuck together in the mornings.

Fever

HEAT alternating with chills; dry; burning.
Better for hot drinks.
Worse at night/evening/mid-morning; for movement; cold drinks; for being uncovered.

Sweats from the slightest exertion, as well as when lying in bed asleep, and sweats all over except for head. Urinates frequently while sweating. May get chilled after being hot and sweaty, when any movement or uncovering will bring on chilliness. Warmth helps the chilliness. Fever may be one-sided. May feel as though hot water is running through the blood vessels.

Flu

PAIN in bones; in eyes; in joints; in legs; aching; shooting; sore, bruised. With EXHAUSTION (see p. 245); FEVER (see above); SNEEZING.

Headache

PAIN in back of head; rheumatic; violent.
Better for gentie walking; for wrapping up head; for movement.
Cause change of weather; cold air/wind; damp weather; getting wet; lifting.

Hives

RASH burning; itching; stinging. With JOINT PAIN (see below).
Worse for cold; after scratching.
Cause getting wet/chilled; cold air; during fever.

Insomnia

SLEEP restless; sleepless after midnight.

Vivid, work-related dreams, caused by working too hard.

Joint pain

PAIN aching; sore, bruised; shooting; tearing. With HEAVINESS; LAMENESS; STIFFNESS.
Better for continued movement; for external heat; for walking; for warm compresses; for warmth of bed.
Worse for damp weather; during fever; on beginning to move; at night; for sitting down; for getting chilled.

Pains are worse for rest and on beginning to move; improve temporarily but gets worse again after a while. Can be brought about by over-exertion, for example, spring-cleaning or gardening.

Mumps

GLANDS swollen/painful. With FEVER (see opposite).
Better for heat.
Worse for cold; on left side.

Left side often becomes swollen first. This is a major mumps remedy, indicated by hard, swollen glands that often feature in *Rhus-t.* acute illnesses.

Nappy rash

BURNS. ITCHES. Becomes FLAKY.
Better for covering.
Worse for cold.

Phlebitis

With *Rhus-t.* general symptoms and emotional state.

Prolapse

Cause over-exertion.

Strained ligaments, from too much pushing in second stage of labour.

Restless legs

In PREGNANCY; in BED.

Scarlet fever

RASH itches and burns.

With *Rhus-t.* general symptoms and emotional state.

Sciatica

Better for movement; for walking; for heat.
Worse for cold; for cold compresses; on beginning to move; for lying on painful part; for washing in cold water; for wet weather.

Sore throat

THROAT dry. Tickling LARYNX. VOICE hoarse.
Worse for cold drinks; for swallowing; for uncovering throat.
Cause straining voice.

Voice is hoarse, or strained, from too much talking or singing, but improves after continued use (as do *Rhus-t.* joints).

Sprains

FOOT. ANKLE. WRIST. With STIFFNESS; TREMBLING.
Cause falling; lifting; twisting.

Use *Arnica* first after injury or a sprain to deal with bruising and swelling. Then give *Rhus-t.* if the sprain is accompanied by the typical general symptoms.

Stiff neck

Cause draughts; getting chilled; lifting.

Strains

With STIFFNESS; TREMBLING.
Better for continued movement.
Worse for beginning to move.

Gardening or spring-cleaning can cause stiffness in joints. Worse when getting up after a rest and better for gentle exercise (whereas *Arnica* stiffness and soreness stays in spite of gentle exercise).

RUMEX CRISPUS (Rumex)

Other name: yellow dock

Physical complaints
Cough

In fits; constant; dry; irritating; tickling. PAIN IN CHEST burning; sore, bruised; stitching. LARYNX raw.
Worse for lying down; for breathing in cold air; for fresh air; for change of temperature from warm to cold; for becoming cold; for cold air; on left side of body; in morning on waking; for talking; for uncovering; for walking in the cold air.

Cough causes pains in the chest, usually on the left side or in the left lung, or under the sternum. Pains are worse on breathing in cold air, so the mouth is covered with a scarf to allow only warm air through. Rawness and tickling in the larynx make the cough worse. Hawks up mucus from the back of the throat, where it gets stuck.

Sore throat

THROAT raw; sore; irritated. AIR PASSAGES irritated. VOICE lost.
Worse for breathing in cold air.

RUTA GRAVEOLENS (Ruta)

Other name: common rue

General symptoms

Pains in bones; in parts lain on; sore, bruised.

Better for movement.
Worse for lying on painful part.

Like *Rhus toxicodendron*, *Ruta* is for sprains, but *Rhus-t.* is for damaged ligaments and *Ruta* for injuries to the tendons and the periosteum (the covering of the bones). It can be hard to differentiate so use *Rhus-t.*'s clear general symptoms to guide you. *Ruta* is indicated for sore, bruised joint pains that feel worse if lain on. There may be restlessness but not nearly so marked as in *Rhus tox*.

Emotional state

Fearful of death. **Weary**.

The emotional symptoms are not strong, but during fever there may be some fear and mild depression.

Physical complaints
Abdominal pain

In PREGNANCY.
Worse as uterus expands towards end of pregnancy. With stiffness in lower abdomen.
Cause ligaments of uterus stretching.

Backache

PAIN sore, bruised. With LAMENESS.
Better for lying on back.

Eye strain

EYESIGHT dim; weak. PAIN aching; burning; strained.
Worse during evening; at night; for poor light; for using eyes; for close work.
Cause too much close work.

Ruta stimulates and strengthens the eye muscles and restores the sight when it has become weak and dim after straining the eyes with fine work or too much reading (where the letters on the page seem to run together, for example). For people who do a great deal of close work. It is not a remedy for eye inflammation.

Headache

PAIN in sides of head; sore, bruised. With EYE STRAIN (see above).
Cause eye strain.

Head feels as though beaten or crushed.

Injuries

CUTS/WOUNDS to shins; PAIN bruised, sore.

Ruta is indicated for bruises to the periosteum (the covering of the bone), in particular on the shins. These can be very painful.

Joint pain

PAIN in hands; in feet; in lower back; in parts lain on; in bones; sore, bruised. With LAMENESS.
Worse for walking.

Sprains/strains

PAIN bruised; constant; in ANKLE; in PERIOSTEUM; in TENDONS; in WRIST. With EXHAUSTION; LAMENESS.
Worse for exercise; for pressure; for standing; for walking.

Hands and feet feel cold. Injured part feels lame and bruised (even after *Arnica* has brought down the swelling) and the pains are constant – movement does not relieve pain (like *Rhus-t.*). Pressure is also painful. Feels generally weak and weary.

Tennis elbow

PAIN bruised, sore.
Worse for exercise.

These injuries need a lot of time to heal in case the tendon is torn. *Ruta* helps to heal a damaged tendon, provided the joint is bandaged tightly and completely rested.

SABINA (Sab.)

Other name: savine

Physical complaints

Afterpains

PAIN spreads from the lower back to the thighs, to the pubic bone. Discharge of blood with every pain.

Bleeding (vaginal) in pregnancy

FLOW OF BLOOD bright red; clotted; flows more with slight exertion. In EARLY PREGNANCY. With PAIN in legs; PAIN in lower back that spreads to pubic area.

The bleeding starts off brown with clots and labour-like pains, then a bright red flow of blood starts.

SARSAPARILLA (Sars.)

Other name: wild liquorice

Physical complaints

Breast(feeding) problems

NIPPLES inverted.

If there are no indications for another remedy, give *Sarsaparilla* to help establish breastfeeding.

Cystitis

DESIRE TO URINATE ineffectual. PAIN cutting. URINATION slow; dribbling; can only pass urine while standing. URINE green; pale; with mucus; with sediment.
Worse at end of urination; during menstrual period.
Cause getting chilled; cold, wet weather.

May pass urine without feeling pain until the very end, when yells with pain. Urinating is difficult while sitting, and may only be possible while standing. Even then she may manage only a feeble stream. Kidneys may also be painful (right more so than left) and inflamed (with cutting pains) – it is advisable to seek professional help before this point, but *Sarsaparilla* will help relieve pain in meantime.

SECALE (Sec.)

Other name: ergot

General symptoms

Better for cold bathing.
Worse for heat.

Secale people feel the cold but are much worse for heat – hot stuffy rooms, the heat of bed, warm compresses etc. They don't want to be covered up. This is a small remedy, invaluable for pregnancy and birth. Be guided by specific indications, rather than the general symptoms.

Emotional state

Anxious. Stupor.
In labour women fall into a sort of stupor. With complaints that come after the birth (or in pregnancy) there may be anxiety.

Physical complaints

Afterpains

In women who have had many children. Long-lasting.

Bleeding (vaginal) in pregnancy

With absence of PAIN. In EARLY pregnancy. FLOW OF BLOOD dark brown or black; scanty.

Breast(feeding) problems

MILK SUPPLY low. PAIN stinging in breasts.

In exhausted women with severe afterpains. Breasts remain small.

Colic

In BABIES. ABDOMEN/STOMACH feels bloated. With DIARRHOEA.
Cause syntometrine.

Sometimes the baby reacts to the syntometrine injection given to expel the placenta. It causes a colic where the abdomen becomes bloated and tight like a drum. Baby is better with the nappy off. Stools are watery and olive-green.

Effects of drugs taken during or after labour

Cause syntometrine.

Labour

SLOW. LABOUR PAINS ineffectual (cervix doesn't soften); long (each contraction lasts a long time); stopping or slowing down; weak. With FAINT FEELING; with EXHAUSTION; TREMBLING if contractions stop.

Lochia

Flow is DARK (brown); SMELLY; lasts too long; SCANTY.

Prolapse

Cause too much straining in labour; forceps delivery.

Retained placenta

With BEARING DOWN sensation.

Muscles feel weak and exhausted.

SEPIA (Sep.)
Other name: cuttlefish ink

General symptoms

Appetite lost in pregnancy. **Catches colds easily**. **Complaints from** getting wet. **Craves** vinegar. **Discharges** yellow. **Dislikes** bread in pregnancy; food in general; smell of food; thought of it in pregnancy; milk; meat. **Face** pasty. **Likes** sour foods (pickles) in pregnancy. **Pains** pressing. **Palpitations** in pregnancy. **Sweat** cold; hot; profuse; smelly; sour; worse after slightest physical exertion; from mental exertion; from pain; on single parts of body. **Symptoms** left-sided.

Better after eating; for vigorous exercise; for running; for walking fast.

Worse before/during/after menstrual period; at night; for cold; for fasting; for getting wet; for rest; for frosty air; for sweating; for touch; for walking in wind; for mental/physical exertion; for writing.

These are chilly types, with cold hands and feet, extremely sensitive to cold. They sweat easily and profusely, with any exertion of body or mind or when experiencing strong emotions. Coughing can also make them sweat. The sweat smells sour and makes them feel worse.

They feel exhausted and run down, have no muscle tone, feel and look saggy, and feel as though something heavy inside is dragging them down. The typical *Sepia* face is yellow, earthy and pale, with marked yellowness across saddle of nose and dark rings under eyes. They are generally better for exercising vigorously – this energises them even if they are feeling unwell or exhausted. Eating helps temporarily (they are much worse for missing meals). They do not want to be touched or massaged.

Emotional state

Angry from contradiction. **Anxious** during fever; worse in evening. **Apathetic** towards children or relatives. **Aversion** to partner. **Confused**. **Depressed**. **Desires** to be alone. **Despair** during labour. **Dislikes** company; consolation; contradiction. **Forgetful**. **Indifferent** to own children; to family; to loved ones; to work. **Irritable** generally; worse for consolation. **Loss of libido**. **Sensitive** to music; to noise; to pain. **Sluggish**. **Tearful**. **Weepy**.

These types are prone to dreadful emotional troughs. The classic *Sepia* picture is too many babies too quickly, but women may also be worn out from too much to do and not enough resources to see them through it. In this state, they sag mentally and physically; sit silently, feel empty and enjoy nothing; feel indifferent to things that formerly gave enjoyment including partners and children. They respond badly to sympathy, preferring to be alone. Thinking is difficult and brains seem to have ground to a halt.

They feel much better if they drag themselves out of their torpor to do something strenuous, such as exercise, dancing or even spring-cleaning.

Physical complaints

Backache

In LOWER BACK. PAIN aching; dragging down.
Better for pressure.
Worse during the afternoon; at night; before/during menstrual period; for bending down; for sitting.

Lower back feels weak and tired, as if hit with a hammer.

Bleeding (vaginal) in pregnancy

In MID-PREGNANCY. FLOW OF BLOOD is dark. With bearing-down PAIN.

Feels as if everything will fall out.

Breast pain

In pregnancy.

With *Sepia* general and emotional state.

Breast(feeding) problems

NIPPLES cracked/sore; with ITCHING.

Cracks may get so bad they bleed, but they'll itch first.

Carpal Tunnel Syndrome

In pregnancy.

With tingling/numbness in fingers.

Common cold

NASAL CATARRH green; dirty yellow; yellow-green; drips down back of throat. SENSE OF SMELL lost.

Constipation

ABDOMEN/STOMACH feels full. STOOLS hard; large. STRAINING ineffectual.
Worse during period.
Cause pregnancy.

For acute constipation that accompanies pregnancy. Strains to pass a large, hard stool but is unable to.

Cough

BREATHING fast. COUGH constant when lying down at night; dry; exhausting; hacking; irritating; loose; must sit up to cough; rattling; short; disturbs sleep; tickling; violent; wakens at night. MUCUS copious; yellow; white; tastes salty.

Better for sitting up.
Worse at night; during evening in bed; for lying down.

Coughs up lots of salty white or yellow mucus. Chest feels constricted (tight) or oppressed and the ribs may hurt from coughing. The air passages feel irritated; the cough seems to come from the stomach and is violent, especially after lying down at night. Sweats after coughing and feels worse for it.

Cramp

In PREGNANCY. In CALF/LEG.

Cystitis

DESIRE TO URINATE constant with dragging-down pain in pelvis; urgent. PAIN pressing. URINATION frequent; slow (takes a long time to start). URINE cloudy; dark brown; red; scanty; smelly; with sediment.

Common after childbirth. Constant dragging-down sensation in the pelvis. Has to rush to pass urine or it escapes involuntarily because of saggy muscles in the pelvic area, then has to wait for it to start once sitting on the toilet.

Exhaustion

NERVOUS; SUDDEN. In PREGNANCY.
Worse on getting up in morning; during a menstrual period; for slightest exertion; for sweating; for walking.
Cause breastfeeding; sweating.

Legs feel stiff and weak. Also accompanies *Sepia* hot flushes, or pregnancy.

Eye inflammation

EYES burning. EYELIDS glued together; swollen.
Worse after walk; during evening; for reading.

Eyes feel sore, as if there's sand in them.

Faintness

With HEAT. COLDNESS after faint. In PREGNANCY.
Worse for exercise; during fever; in stuffy room.

Sepia types feel faint easily and are always worse for standing for any length of time.

Fever

With ANXIETY; SWEATING (see General symptoms).
Worse in autumn; for sweating; for covering.
Cause anger.

Fever accompanying flu or other infection is often severe with external heat and internal chilliness. External heat is followed by chills with shaking and no thirst. Covering up warmly makes them uneasy (an unusual and helpful symptom) even when chilled. Characteristic *Sepia* general and emotional symptoms are also present.

Hair loss

After childbirth.

Headache

EXTREMITIES icy-cold. PAIN in bones; bursting; pressing; shooting; tearing; throbbing; in waves. In PREGNANCY.
Better after eating; for fresh air.
Worse for bending down; for getting head cold; for travelling.
Cause artificial light; breastfeeding.

Pains can be almost anywhere in the head, although the left side is often more affected.

Incontinence

In PREGNANCY.
Worse for coughing; laughing; sneezing; walking.

Insomnia

WAKING around 3 a.m. With SLEEPINESS.

Wakes but can't get back to sleep, and may lie awake thinking dismal thoughts. By morning, feels exhausted.

Labour

PAIN in back; distressing; severe (violent); stopping or slowing down. With EXHAUSTION.

Anxious, despairing and irritable in labour; may take dislike to their partner. The pains drag down and are much better for vigorous exercise.

Nausea

INTERMITTENT. ABDOMEN/STOMACH feels empty. PAIN gnawing. With VOMITING (see below).
Worse after eating; before breakfast; during morning; for milk; for pork.

Cause pregnancy.

Empty, sinking feeling in the stomach, only temporarily relieved while eating. Often accompanied by a headache and worse when thinking about food or eating.

Nosebleeds

In PREGNANCY.

Prolapse

With CONSTIPATION; BEARING-DOWN SENSATION.
Better for sitting with legs crossed.

Too many children too close together can cause a prolapse, with a feeling as if everything will fall out.

Skin complaints in pregnancy

BROWN PIGMENTATION in patches on face.

Thrush (genital)/Yeast infection

DISCHARGE burning; copious; like cottage cheese; lumpy, like egg white; smelly; yellow. With DRYNESS; ITCHING. In PREGNANCY.

Simple thrush which occurs during pregnancy. Feels exhausted and worn down.

Toothache

PAIN radiates to the ears; pulling; stitching; tearing; throbbing.
Worse for biting teeth together; for cold drinks/food; during pregnancy; for touch; for hot drinks.

Travel sickness

With BILIOUSNESS; HEADACHE (see opposite); NAUSEA (see opposite).
Worse after eating; during morning.
Cause pregnancy.

Vomiting

VOMIT bile; smelly.
Worse after eating; during morning.
Cause pregnancy.

May feel better for eating, but improvement is temporary.

SILICA (Sil.)

Other name: pure flint

General symptoms

Catches colds easily. **Complaints from** getting feet wet; change of weather to cold. **Dislikes** meat. **Glands** swollen. **Pains** stinging. **Sweat** worse at night, during sleep; profuse; smelly; sour. **Thirsty**. **Weight gain** poor in babies.
Better for heat; for wrapping up head.
Worse for change of weather; for cold; for damp; for draughts; for fresh air; for getting feet wet; for touch; for uncovering; for wet weather.

Silica types feel the cold intensely. They are easily tired and chilled, such as by going out into the cold air after swimming, and are sensitive to draughts and changes of weather. They are prone to catching colds, especially if they get a thorough soaking. They are always better for warmth and being wrapped up well, especially the head.

They sweat at night, particularly on the back of the head and neck (like *Calcarea carbonica*, but not so profuse). The sweat smells sour. Their feet are cold, sweaty *and* smelly. They have trouble assimilating food and their bones do not always form as well as in other children. They can be slow learning to walk and in teething. Their fontanelles close slowly.

Emotional state

Anxious. **Aversion** to being touched/examined; to consolation. **Complaints from** mental strain; shock. Poor **concentration**. **Confused**. **Conscientious**. **Irritable** generally; worse for consolation (babies). **Jumpy**. **Lack of self-confidence**. **Mild**. **Play** – babies don't want to. **Restless**. **Sensitive** to noise; to pain. **Shy**. **Sluggish**.
Worse for being consoled.

These are people who typically lack stamina both mentally and physically – who lack 'grit'. They become worn out easily from too much work (usually mental). Alternatively they *can* be 'gritty' and conscientious under pressure, able to sustain superhuman feats of endurance, collapsing only when the job in hand is done.

They are very shy, and anxious about appearing in public because of fear of failure. Unassertive, lacking in confidence, they give way rather than take a position and fight for it. Conversely can be stubborn, wilful and develop fixed ideas. Irritable if consoled when feeling low. Restless and nervous inside, oversensitive to noise, especially small noises, and startle easily.

Physical complaints

Abscesses

Of GLANDS; of ROOTS OF TEETH.

Silica brings abscesses that are forming to a head.

Afterpains

PAIN in hips.
Worse when baby nurses.

Athlete's foot

Cracks between toes. With sweat on feet; profuse; smelly.

Backache

PAIN sore, bruised; stitching. With LAMENESS; STIFFNESS; WEAKNESS.
Worse on getting up from sitting; breastfeeding; at night; for pressure; for sitting.
Cause falling on back; injury to coccyx; manual labour.

Blocked tear duct

In babies.

This remedy will clear simple blockages of the tear duct.

Breast(feeding) problems

BREAST inflamed; painful; lumpy. NIPPLES cracked/ sore, with bleeding; inverted. PAIN in breast; cutting; stitching. BREAST ABSCESSES.
Worse while nursing; in left breast.

Sudden sharp pains while the baby is nursing and cracks become bad so quickly they bleed. Back may ache while nursing.

Broken bones

SLOW TO MEND.

Common cold

NASAL CATARRH dry; hard crusts; smelly; thick. SINUSES painful. SENSE OF SMELL/TASTE lost. SNEEZING difficult.

Sinuses blocked, nose dry and blocked, nostrils sore and ulcerated.

Constipation

Ineffectual STRAINING. PAIN burning after stool. STOOL hard; knotty; large; 'shy'.
Worse before/during menstrual period.

Muscles in bowel are weak. Stools are painfully expelled and then slip back.

Cough

Irritating. MUCUS lumpy; thick; yellow.
Better for hot drink.
Worse on waking in morning; for becoming cold; for uncovering feet or head.

Lingering winter coughs that started after getting chilled, or wet and chilled, that do not clear up easily with indicated remedy.

Diarrhoea

In TEETHING babies (see p. 254). FLATULENCE smelly (see opposite).
Better for heat; for wrapping up warmly; for warmth of bed.
Cause teething.

Dizziness

HAS TO LIE DOWN. With HEADACHE (see opposite).

Earache

With BLOCKED FEELING IN EAR. PAINS behind ear; tearing.

Eustachian tube is itchy and full of mucus. Any discharge is bloody, smelly and thick.

Exhaustion

NERVOUS.
Cause diarrhoea; breastfeeding.

Eye inflammation

DISCHARGE yellow. EYES sore.
Worse for cold air.
Cause foreign body in the eye.

If a foreign body is still in the eye, *Silica* taken internally will help expel it.

Fever

Worse for movement; for being uncovered; in the evening; at night.

Feels icy cold and shivery all day; this may be one-sided. Sweat is profuse and sour-smelling; if it is suppressed the conditions are exacerbated.

Fingernails

Split easily; weak. With WHITE SPOTS.

Flatulence

GAS smelly; obstructed (difficult to expel). ABDOMEN/STOMACH rumbling.

Headache

PAIN in back of head; in forehead; spreading to top of head/to eyes/to right eye; in sinuses; burning; hammering; pressing; sore, bruised; throbbing; violent.
Better for closing eyes; for lying in quiet, dark room; for heat; for wrapping up head.
Worse for getting chilled; for getting feet/head cold; for daylight; for getting up from lying down; for jarring movement; for walking upstairs/heavily.
Cause cold air; damp weather; draughts; eye strain; overwork; working in artificial light; travelling (car, coach, train, etc.).

Often a result of sinus catarrh; it settles over the eyes, forehead feels heavy. Head and feet feel cold.

Inflammation of navel

In newborn babies.

Injuries

CUTS/WOUNDS slow to heal; inflamed; painful; with pus inside; with dirt/splinter still inside; suppurate. SCARS become lumpy; are painful; break open.
Cause episiotomy; splinter; surgery.

Silica cuts and wounds become infected easily and heal slowly; skin looks unhealthy.

Insomnia

DREAMS, NIGHTMARES VIVID. SLEEP restless.
Worse after midnight; after waking.

Lochia

FLOWS while the baby breastfeeds.

Mumps

GLANDS painful; swollen.
Better for heat.
Worse for cold.

Sore throat

THROAT dry. GLANDS swollen. PAIN stitching. TON-
SILS swollen/inflamed. With HAIR SENSATION at
back of tongue.
Worse for getting cold; for swallowing; for
uncovering throat.

Splinters

WOUND inflamed.

Helps push out splinters especially if the wound has
become inflamed. It heals wound once pus has
started discharging.

Spots

In babies.

In skinny, chilly, sweaty babies.

Teething

PAINFUL in babies. DIFFICULT. SLOW. With DIAR-
RHOEA (see p. 253).

Silica types are slow to produce teeth and will get
coughs, colds and diarrhoea during this time. *Silica*
will help push the teeth out.

Vomiting

In BREASTFED BABIES.
Worse for milk.

Babies who refuse mother's milk and/or vomit (posset) it up. Bottled milk may be no better.

SPONGIA TOSTA (Spo.)

Other name: sea sponge

General symptoms

Worse after sleep; for cold wind; for movement; for
tight clothing; for tobacco.

Feels worse when excited or on exertion. Wakes from
sleep with a sense of suffocation and anxiety, and
finds it difficult to catch the breath. Is intolerant of
tight clothing because of difficulty in breathing.

Emotional state

Anxious on waking. **Tearful** during a fever.

May wake up with a start and be anxious and tearful.

Physical complaints
Cough

Barking; constant; dry; hollow; in fits; irritating; tickling. BREATHING difficult; rough. PAIN IN CHEST
burning; sore, bruised. VOICE HOARSE.
Better for drinking/eating.
Worse daytime; for excitement.

Cough may even have been caused by too much
excitement. Eating sweets may aggravate the cough
but it is generally better for eating and drinking,
especially warm things. The chest is sore and bruised
from coughing. Breathing is difficult and may sound
loud between bouts of coughing. It is worse after
sleep and for exercise, and sometimes also for talking. Voice is crowing and hollow.

Croup

With COUGH (see above).

This is one of the main croup remedies, though it
may be difficult to differentiate between *Aconite* croup
and *Spongia* croup as both have acute anxiety, but
Aconite croup is worse at night, around midnight.
Even so, if *Aconite* is indicated and fails to help,
Spongia will usually help.

Exhaustion

Worse for slightest exertion; for movement.

Sore throat

THROAT dry. PAIN burning; sore. VOICE hoarse.
Worse for coughing; for singing; for swallowing; for
sweet drinks/food; for talking; for touch.

The larynx is sore and sensitive to touch, the voice
hoarse and hollow-sounding; the throat feels raw,
rough and sore, and swollen – as if there is a plug in
it.

STAPHYSAGRIA (Stap.)

Other name: palmated larkspur

General symptoms

Anaemia. **Dislikes** milk; tobacco; water. **Gums**
bleeding; pale. **Sweat** worse for mental exertion.

Worse for exertion; for fasting; for tobacco; for touch.

These individuals are extremely sensitive, physically and emotionally, and suffer pain acutely. Wounds and cuts are unusually painful, especially if there is a feeling of having been assaulted. They feel generally worse for exercise, smoky rooms and missing meals, and are especially irritable after an afternoon nap.

Emotional state

Violently **angry**. **Anxious** about others. **Apathetic**. **Capricious**. **Complaints from** disappointed love; excitement; grief; humiliation; indignation; mental strain; reprimands; suppressed anger/emotions. **Disappointment**. **Forgetful**. **Irritable** generally, babies. **Resentful**. **Sensitive** to pain; to rudeness. **Sluggish**.

These are sensitive, touchy people who are easily offended. They don't tolerate rudeness in others although they may be rude themselves. They suppress their feelings, brood and let little out. In particular, anger is suppressed; they fume inside and may even appear sweet and compliant outside. Afterwards, they quickly become exhausted and may feel shaky; cannot sleep, work or speak; and may get a headache. Suppression of anger can turn into an active and acid resentment. Complaints are accompanied by sense of violation or humiliation with ensuing indignation and resentment. These people do not want to be touched when feeling low or upset.

These people cannot say no and allow pressure to build up inside. This ends in violent outburst, or getting sick, or both. In this state they may throw things (as do *Chamomillas*).

Physical complaints

Abdominal pain

In PREGNANCY. PAINS sudden; with SHOCK AND ANGER.
Cause sudden, unexpected kick by the baby.

Some babies can deliver a kick that hurts and shocks.

Bites/stings

Painful; sensitive to touch.

Colic

PAIN cramping.
Worse after drinking.
Cause indignation; vexation.

Cough

Tickling.
Cause suppressed anger.

Larynx and air passages feel irritated.

Cystitis

DESIRE TO URINATE frequent. URINATION frequent; involuntary. URINE scanty.

Often follows a sense of assault physically or emotionally, where strong feelings and/or needs were not expressed.

Exhaustion

NERVOUS. With TREMBLING.

For people worn out, anaemic, trembly and exhausted from suppressing feelings.

Eye injuries

WOUND punctured.
Worse for touch.

Headache

PAIN in back of head; in forehead; pulling; pressing; sore, bruised.
Worse for touch.
Cause emotion; excitement; grief; vexation.

Headaches of people who suppress their emotions.

Injuries

CUTS/WOUNDS lacerated; painful; to nerve-rich parts of the body. PAIN tearing.
Worse for touch.
Cause accident; childbirth; circumcision; episiotomy; surgery.

Wounds or injuries with feelings of humiliation, indignation and anger. Might be caused by an operation to sphincter (anus, urethra, stomach, etc.), or any operation, especially if more was done than expected, or after a mechanical childbirth with pain afterwards and possibly stitches. May simply be pain following unpleasant examination. Babies may be seriously aggrieved after circumcision.

Piles

Worse for touch.

After a difficult birth or forceps delivery everything

hurts/feels sensitive and piles are excruciatingly painful.

Retention of urine (after labour)

After a difficult birth or a forceps delivery.

Shock

With ANGER, INDIGNATION.
Cause injury; surgery.

With typical emotional state.

Styes

Sensitive to touch.

Travel sickness

With INDIGNATION.

Where the individual is extremely difficult and irritable.

STRAMONIUM (Stram.)
Other name: thorn-apple

General symptoms

Better for light.
Worse for dark.

These types feel worse emotionally and physically at night when it gets dark.

Emotional state

Anxious about strangers (babies); at night (babies). **Apathetic** uncomplaining. **Clingy**. **Complaints from** childbirth. **Confused** (sense of unreality). **Fear** of the dark. **Hyperactive**. **Indifferent**. **Lonely**. **Mischievous**. **Rage** during labour; in babies on being picked up. **Restless** wanders aimlessly. **Shock**. **Tantrums**. **Terror** of glittering surfaces.

Babies are terrified of the dark and wake up with frightful nightmares, knowing no one. They have a strange fear of water and glittering surfaces such as mirrors; may become hysterical if you try to encourage them to swim. They are prone to tantrums as soon as they are mobile; may hit and bite.

Women take a long time to recover from childbirth, feel they have lost touch with reality, and are confused and apathetic. After a shock someone needing this remedy becomes anxious and fright-

ened; babies become hyperactive and aimlessly restless.

Physical complaints
Convulsions

With RAGE.
Cause over-excitement.

Eyes glitter and pupils become large.

Shock

With FEAR.
Cause childbirth; surgery.

The fear can border on terror and is accompanied by nightmares or a sense of the birth having been a nightmare.

SULPHUR (Sul.)
Other name: flowers of sulphur

General symptoms

Anaemia. **Aversion (babies)** to being washed/bathed. **Breath** smells. **Complaints from** change of weather from cold to warm. **Discharges** smelly; sour; watery. **Dislikes** bread; eggs; meat. **Face** red; sallow; red in spots. **Glands** swollen. **Hot flushes** in pregnancy. **Likes** spicy food; sweets. **Lips** cracked; dry; red. **Pains** burning. **Sweat** profuse; smelly; sour; from slightest physical exertion. **Symptoms** left-sided. **Taste** in mouth bitter; bad. **Thirsty** extreme; for large quantities; for water. **Tongue** white coated; red-edged and red-tipped.
Better for fresh air.
Worse for bathing; for change of weather to warm; for draughts; for exertion; for fasting; for heat; for milk; around 10–11 a.m.; for standing; in stuffy rooms; for warmth of bed.

Sulphur types always look untidy and/or unwashed, no matter what they do. They are usually given away by an odd sock, a hem coming down, or a collar escaped from inside a jumper (things no self-respecting *Arsenicum* would put up with!). Often indifferent to how they look, or simply do not notice. They are warm-blooded and have hot feet; can wear sandals all year round. They are lazy about washing; often feeling worse for it. They slump when sitting and stoop when walking and are always worse for having to stand up for long. They have markedly red faces and red lips which can become dry and cracked during illness. The tongue is often white-coated with red edges and tip. They are thirsty types; consuming large quantities of water whether sick or well.

They are sensitive to heat and always worse for being in a stuffy room; and better for fresh air. Discharges are usually hot, smelly and burning. They sweat profusely and feel worse while sweating.
NB This remedy is hailed for its effect on eczema and skin rashes, but I strongly advise you not to prescribe for these complaints without consulting a professional homeopath, as the aggravations can be severe and need to be monitored carefully.

Emotional state

Angry. **Anxious** worse in evening; about others. **Confused**. **Critical**. **Depressed**. **Despair**. **Discontented**. **Impatient**. **Indifferent** to personal appearance. **Irritable**. **Lazy**. **Quarrelsome**. **Restless** generally; babies. **Sluggish** in babies.

Sulphur people have many ideas which may owe more to dreams than reality. They can be successful academics or unrealistic dreamers – so-called 'ragged philosophers'. They may start many things and finish nothing; the further away they are from realising their ideas, the sicker they become.

They are sloppy, lazy and disorganised; they feel constantly rushed and hurried; would rather not work at all. Mess doesn't bother them, although they may get periodical cravings for a limited external order. They are hoarders; cannot throw anything away.

Sulphur types are basically self-centred, impatient and irritable; critical of others and how they run their lives, with lots of ideas about how they could do it better themselves. Suffer from worries which plague them in evening and stop them sleeping at night. They worry about those closest to them and become depressed and despairing when ill. *Sulphur* babies are restless, always on the go and impatient. When ill, they become sluggish but never lose their restlessness.

Physical complaints
Backache

Back feels weak/tired. PAIN in LOWER BACK; aching; sore, bruised. With STIFFNESS; WEAKNESS.
Worse after period of long sitting; for bending down; on getting up from sitting; at night; for standing; for walking.

Breast(feeding) problems

NIPPLES cracked/sore; itching; burn and itch after nursing. BREAST ABSCESS inflamed. BREAST red, may be itchy.

Breathless

In PREGNANCY.
Better for fresh air.
Worse for exertion.

Chickenpox

See MEASLES.

Common cold

NASAL CATARRH smelly; dirty yellow. NOSE dry; itching. With frequent SNEEZING; EYE INFLAMMATION (see p. 258).

The nose is dry and itchy and the tip is red. It may bleed when blown. May be constantly aware of unpleasant smells.

Constipation

In PREGNANCY. With BURNING; REDNESS; ITCHING around anus.

Cough

BREATHING fast. COUGH disturbs sleep; dry during evening/at night, loose by day/in morning; painful; irritating; racking; suffocative. CHEST congested. LARYNX raw. MUCUS green.
Worse for coughing; during evening in bed; during morning; at night; for lying down.

Wakes from the cough and sides will hurt from coughing. Larynx feels irritated and raw, as if dusty. Difficulty breathing in a warm room, may be better for fresh air; usually wants the window open.

Cradle cap

Dry; itchy.

May smell. In restless sulphur-type babies.

Cramp

In THIGHS; in LEG; in CALF; in SOLE OF FOOT.
Worse at night; in bed; when walking.

With typical general symptoms and emotional state.

Cystitis

DESIRE TO URINATE frequent; urgent. PAIN burning. URINE burning; brown like beer; copious; scanty; smelly.
Worse on getting up in the morning; at night; while urinating.

Hurries to pee to prevent it escaping, but then passes only a few drops and dribbles each time.

Diarrhoea

In BABIES. During morning only; drives person out of bed; painless. FLATULENCE smelly. PAIN burning; cramping. STOOLS slimy; smelly; sour-smelling; watery.
Better for passing wind.
Worse around 5 a.m.; at night; for standing.

Wakes early with an urge to pass a stool which forces them out of bed. There is rumbling before passing stool; pains are felt in the belly before, during and even after passing one. The anus becomes sore and red after passing a stool, especially in babies.

Dizziness

Worse for getting up from lying/sitting; for stooping.
Cause high places.

Earache

PAIN aching; lacerating; stitching; tearing. With painful NOISES IN EAR.
Worse in left side; for noise.

Roaring and ringing noises in the ear are more noticeable when in bed. The external parts of the ear itch.

Exhaustion

Worse during the afternoon; for the heat of the sun; for talking.
Cause diarrhoea; flu; hunger; talking; walking; pregnancy; breastfeeding.

Eye inflammation

EYES burning; gritty; sensitive to light; itching; stitching; watering. EYELIDS itching in daytime only; burning; red.
Worse for washing eyes.

Eyes are glued together in the mornings; may be dry, feel sandy. Water easily in the fresh air, and are sensitive to bright sunlight.

Fever

HEAT alternating with chills. With SWEATING (see General symptoms); SHIVERING.
Worse at night; for thinking.

Feels worse while sweating, and hot, especially on soles of the feet, which are poked out of bed.

Flatulence

ABDOMEN/STOMACH bloated; gurgling; rumbling. GAS smelly; of rotten eggs.
Better for passing wind.

Hair loss

Cause childbirth.

Headache

HEAD feels constricted, full/hot. PAINS in forehead; burning; bursting; hammering; pressing; in top of head; throbbing. With NAUSEA (see p. 259).
Better for cold.
Worse after eating; for bending down; for blowing nose; for coughing; on getting up; during morning; for sneezing; for walking.
Cause damp weather; excited conversation; winter.

Feels like a band is tied around the head and head feels full and hot, especially in bed or a stuffy room. Headache may recur weekly, especially on the day a person tries to relax.

Indigestion

ABDOMEN/STOMACH feels bloated; feels empty around 11 a.m. BELCHES empty; sour. With FLATULENCE wind smells of rotten eggs. PAIN in the stomach burning.
Worse after eating; after drinking milk.

May feel suddenly hungry mid-morning after not wanting breakfast; feels faint, weak and headachey. Appetite may, however, vanish at the sight of food. Stomach feels full and heavy after eating, and rumbles and gurgles.

Insomnia

DREAMS unpleasant; NIGHTMARES. SLEEP disturbed; unrefreshing; restless. WAKING frequent; late.
Better for short naps.
Worse after 3, 4, or 5 a.m.

The *Sulphur* insomniac always wakes tired. Feels sleepy in the daytime and may be refreshed by a catnap. At night feet get hot and burn in bed; have to be poked out of bed to cool them down. Wakes in early hours, often from cold, and may be unable to get back to sleep. Restless, and has nightmares when lying on the back. May have to get out of bed around 5 a.m. to pass a stool.

Joint pain

PAIN burning; tearing.
Worse for walking; for warmth of bed.

Feeling of heat in the joints, and general restlessness.

Measles

SKIN RASH red; burns; itches maddeningly; slow to appear. With COUGH (see p. 257); FEVER (see p. 258).
Worse for heat.

Often needed where recovery is slow from a childhood illness. Can help relieve the itching of measles, German measles or chickenpox if severe, very red and much worse for heat (of bed or a bath). Babies will be restless, feverish and sweaty, and should fit the general picture. Will also be thirsty and hungry but eat very little. Rash becomes crusty, smelly and weeps after scratching.

Nappy rash (Diaper rash)

Skin red, itchy, burns. Becomes red raw and bleeds.
Better for uncovering.
Worse for washing/bathing; heat.

Nausea

In PREGNANCY. With VOMITING.

Nosebleeds

Worse for blowing nose.

Piles

Painful; in pregnancy; bleeding; burning; itching; large; external or internal. With CONSTIPATION (see p. 257).
Worse for touch; standing/walking.

Prickly heat

With typical general symptoms and emotional state.

Restless legs

In pregnancy.
Worse for heat.

Skin complaints of pregnancy

ITCHING without a rash.
Towards the end of pregnancy the stretched skin across the abdomen may itch, and this can spread all over the body. There is no rash.

Sore throat

THROAT dry; raw. CHOKING sensation. PAIN burning; raw; sore; stitching. TONSILS swollen. VOICE HOARSE.
Worse for coughing; for swallowing.

Larynx is dry, dusty. Voice is most hoarse in mornings.

Spots

In babies. Newborn babies become covered in a 'milk' rash.

Vomiting

In BREAST-FED babies.

SULPHURIC ACID (Sul-ac.)

Other name: oil of vitriol

General symptoms

Anaemia.
Worse for heat; during the evening; mid-morning.

Sulphuric acid people are anaemic, chilly types who feel hurried and trembly inside.

Emotional state

Irritable. Feeling of being **hurried** while eating; at work; while writing; while walking. **Moody**.

In spite of feeling exhausted, these types feel rushed and hurried inside and do everything 'at a pace'; they bolt their food, walk quickly, and work frantically, including writing quickly. They feel driven inside and cannot do things fast enough. Their moods may be changeable, swinging from reasonable and agreeable to irritable.

Physical complaints

Bruises

Bluish-black; slow to heal.

Sulphuric acid finishes the healing of bruises that turn bluish-black and do not clear up in spite of taking *Arnica* and/or *Ledum*.

Diarrhoea

BELCHES sour. STOOLS soft; stringy; yellow. VOMIT sour.

Stools are bright yellowy-orange, like saffron; feeling of emptiness and weakness after passing a stool. The upset stomach causes sour belches and vomiting.

Exhaustion

With TREMBLING.
Worse after passing a stool.

Extreme lassitude which may not be visible on the surface, but they feel trembly inside.

Thrush (oral)

In babies. Of TONGUE/GUMS.

SYMPHORICARPUS RACEMOSA (Symph-r.)
Other name: snowberry

Physical complaint
Vomiting

In PREGNANCY. Constant. Violent. With nausea; retching.
Better lying on back.
Worse movement.

Appetite is lost – the smell or thought of food aggravates but whereas *Asarum* nausea is worse for noise this one is worse for movement.

SYMPHYTUM (Symph.)
Other name: comfrey

Physical complaints
Broken bones

PAIN sticking.

Eases the pain and speeds up the healing of broken and fractured bones – after being set, of course.

Eye injuries

PAIN in eyeballs; sore, bruised.
Cause a direct blow to eyeball.

For an injury to the eyeball or the bones surrounding the eye (resulting from, for example, a stray fist or tennis ball) where pain persists after *Arnica* has been given and has dealt with the swelling.

TABACUM (Tab.)
Other name: tobacco

Physical complaints
Heartburn

In PREGNANCY. With WATERY BELCHES.

Nausea

DEATHLY; INTERMITTENT; VIOLENT. With VOMITING (see below).
Better for fresh air.
Worse in a stuffy room; for fasting; before breakfast.
Cause pregnancy; travelling.

Nausea is better for fresh air, although dizziness is worse for it. Empty, sinking feeling in the stomach. May also feel sluggish and confused or anxious and restless.

Travel sickness

With NAUSEA (see above); VOMITING (see below).
Better for fresh air.
Worse for stuffy room; for movement; for tobacco.

Nausea is more acute when travelling by boat and the vomiting is worse when travelling by car or train (although vomiting on a boat is also possible).

Vomiting

EXHAUSTING. VOMIT sour; violent.
Worse before breakfast; for movement.
Cause pregnancy; travelling.

Face is pale and drawn.

THIOSINAMINUM (Thios.)
Other name: mustard seed oil

Physical complaint
Scars

Lumpy. Adhesions.

Where the scar, i.e. of an episiotomy, leaves lumps (keloids); if there is pain after a Caesarean because of adhesions (poor healing of scars *inside* the body); or if the foreskin of a baby has become stuck to the glans of the penis because it has been retracted accidentally. Short courses of this remedy in a low potency (6X) will help – it can be taken three times a day for up to a week and repeated every two or three weeks for as long as it is helping.

THUJA OCCIDENTALIS (Thu.)

Other name: white cedar

Physical symptoms

Birthmarks

In babies.

Use this remedy cautiously (see below).

Warts

BLEEDING; LARGE; STINGING.

Indicated for warts that grow in a cauliflower shape, which may appear anywhere on the body (hands, feet, face, etc.). Use the remedy cautiously: do not take it for longer than a week at a time; one week on and one week off for a couple of months is ideal. If there is no alleviation of the symptoms, seek professional help.

This is a deep-acting remedy best prescribed by a competent homeopath. I have included it here because it is available in most chemists and wholefood shops that stock homeopathic medicines.

URTICA URENS (Urt-u.)

Other name: common nettle

Physical complaints

Bites/stings

ITCHING. PAIN biting; burning; stinging.

Breastfeeding problems

MILK SUPPLY low; overabundant.

Useful remedy to help establish good supply of milk in early days of feeding where it is slow without an obvious cause. Give where there are no obvious general or emotional/mental symptoms that would guide you to another remedy. Can also help where there is overabundance of milk and no desire to express and store it but wants it to be geared more to demand.

Burns

MINOR. PAIN burning; stinging.

Useful in everyday minor scalds and burns, especially where there are burning, stinging pains afterwards.

Hives

RASH biting; burning; itching; stinging. With JOINT PAIN.
Better for rubbing
Worse at night; for heat; for exercise.
Cause stinging nettles; insects.

Rash appears as red, raised blotches. It may accompany a rheumatic flare-up, or may be a reaction to eating shellfish. There is a constant desire to rub the skin.

Prickly heat

With symptoms of HIVES (see above).

Feels as though stung by stinging nettles.

VERATRUM ALBUM (Ver-a.)

Other name: white hellebore

General symptoms

Appetite increased in pregnancy. **Breath** cold. **Collapse** after diarrhoea. **Expression** anxious. **Face** blue; pale. **Hot flushes** in pregnancy. **Likes** cold foods; sour and salty food in pregnancy; cold drinks; fruit; ice-cream; refreshing things; sour food. **Saliva** increased. **Sweat** clammy; cold; profuse; sour. **Thirsty** for large quantities. **Tongue** cold.
Worse after eating fruit.

This remedy is indicated for the exhaustion with faintness that may accompany an acute illness, usually a 'tummy bug', such as gastroenteritis, dysentery or food poisoning. Acute illnesses are accompanied by a general coldness of breath, tongue and skin (which is cold to touch). Icy-cold sweat is another general symptom, and these types feel worse while sweating. There is an increase of saliva in the mouth and a ferocious thirst for large quantities of cold or icy-cold drinks, which may be vomited immediately in gastric troubles. Eating fruit causes a general aggravation.

Emotional state

Anxious after shock. **Apathetic. Aversion** to partner and children. **Broody. Confused**/dull. **Depressed. Desires** in pregnancy. **Despair. Forgetful. Hyperactive. Tearful. Uncommunicative.**

These types may appear distressed, restless (*have* to be up and doing something), and prone to weeping and wailing and incessant talking. Alternatively, they may be totally withdrawn, silent and inactive.

Physical complaints

Cough

Deep; hollow.

Breathing is difficult and may be louder than usual. Feeling of tightness in the chest, and the cough is accompanied by the characteristic cold sweat.

Cramp

In PREGNANCY. In CALF/LEG; preventing sleep.

Diarrhoea

EXHAUSTING; INVOLUNTARY; VIOLENT. PAIN burning; cutting; dull/aching. STOOLS copious; frequent; green; watery. With ICY-COLD HANDS AND FEET; SWEATING (see General symptoms) during and after passing stool; VOMITING (see below).
Worse after drinking; for movement.
Cause fruit; getting chilled.

May be accompanied by a ravenous appetite, with a feeling of emptiness not relieved by eating. Has trouble passing wind, and when able to do so may involuntarily pass stool. Stools shoot out and have to be passed frequently. Hands and feet are icy cold.

Exhaustion

PARALYTIC; SUDDEN. With COLD EXTREMITIES. In pregnancy.
Worse after passing stool.
Cause diarrhoea.

Fever

With SWEATING (see General symptoms).
Worse for sweating.

The skin is pale and icy cold to touch over whole body or in spots or patches. With diarrhoea sweating is worse (during and after passing stools).

Labour

With FAINT FEELING; EXHAUSTION (see above); VOMITING (see below); NAUSEA.

Nausea

In PREGNANCY. With VOMITING (see below).

Vomiting

ABDOMEN/STOMACH feels cold. PAIN IN STOMACH cramping/griping. VOMIT of bile; of mucus; sour; watery; yellow. VOMITING violent. With DIARRHOEA (see opposite); DIZZINESS; HICCUPPING after vomiting.
Worse after drinking; after eating.

Often accompanies the diarrhoea and is one of the most severe forms of diarrhoea and vomiting. May vomit and pass diarrhoea simultaneously.

ZINCUM METALLICUM (Zinc.)
Other name: zinc

General symptoms

Face pale. **Gums** bleeding; pale. **Oedema** (swelling) of ankles/feet. **Taste** in mouth metallic. **Trembling. Twitchy.** White spots on **fingernails**.
Worse after eating; during evening; at night; for wine.

For people of any age who are weary and run-down from stress and overwork. May tremble, twitch and jerk. Symptoms tend to be worse at night, from drinking wine and after eating, although they may feel better during eating. Like *Sulphur* types, they have an empty feeling in the stomach around 11 a.m. Keynote symptom is restlessness and twitchiness in legs; these types feel exhausted but fidgety and must keep their legs constantly on the move. Worse in the evenings in bed; legs will carry on twitching during sleep.
   In childhood illness such as measles where rash does not appear properly, baby may be weak and twitchy, and possibly chesty. *Zincum* will help.

Emotional state

Depressed. Irritable. Moody. Screaming on waking (babies). **Sensitive** to noise. **Sluggish. Uncommunicative.**

Nervous exhaustion makes for difficulty in thinking: thoughts wander, is slow to answer, repeats questions, and forgets what they are saying halfway through a sentence. They are depressed, irritable and generally worn out.

Physical complaints

Backache

In COCCYX; in neck; in spine. PAINS aching; sore, bruised. With WEAKNESS.
Worse for sitting, for writing.

Whole back feels sore and weak from too much stress.

Constipation

In BABIES. In NEWBORN BABIES.

For newborn babies who are nervous and twitchy and find it difficult to establish a regular bowel movement.

Exhaustion

LEGS restless (see opposite); weak.
Cause loss of sleep (broken nights).

Legs feel weak and twitchy, especially in bed at night.

Eye inflammation

EYES: sore; gritty; burning.
Worse during evening; at night.

Eyes feel particularly sore in inner corners. May water during the evening and at night.

Headache

NERVOUS. PAIN in forehead; in sides of head; in temples; bursting; tearing.
Better for fresh air.
Cause overwork.

May be on both sides of the head or on one side only.

Heartburn

In PREGNANCY. With sweetish BELCHES.

Restless legs

In pregnancy.
Worse in the evening.

Varicose veins

In PREGNANCY. Of LEG/THIGH/VULVA. Painful.

INTERNAL REPERTORY

See page 300 for list of remedies and abbreviations

Abdominal pain in pregnancy *Arn., Bell-p., Bry.,
Cimi., Nux-v., Rhus-t., Ruta., Stap.*
  Pains:
    sore and bruised: *Arn.*
    move about (wandering): *Cimi.*
    sudden: *Bell-p., Stap.*
    uterus feels sore: *Bell-p.*
  With:
    nausea (morning sickness): *Nux-v.*
    shock and anger: *Stap.*
    stiffness in lower abdomen: *Bell-p., Bry., Rhus-t.,
      Ruta.*
  Worse:
    as uterus expands (towards end of pregnancy):
      Bell-p., Bry., Rhus-t., Ruta.
  Caused by:
    an active baby: *Arn.*
    a sudden, unexpected kick (by the baby): *Stap.*
    ligaments of uterus stretching: *Bell-p., Bry.,
      Rhus-t., Ruta.*
Abscesses *Calc-s., Hep-s., Merc-s., Sil.*
  Discharging pus: *Calc-s.*
  Pains see **Pains**
  Of glands: *Calc-s., Hep-s., Merc-s., Sil.*
  Of roots of teeth: *Hep-s., Merc-s., Sil.*
Absent-minded (see also **Confused**; **Forgetful**)
  Caust., Nat-m.
Accidents see **Broken bones**; **Bruises**; **Burns**; **Bites/
  stings**; **Eye injuries**; **Injuries**; **Sprains**; **Strains**
Affectionate *Phos., Puls.*
Afraid see **Fearful**
Afterpains *Arn., Cham., Cimi., Cupr., Hyp., Kali-c.,
  Nux-v., Puls., Rhus-t., Sab., Sec., Sil.*
  Pains:
    cramping: *Cupr.*
    frequent: *Rhus-t.*
    in groin: *Cimi.*
    in hips: *Hyp., Sil.*
    in lower back radiating to thighs: *Hyp., Sab.*
    in lower back radiating to pubic bone: *Sab.*
    in women who have had many children: *Cupr.,
      Sec.*
    long lasting: *Sec.*
    shooting down into hips, buttocks and/or legs:
      Kali-c.
    sore, bruised: *Arn.*
    stitching: *Kali-c.*
    unbearable: *Cham., Cimi.*
  With:
    cramps in fingers or toes: *Cupr.*
    desire to pass a stool with every pain: *Nux-v.*

faint feeling after the pains: *Nux-v.*
headache: *Hyp.*
restlessness: *Rhus-t.*
  Worse:
    when the baby nurses: *Arn., Cham., Sil.*
  Cause:
    forceps delivery: *Hyp.*
Anaemia *Ars., Calc-c., Calc-p., Carb-v., Chin.,
  Ferr-m., Kali-c., Kali-p., Merc-s., Nat-m., Nit-ac.,
  Pho-ac., Phos., Puls., Stap., Sul., Sul-ac.*
  After acute illness: *Calc-p.*
  Lips pale: *Ferr-m.*
  With exhaustion: *Calc-p., Ferr-m.*
  Causes:
    loss of blood (haemorrhage, pregnancy, etc.):
      Chin., Ferr-m., Pho-ac.
Angry (see also **Complaints from** anger; **Irritable**)
  *Ars., Bell., Bry., Cham., Hep-s., Ign., Kali-c., Kali-s.,
  Lyc., Nat-m., Nit-ac., Nux-v., Sep., Stap., Sul.*
    Babies: *Ant-c., Ant-t., Cham., Cina, Lyc., Puls.*
    During labour: *Bell., Cham.*
    From contradiction: *Ign., Lyc., Sep.*
    Raging: *Bell., Cham.*
    Violently: *Cham., Hep-s., Nit-ac., Nux-v., Stap.*
    When has to answer questions: *Nux-v.*
Antisocial see **Desires to be alone**
Anxious *Aco., Arg-n., Ars., Bar-c., Bell., Bry.,
  Calc-c., Calc-p., Calc-s., Carb-v., Caust., Chin., Cocc.,
  Con., Kali-c., Kali-p., Kali-s., Lyc., Mag-c., Mag-m.,
  Nat-c., Nit-ac., Nux-v., Phos., Puls., Rhus-t., Sec.,
  Sep., Sil., Spo., Stram., Sul.*
  About health: *Calc-c., Nit-ac., Phos.*
  About others: *Ars., Nux-v., Pho-ac., Stap., Sul.*
  About strangers: *Stram.*
  After shock: *Ign., Ver-a.*
  Anticipatory: *Arg-n., Gels., Lyc.*
  At night: *Ars., Bor., Calc-c., Cina, Kali-p., Puls., Stram.*
  Babies: *Bor., Cina, Gels., Kali-c.*
  During a fever: *Aco., Ars., Bar-c., Ip., Sep.*
  During labour: *Aco., Ars., Kali-c., Lyc., Sep.*
  During pregnancy: *Aco., Ign.*
  On waking: *Ars., Lach., Spo.*
  When chilled: *Aco.*
  When indoors: *Kali-s., Lyc., Puls., Rhus-t.*
  When overheated: *Kali-s.*
  Better for:
    fresh air: *Kali-s., Puls.*
  Worse:
    after midnight: *Ars.*
    around 3 a.m.; *Ars.*
    evening: *Calc-c., Calc-s., Carb-v., Sep., Sul.*

in bed: *Ars., Carb-v., Mag-c., Rhus-t.*
when alone: *Ars., Phos.*
from downward motion: *Bor.*
heat: *Kali-s.*
indoors: *Lyc., Puls., Rhus-t.*
night: *Ars., Bor., Puls.*
on waking: *Ars., Lach., Spo.*

Apathetic   (see also **Sluggish**) *Alu., Ant-t., Ap., Carb-v., Chin., Con., Gels., Lil-t., Nat-c., Nat-m., Nat-p., Nux-m., Op., Pho-ac., Phos., Puls., Sep., Stap., Stram., Ver-a.*
About anything being done for them: *Lil-t.*
Doesn't complain: *Op., Stram.*
During fever: *Op.*
During labour: *Gels., Op., Puls.*
To her own children or relatives: *Phos., Sep.*

Appetite
Alternating with hunger: *Cina, Ferr-m.*
Increased during pregnancy: *Ver-a.*
Lost: *Chin., Cina, Ferr-m.*
Lost during pregnancy: *Caust., Nat-m., Sep.*

Apprehensive   see **Anxious** anticipatory
Argumentative   see **Quarrelsome**
Arthritis   see **Joint pain**
Athlete's foot   *Sil.*

Aversions   (see also **Dislikes**)
Being alone: *Kali-c., Lyc.*
Being examined: *Bell., Chin., Cina, Lach., Sil.*
Being hugged: *Cina*
Being looked at: *Ant-c., Cham., Cina*
Being spoken to: *Cham.*
Being touched: *Ant-c., Ant-t., Arn., Bell., Cham., Chin., Cina, Kali-c., Lach., Sil.*
Being washed (babies): *Sul.*
Company see **Desires** to be alone
Consolation: *Ign., Lyc., Nat-m., Nux-v., Sep., Sil.* (see also **Quarrelsome**)
Fresh air: *Cocc., Ign.*
Her own children: *Lyc.*
Her partner: *Sep.*
Her partner and her children: *Ver-a.*
Strangers: *Bar-c., Bor.*

Awkward   see **Clumsy**

Backache   *Aesc., Bell., Bry., Calc-c., Calc-f., Cimi., Dulc., Ferr-m., Hyp., Kali-c., Kali-p., Lyc., Merc-s., Nat-m., Nat-s., Nux-v., Phos., Puls., Rhod., Rhus-t., Ruta., Sep., Sil., Sul., Zinc.*
Between shoulder blades: *Phos.*
Coccyx: *Hyp., Zinc.*
Lower back: *Bry., Calc-c., Calc-f., Dulc., Ferr-m., Hyp., Kali-c., Lyc., Merc-s., Nat-m., Nux-v., Phos., Puls., Rhod., Rhust-t., Sep., Sul.*
Neck: *Rhod., Rhus-t., Zinc.*
Small of back: *Puls., Rhus-t.*

Spine: *Kali-p., Zinc.*
Pains:
aching: *Calc-c., Dulc., Nat-m., Nux-v., Puls., Rhus-t., Sep., Sul., Zinc.*
back feels broken: *Nat-m., Phos.*
burning: *Merc-s., Phos.*
dragging down: *Bell., Kali-c., Nux-v., Puls., Rhus-t., Sep.*
pressing: *Nux-v., Puls.*
rheumatic: *Cimi., Rhod., Rhus-t.*
shooting: *Hyp., Merc-s.*
sore, bruised: *Dulc., Hyp., Kali-c., Kali-p., Nat-m., Nat-s., Nux-v., Rhod., Rhus-t., Ruta., Sil., Sul., Zinc.*
feels sprained: *Calc-c.*
stitching: *Bry., Kali-c., Sil.*
tearing: *Hyp.*
With:
lameness: *Dulc., Ruta., Sil.*
stiffness: *Lyc., Rhus-t., Sil., Sul.*
weakness: *Sil., Sul., Zinc.*
Better for:
continued movement: *Calc-f.*
gentle exercise: *Puls.*
heat: *Rhus-t.*
lying on back: *Ruta.*
lying on a hard surface: *Kali-c., Nat-m., Rhus-t.*
massage: *Phos.*
movement: *Dulc., Kali-p., Lyc., Rhod., Rhus-t.*
passing wind: *Lyc.*
pressure: *Kali-c., Sep.*
rubbing: *Phos.*
urinating: *Lyc.*
walking: *Dulc., Rhus-t.*
walking slowly: *Ferr-m., Puls.*
Worse:
afternoon: *Sep.*
around 3 a.m.: *Kali-c.*
in bed: *Nux-v.*
bending down: *Sep., Sul.*
beginning to move: *Calc-f., Ferr-m., Lyc., Puls., Rhus-t.*
breastfeeding: *Sil.*
breathing: *Merc-s.*
coughing: *Bry., Merc-s.*
damp: *Calc-c.*
before a menstrual period: *Kali-c., Puls., Sep.*
during a menstrual period: *Bry, Puls., Sep., Sul.*
morning: *Nux-v.*
movement: *Nux-v.*
slightest movement: *Bry.*
night: *Sep., Sil., Sul.*
passing a stool: *Lyc.*
pressure: *Sil.*
reaching up: *Rhus-t.*
sitting: *Sep., Sil., Zinc.*

after long sitting: *Kali-c., Sul.*
getting up from sitting: *Calc-c., Lyc., Merc-s.,*
Phos., Puls., Rhus-t., Sil., Sul.
standing: *Sul.*
sweating: *Merc-s.*
walking: *Kali-c., Sul.*
wet weather: *Dulc., Rhod., Rhus-t.*
writing: *Zinc.*
Causes:
change of weather: *Dulc.*
childbirth: *Hyp., Nux-v., Phos.*
childbirth where baby was 'posterior':
Kali-c.
damp weather: *Dulc., Rhus-t.*
draughts: *Rhus-t.*
epidural: *Hyp.*
forceps delivery (childbirth): *Hyp.*
falling on the back: *Sil.*
getting cold: *Dulc., Nux-v.*
getting wet: *Dulc.*
injury: *Rhus-t.*
injury to coccyx: *Hyp., Sil.*
injury to spine: *Hyp., Nat-s.*
lifting: *Calc-c., Lyc., Rhus-t.*
manual labour: *Nat-m., Sil.*
pregnancy: *Aesc., Bell., Cimi., Kali-c., Nux-v.,*
Puls., Rhus-t.
sprain: *Rhus-t.*
Bad tempered see **Angry; Irritable**
Better (generally)
Bathing: *Asar., Puls.*
Changing position: *Rhus-t.*
Cold applications: *Glon.*
Cold bathing: *Led., Sec.*
Cold drinks: *Caust., Cupr., Phos.*
Cold drinks/food: *Asar.*
Cold/dry air/weather: *Asar.*
Company: *Arg-n.*
Constipation: *Calc-c.*
Crying: *Puls.*
Damp: *Caust.*
After eating: *Ign., Nat-c., Phos., Sep.*
While eating: *Lach.*
Fanning: *Carb-v.*
Firm pressure: *Bry., Chin., Mag-p.*
Fresh air: *Aco., Arg-n., Asar., Bor., Carb-v., Kali-s.,*
Lach., Lyc., Mag-c., Mag-m., Nat-s., Puls.,
Rhus-t., Sul.
Heat: *Ars., Calc-c., Caust., Hep-s., Ign., Kali-p.,*
Mag-p., Nux-m., Nux-v., Sil.
Hot drinks: *Ars., Nux-v., Rhus-t.*
Light: *Stram.*
Lying down: *Ars., Asar., Bell., Calc-c., Cocc.,*
Nat-m., Nit-ac., Nux-v.
Lying still: *Bry.*
Massage: *Nat-c., Phos.*

Movement: *Dulc., Phos., Puls., Pyr., Rhod.,*
Rhus-t., Ruta.
Pressure: *Mag-m., Puls.*
Rest: *Asar., Kali-p.*
After a rest: *Nat-m.*
After a good sleep: *Pho-ac., Phos.*
Running: *Sep.*
Sitting down: *Colch., Con., Nux-v.*
Sweating: *Gels., Nat-m., Rhus-t.*
Uncovering: *Cham.*
Urinating: *Gels.*
Vigorous exercise: *Sep.*
Walking: *Dulc.*
Walking fast: *Sep.*
Walking in fresh air: *Puls.*
Walking slowly: *Ferr-m.*
Warmth of bed: *Ars., Caust., Hep-s., Kali-c., Lyc.,*
Rhus-t.
Wrapping up: *Hep-s.*
Wrapping up the head: *Sil.*
Birthmarks   *Thu.*
Bites/stings   *Ap., Hyp., Lach., Led., Stap., Urt-u.*
Blue: *Lach.*
Inflamed: *Hyp.*
Itching: *Ap., Urt-u.*
Pains:
biting: *Urt-u.*
burning: *Ap., Urt-u.*
shooting: *Hyp.*
stinging: *Ap., Urt-u.*
tearing: *Hyp.*
Red/swollen: *Ap.*
Better for:
cold: *Ap., Lach., Led.*
Worse for:
heat: *Ap., Led., Lach.*
Causes:
animal/insect bites: *Ap., Hyp., Lach., Led.*
Biting   *Bell.*
Black eye   *Led.*
Bleeding   *Arn., Bell., Ip., Phos.*
Bright red; occurs easily; profuse: *Phos.*
profuse after labour: *Bell., Ip., Phos.*
bright red flow: *Ip., Phos.*
dark red, clotted flow: *Bell.*
Bleeding gums   see **Gums**, bleeding
Bleeding (vaginal) in pregnancy   *Aco., Arn., Bell.,*
Caul., Ign., Kali-c., Kreos., Op., Puls., Rhus-t., Sab.,
Sec., Sep.
In early pregnancy: *Kreos., Sab., Sec.*
In mid pregnancy: *Sep.*
Flow:
black: *Kreos., Sec.*
bright red: *Bell., Sab.*
brown: *Sab., Sec.*
changeable: *Puls.*

clotted: *Bell., Kreos., Puls., Rhus-t., Sab.*
dark, red: *Bell., Sep.*
scanty: *Caul., Sec.*
smelly: *Kreos.*
stops and starts: *Puls.*
sudden gushes: *Bell.*
With:
  an absence of pain: *Sec.*
  anxiety: *Aco.*
  back pain: *Caul., Kali-c., Sab.*
    spreading down into buttocks and thighs:
      Kali-c.
    spreading to the pubic area: *Sab.*
  bearing down pains: *Caul., Sep.*
  labour-like pains: *Rhus-t., Sab.*
  pains in the legs: *Sab.*
  shooting pains: *Bell.*
  sore, bruised pains: *Arn.*
  weakness and trembling: *Caul.*
Cause:
  emotional shock: *Ign.*
  fright: *Aco., Op.*
  grief: *Ign.*
  injury: *Arn.*
  over-exertion: *Rhus-t.*

Blisters *Caust., Lyc., Nat-m.*
Burning: *Lyc.*
Painful: *Caust.*
Tip of tongue: *Caust., Lyc., Nat-m.*

Bloated see **Indigestion**
Blocked tear duct: *Bar-c., Sil.*
Blood blisters *Arn.*
Blood poisoning *Pyr.*
Bossy see **Dictatorial**
Braxton Hicks Contractions *Bell., Calc-c., Caul.,*
Cimi., Cham., Gels., Puls., Sec.
Breast (feeding) problems
Breast abscess (Mastitis): *Hep-s., Merc-s., Phyt.,*
  Sil., Sul.
Breasts:
  engorged: *Bell., Bry.*
  hard/hot: *Bell., Bry.*
  inflamed: *Bell., Bry., Hep-s., Phyt., Sil., Sul.*
  lumpy: *Con., Phyt., Sil.*
    worse in right breast: *Con.*
  painful: *Bell., Bor., Bry., Merc-s., Sep., Sil.*
  painful in pregnancy: *Bell., Bry., Calc-p., Sep.*
    with inflammation: *Bell., Bry.*
  pains:
    aching after nursing: *Bor.*
    while nursing: *Phyt., Puls., Sil.*
    cutting/stitching: *Sil.*
    in opposite breast whilst nursing: *Bor.*
    slightest movement: *Bry.*
    throbbing: *Bell.*
    worse: left breast, while nursing: *Sil.*

pale: *Bry.*
red: *Sul.*
red-streaked: *Bell.*
Milk supply:
  low: *Calc-c., Caust., Dulc., Lac-d., Sec., Urt-u.*
    in chilly women: *Dulc.*
  over-abundant: *Bell., Bry., Calc-c., Puls., Urt-u.*
Nipples:
  cracked/sore: *Cast., Caust., Phyt., Sep., Sil., Sul.*
    and bleeding: *Sil.*
    and itching: *Sep., Sul.*
  inverted (retracted): *Sars., Sil.*
  pains when the baby nurses: *Phyt.*
Weaning:
  to dry up milk: *Lac-c., Puls.*

Breath
Cold: *Ver-a.*
Smelly: *Arn., Carb-v., Lach., Merc-c., Merc-s.,*
  Nit-ac., Phyt., Puls., Sul.

Breathing difficulties in newborn babies *Ant-t.,*
Carb-v.
Breathless *Ars., Calc-c., Carb-v., Ferr-m., Puls., Sul.*
Better:
  fresh air: *Puls., Sul.*
  gentle exercise: *Ferr-m.*
Worse:
  burping: *Carb-v.*
  exertion: *Ars., Calc-c., Puls., Sul.*
  lying down: *Ars., Carb-v.*
  at night in bed: *Ars.*
  walking uphill or upstairs: *Ars., Calc-c., Carb-v.*
Breech baby *Puls.*
Broken bones *Arn., Bry., Calc-c., Calc-p., Sil., Symph.*
Pains:
  sticking: *Symph.*
  stitching: *Bry.*
Slow to mend: *Calc-c., Calc-p., Sil.*
With swelling/bruising: *Arn.*
Worse:
  slightest movement: *Bry.*
Broody (see also **Introspective**; **Moody**) *Ign.,*
Pho-ac., Ver-a.
Bruises (see also **Injuries**) *Arn., Bell-p., Led., Sul-ac.*
Bluish-black: *Sul-ac.*
Pains:
  sore, bruised: *Arn., Bell-p.*
Slow to heal: *Sul-ac.*
With:
  bumps, lumps remaining: *Bell-p.*
  discolouration: *Led.*
  swelling (no discolouration): *Arn.*
Causes:
  childbirth: *Arn., Bell-p.*
  injury: *Arn., Bell-p., Led.*
  over-exertion: *Bell-p.*
  surgery: *Arn., Bell-p.*

Burns *Ars., Canth., Caust., Kali-b., Urt-u.*
 Deep: *Kali-b.*
 Minor: *Urt-u.*
 Pains:
  burning: *Ars., Canth., Caust., Urt-u.*
  stinging: *Urt-u.*
 Second degree: *Canth.*
 Slow to heal: *Kali-b.*
 Third degree: *Caust.*
 With blisters: *Ars., Canth., Caust.*
 Better for:
  cold compresses: *Canth.*
  heat: *Ars.*

Capricious *Bry., Cham., Cina, Ip., Kreos., Puls., Rhe., Stap.*
Carpal Tunnel Syndrome *Ap., Ars., Calc-c., Lach., Lyc., Rhus-t., Sep.*
Carried see **Desires** to be
Catches colds easily *Ars., Bar-c., Calc-c., Calc-p., Dulc., Hep-s., Kali-c., Nat-m., Nux-v., Sep., Sil.*
Changeable see **Moody**
Cheerful *Coff., Lach., Nat-c.*
Chickenpox *Aco., Ant-c., Ant-t., Bell., Merc-s., Puls., Rhus-t., Sul.*
 First stage: *Aco.*
 Skin rash:
  itches maddeningly: *Rhus-t., Sul.*
  slow in coming out: *Ant-t.*
  suppurates: *Merc-s.*
 With:
  cough: *Ant-c., Ant-t., Puls.*
  fever: *Aco., Bell.*
  headache: *Bell.*
Chilblains *Agar.*
Circumcision *Staph.* see also **Shock; Injuries**
Clingy *Ant-t., Bor., Gels., Phos., Puls., Stram.*
Clumsy *Agar., Ap., Calc-c., Caust.*
 Drops things: *Ap.*
 During pregnancy: *Calc-c.*
 Trips easily while walking: *Agar., Caust.*
Cold sores *Nat-m.*
Colds see **Common cold**
Colic (see also **Indigestion; Heartburn**) *Cham., Coloc., Cupr., Dios., Ip., Mag-m., Mag-p., Nat-p., Nat-s., Nux-v., Sec., Stap.*
 In babies: *Cham., Coloc., Dios., Mag-m., Sec.*
 Abdomen/stomach feels:
  bloated: *Cham., Coloc., Nat-p., Sec.*
  rumbling/windy: *Dios.*
 Pains:
  aching: *Ip.*
  around the navel: *Dios.*
  cramping: *Cupr., Dios., Ip., Mag-m., Mag-p., Nux-v., Stap.*

  cutting: *Coloc., Dios.*
  drawing: *Mag-p.*
  griping: *Coloc., Dios., Ip., Nux-v.*
  pressing: *Nux-v.*
  sore, bruised: *Mag-m., Nux-v.*
  tearing: *Coloc.*
  twisting: *Dios.*
  violent: *Coloc., Cupr.*
  in waves: *Coloc.*
 With:
  constipation: *Mag-m.*
  diarrhoea: *Cham., Coloc., Mag-m., Nat-p., Sec.*
  indigestion: *Mag-m., Nat-s.*
  nausea: *Coloc., Cupr.*
  vomiting: *Coloc., Cupr.*
  sour vomit: *Nat-p.*
 Better:
  bending back/stretching out: *Dios.*
  bending double/pressure: *Coloc., Mag-p.*
  hot drinks/warmth of bed: *Nux-v.*
  passing a stool: *Coloc., Nux-v.*
  passing wind: *Nux-v.*
  pressure: *Coloc.*
  stretching out: *Dios.*
  warmth: *Mag-p.*
  warmth of bed: *Nux-v.*
 Worse:
  after drinking: *Coloc., Stap.*
  after eating: *Nux-v.*
  after eating fruit: *Coloc.*
  bending forward: *Dios.*
  cold drinks when overheated: *Coloc.*
  coughing: *Nux-v.*
  during a fever: *Nux-v.*
  before a stool: *Coloc.*
  after drinking milk: *Mag-m.*
  in the morning: *Dios., Nux-v.*
  for movement: *Ip.*
  tight clothing: *Nux-v.*
 Causes:
  anger: *Cham., Coloc.*
  drinking milk: *Mag-m.*
  excitement: *Coloc.*
  fruit: *Coloc.*
  indignation: *Stap.*
  syntometrine: *Sec.*
  teething: *Mag-m.*
  vexation: *Coloc., Stap.*
Collapse
 After diarrhoea: *Ver-a.*
Common cold (see also **Snuffles**) *Aco., All-c., Ars., Bar-c., Bell., Bry., Calc-c., Calc-f., Calc-p., Calc-s., Carb-v., Dulc., Euphr., Hep-s., Kali-b., Kali-m., Kali-s., Lyc., Mag-m., Merc-s., Nat-c., Nat-m., Nit-ac., Nux-v., Pho-ac., Phos., Puls., Sep., Sil., Sul.*

Eyes:
 dry/burning: *Ars.*
 streaming: *All-c., Euphr.*
Discharge from eyes:
 burning: *Euphr.*
 watery: *All-c., Nat-m., Nux-v.*
Eyelids:
 red/puffy: *Ars.*
Glands:
 swollen: *Bar-c.*
Nasal catarrh:
 bland (not irritating): *Euphr., Puls.*
 blood-streaked: *Calc-s., Phos.*
 bloody: *Merc-s., Nit-ac.*
 burning: *All-c., Ars., Merc-s., Nit-ac., Nux-v.*
 crusty: *Kali-b.*
 drips down back of throat: *Hep-s., Kali-b., Nat-c.,
  Nat-m., Sep.*
 dry (stuffed up/congested without discharge):
  Calc-c., Calc-f., Kali-b., Phos., Sil.
 dry at night, profuse during the day: *Nux-v.*
 dry alternating with profuse: *Puls.*
 like egg-white: *Nat-m.*
 green: *Kali-b., Merc-s., Puls., Sep.*
 hard crusts: *Kali-b., Sil.*
 one-sided: *All-c., Phos.*
 profuse: *All-c., Ars., Kali-s., Nat-m., Phos.*
 smelly: *Calc-c., Calc-s., Hep-s., Kali-b., Merc-s.,
  Nat-c., Puls., Sil., Sul.*
 sticky/stringy: *Kali-b.*
 thick: *Calc-s., Dulc., Kali-b., Kali-s., Nat-c., Puls.,
  Sil.*
 thin: *Nit-ac.*
 watery: *All-c., Ars., Euphr., Merc-s., Nit-ac., Nux-v.*
 watery, alternating with blocked up nose: *Nat-m.*
 watery in the fresh air: *Nit-ac., Puls.*
 white: *Kali-m., Nat-m.*
 yellow: *Calc-c., Calc-s., Dulc., Hep-s., Kali-b.,
  Kali-s., Lyc., Merc-s.*
 dirty yellow: *Nit-ac., Puls., Sep., Sul.*
 yellow-green: *Kali-b., Merc-s., Puls., Sep.*
Nose:
 blocked: *Calc-c., Carb-v., Dulc., Lyc., Nat-c.,
  Nit-ac.*
 dry: *Bar-c., Lyc., Sul.*
 itching: *Sul.*
 runs during day, blocked at night: *Nux-v.*
 streaming: *All-c.*
Sinuses:
 blocked/painful: *Ars., Kali-b., Lyc., Merc-s.,
  Nux-v., Puls., Sil.*
 Sneezing: *All-c., Ars., Bry., Carb-v., Eup-p.,
  Hep-s., Merc-s., Nux-v., Puls., Sul.*
  better for sneezing: *Calc-f.*
  frequent sneezing: *Ars., Carb-v., Merc-s.,
   Nux-v., Sul.*

difficult sneezing: *Calc-f., Carb-v., Sil.*
  in a stuffy room: *Puls.*
  slightest uncovering: *Hep-s.*
With:
 cough: *Bar-c., Euphr.*
 deafness after a cold: *Kali-m.*
 dry throat: *Kali-b.*
 eye inflammation: *All-c., Euphr., Sul.*
 fever: *Bell., Merc-s.*
 headache: *Aco., All-c., Bell., Bry., Calc-s., Lyc.,
  Merc-s., Nux-v.*
 hoarseness: *Calc-c., Carb-v., Merc-s., Phos.*
 itching throat: *Carb-v.*
 painless hoarseness: *Calc-c.*
 loss of smell: *Bell., Calc-c., Calc-s., Merc-s.,
  Nat-m., Phos., Puls., Sep., Sil.*
 loss of taste: *Bell., Nat-m., Phos., Puls., Sil.*
 sneezing: *All-c., Ars., Bry., Merc-s.*
 sore throat: *All-c., Merc-s., Nux-v., Phos.*
Better:
 fresh air: *All-c., Kali-s., Nux-v., Puls.*
Worse:
 cold and heat: *Merc-s.*
 after eating: *Nux-v.*
 fresh air: *Nit-ac.*
 after getting up: *Nux-v.*
 morning: *Calc-c., Nux-v.*
 evening: *Ars.*
 night: *Bar-c., Merc-s., Nit-ac.*
 on the right: *Ars., Lyc.*
 for drinking milk: *Calc-s.*
 stuffy room: *All-c., Kali-s., Puls.*
 uncovering: *Hep-s.*
Causes:
 getting chilled: *Aco., Bell.*
 getting chilled when overheated: *Ars.*
 cold wind: *All-c.*
 cold, dry wind: *Aco., Bell.*
 draughts: *Nux-v.*
 getting head wet: *Bell.*
 getting wet feet: *All-c.*
 shock: *Aco.*
 swimming in the sea: *Mag-m.*
 wet weather: *Dulc.*
Complaints from/after   (see also **Worse**)
 Accident/injury: *Arn., Bell-p., Con., Hyp., Nat-s.*
 Anger: *Cham., Cocc., Colch., Coloc., Ign., Ip.,
  Nux-v., Op.*
  suppressed anger: *Ign., Lyc., Stap.*
  anger with anxiety: *Ars., Ign., Nux-v.*
 Bad news: *Gels.*
 Getting chilled: *Aco., Bry., Merc-s., Nux-v., Phos.,
  Rhus-t.*
  when overheated: *Bell-p.*
 Change of weather: *Bry., Caust., Dulc., Kali-s.,
  Phos., Rhod., Rhus-t., Sil., Sul.*

any change: *Phos.*
from cold to warm: *Bry., Kali-s., Sul.*
to cold: *Rhus-t., Sil.*
to damp: *Dulc., Rhus-t.*
to dry (especially dry cold): *Caust.*
to stormy: *Rhod.*
Childbirth: *Cimi., Stram.*
Coffee: *Cham.*
Cold wind: *Aco., Bell., Hep-s., Nux-v., Spo.*
Death of a child: *Ign.*
Disappointed love: *Ign., Nat-m., Pho-ac., Stap.*
Excitement: *Coff., Gels., Pho-ac., Puls., Stap.*
Fear: *Aco.*
Fright: *Ign., Pho-ac., Puls.*
Grief: *Caust., Cocc., Ign., Lach., Nat-m., Pho-ac., Puls., Stap.*
Humiliation (wounded pride): *Coloc., Ign., Lyc., Nat-m., Pho-ac., Stap.*
Indignation: *Colch., Coloc., Stap.*
Injuries to nerves/coccyx: *Hyp.*
Joy: *Coff.*
Loss of body fluids: *Calc-c., Carb-v., Chin., Pho-ac.*
Measles: *Carb-v., Puls.*
Mental strain: *Arg-n., Kali-p., Lach., Lyc., Nat-c., Sil., Stap.*
Overeating: *Ant-c.*
Overwork: *Kali-p.*
Reprimands: *Ign., Op., Stap.*
Shock: *Aco., Arn., Ign., Op., Pho-ac., Puls., Sil.*
Sprains: *Calc-c.*
Sunstroke: *Glon., Nat-c., Nat-m.*
Suppression of emotions: *Ign., Nat-m., Stap.*
Surgery: *Arn., Bell-p., Hyp., Stap.*
Teething: *Cham.*
Vexation: *Ip.*
Weaning: *Bry., Dulc., Puls.*
Getting wet: *Calc-c., Caust., Puls., Rhus-t., Sep.*
Getting feet wet: *Puls., Sil.*
Getting head wet: *Bell.*

Concentration
Poor: *Bar-c., Caust., Lyc., Nux-v., Sil.*
Confidence   see **Self-confidence, Lack of**
Confused   (see also **Absent-minded; Forgetful**)
Arg-n., Bell., Calc-c., Carb-v., Cocc., Glon., Lach., Merc-s., Nat-c., Nat-m., Op., Petr., Rhus-t., Sep., Sil., Stram., Sul.
In the fresh air: *Petr.*
Conjunctivitis   see **Eye inflammation**
Conscientious   *Ign., Sil.*
Constipation   *Aesc., Alu., Calc-c., Caust., Hep-s., Kali-c., Lyc., Mag-m., Nat-m., Nux-v., Op., Puls., Sep., Sil., Sul., Zinc.*
Alternates with diarrhoea: *Nux-v.*
Abdomen/stomach feels full: *Sep.*
In babies: *Alu., Lyc., Mag-m., Nux-v., Op.*
In newborn babies: *Zinc.*

In pregnancy: *Aesc., Alu., Kali-c., Lyc., Nux-v., Puls., Sep., Sul.*
Desire to pass stool:
absent: *Alu., Op.*
constant: *Nux-v.*
ineffectual: *Caust., Lyc., Mag-m., Nat-m., Nux-v., Sep., Sil.*
Pains:
burning after stool: *Aesc., Sil.*
stitching: *Caust.*
Stools:
black balls: *Op.*
changeable: *Puls.*
crumbling: *Mag-m., Nat-m.*
hard: *Aesc., Kali-c., Lyc., Mag-m., Nux-v., Op., Sep., Sil.*
hard at first: *Calc-c.*
knotty: *Lyc., Mag-m., Sil.*
large: *Aesc, Calc-c., Kali-c., Mag-m., Nux-v., Sep., Sil.*
pale: *Calc-c.*
passed with difficulty: *Mag-m.*
like rabbits'/sheep's droppings: *Mag-m., Nat-m., Op.*
'shy' (they recede): *Op., Sil.*
small balls: *Mag-m., Nat-m., Op.*
soft: *Alu., Hep-s.*
sour smelling: *Calc-c.*
With:
burning, redness and itching around anus: *Sul.*
flatulence: *Lyc.*
ineffectual straining: *Aesc., Alu., Mag-m., Nat-m., Sep., Sil.*
unfinished feeling: *Kali-c., Nat-m., Nux-v., Op.*
Better:
being constipated: *Calc-c.*
passing a stool when standing: *Caust.*
Worse:
before a menstrual period: *Sil.*
during a menstrual period: *Nat-m., Sep., Sil.*
Causes:
bottle-feeding: *Alu., Nux-v., Op.*
cow's milk: *Mag-m.*
drinking milk: *Mag-m.*
overeating: *Nux-v.*
pregnancy: *Aesc., Nux-v., Sep.*
sedentary habits: *Nux-v.*
weaning: *Alu., Nux-v., Op.*
Convulsions   *Bell., Cina, Cupr., Stram.*
With:
blue lips: *Cupr.*
coldness of hands and feet: *Cupr.*
rage: *Stram.*
Causes:
over-excitement: *Stram.*
teething babies: *Bell., Cina, Cupr.*

vexation: *Cupr.*
worms: *Cina*

Cough *Aco., All-c., Ant-t., Arn., Ars., Bar-c., Bell.,
Bry., Calc-c., Calc-p., Calc-s., Carb-v., Caust., Cham.,
Cina, Cocc-c., Con., Cupr., Dros., Dulc., Euphr.,
Ferr-m., Hep-s., Ign., Ip., Kali-b., Kali-c., Kali-m.,
Kali-s., Lach., Lyc., Merc-s., Nat-m., Nat-s., Nux-v.,
Op., Pho-ac., Phos., Puls., Rhus-t., Rumex, Sep., Sil.,
Spo., Stap., Sul., Ver-a.*

  Breathing:
  asthmatic: *Ant-t.*
  abdominal/difficult: *Ant-t.*
  difficult: *Ant-t., Ars., Cupr., Dros., Ip., Lyc.,
    Nux-v., Op., Phos., Spo., Ver-a.*
  fast: *Aco., Ant-t., Ars., Bell., Bry., Carb-v., Cupr.,
    Dros., Ip., Lyc., Phos., Sep., Sul.*
  rattling: *Ant-t., Dulc.*
  rough: *Spo.*
  slow: *Bell., Op.*
  snoring: *Op.*
  wheezing: *Ars., Carb-v., Ip., Kali-c.*

  Cough:
  barking: *Aco., Bell., Dros., Hep-s., Kali-m.,
    Spo.*
  choking: *Cocc-c., Ip.*
    as soon as falls into a deep sleep: *Lach.*
  constant: *Caust., Lyc., Rumex, Spo.*
    when lying down at night: *Sep.*
    in the evening: *Puls.*

  croupy see **Croup**
  deep: *Dros., Ver-a.*
  disturbs sleep: *Bry., Kali-c., Lyc., Puls., Sep.,
    Sul.*
  distressing: *Caust., Nux-v.*
  dry: *Aco., Ars., Bell., Bry., Calc-c., Calc-s., Con.,
    Dros., Hep-s., Ign., Ip., Kali-c., Lach., Lyc.,
    Nat-m., Nux-v., Pho-ac., Phos., Rumex, Sep.,
    Spo., Sul.*
  dry in the evening, loose in the morning: *Calc-c.,
    Hep-s., Sul.*
  dry at night: *Ars., Calc-c., Cham., Dros., Hep-s.,
    Phos., Puls., Sul.*
    loose by day: *Sul.*
    loose in the morning: *Calc-c., Puls., Sul.*
  dry during fever: *Aco., Phos., Puls.*
  exhausting: *Ars., Bell., Caust., Sep.*
    night: *Puls.*
  hacking: *All-c., Ars., Dros., Hep-s., Lach., Nat-m.,
    Phos., Sep.*
    evening in bed after lying down: *Ign., Sep.*
    worse for cold air: *All-c.*
    worse after dinner: *Hep-s.*
    from tickling in the larynx: *All-c., Ars., Dros.,
      Lach., Nat-m., Phos.*
  hard: *Bell., Kali-c., Kali-m.*
  hollow: *Bell., Caust., Spo., Ver-a.*

in fits: *Bell., Bry., Carb-v., Cina, Cocc., Cocc-c.,
  Ferr-m., Ip., Puls., Rumex, Spo.*
in long fits at irregular intervals: *Cupr.*
irritating: *Aco., All-c., Bell., Bry., Cham., Cocc-c.,
  Con., Dros., Hep-s., Ign., Ip., Kali-c., Lach., Lyc.,
  Nat-m., Nux-v., Pho-ac., Phos., Puls., Rhus-t.,
  Rumex, Sep., Sil., Spo., Stap., Sul.*
loud: *Ant-t.*
loose: *Ars., Kali-c., Sep.*
painful: *All-c., Bry., Lyc., Sul.*
racking: *Bell., Bry., Carb-v., Caust., Cocc-c., Ign.,
  Kali-c., Merc-s., Nux-v., Phos., Puls., Sul.*
rattling: *Ant-t., Caust., Dulc., Ip., Kali-s., Sep.*
short: *Aco., Ign., Kali-m., Rhus-t., Sep.*
suffocative: *Carb-v., Cina, Cupr., Dros., Hep-s.,
  Lach., Nux-v., Sul.*
tickling see **irritating**
tight: *Phos.*
tormenting: *Ars., Bell., Caust., Dros., Ip.*
uninterrupted: *Cupr.*
violent: *Bell., Carb-v., Caust., Cocc-c., Con., Cupr.,
  Hep-s., Ign., Kali-c., Lach., Pho-ac., Phos., Puls.,
  Sep.*
violent fits: *Dros., Nux-v.*
vomiting with or after cough: *Ant-t., Bry., Dros.,
  Hep-s., Ip., Kali-c.*
wakens from the cough at night: *Caust., Kali-c.,
  Phos., Sep., Sul.*
whooping: *Ant-t., Arn., Carb-v., Cocc-c., Cupr.,
  Dros., Ip., Kali-s.*
Chest congested: *Sul.*
Daytime only: *Euphr., Nat-s.*
Expectoration see **Mucus**
In pregnancy: *Bell., Bry., Calc-c., Caust., Phos.,
  Puls.*
Larynx:
  raw: *Nux-v., Phos., Rumex, Sul.*
  tickling: *All-c., Ars., Cocc-c., Dros., Lach., Nat-m.,
    Phos.*
Mucus:
  bloody: *Ip., Phos.*
  copious: *Ars., Calc-c., Calc-s., Cocc-c., Euphr.,
    Hep-s., Lyc., Phos., Puls., Sep.*
    after each coughing fit: *Cocc-c.*
  difficult to cough up: *Ant-t., Caust., Con., Ip.,
    Kali-b., Kali-s., Puls.*
    has to swallow what comes up: *Caust., Con.,
      Kali-s.*
  egg white: *Nat-m.*
  frothy: *Ars.*
  green: *Carb-v., Lyc., Merc-s., Nat-s., Phos., Puls.,
    Sul.*
  lumpy: *Calc-s., Sil.*
  smelly: *Calc-c.*
  sticky: *Cocc-c., Hep-s., Kali-b., Puls.*
  ropy/stringy: *Cocc-c., Kali-b.*

tastes:
  bitter: *Cham., Puls.*
  sour: *Calc-c., Nux-v.*
  sweet: *Calc-c., Phos.*
  salty: *Ars., Lyc., Phos., Puls., Sep.*
  thick: *Hep-s., Kali-b., Sil.*
  tough: *Calc-c., Hep-s., Kali-b.*
  transparent: *Nat-m., Phos.*
  white: *Lyc., Nat-m., Phos., Sep.*
  yellow: *Calc-c., Calc-p., Calc-s., Hep-s., Kali-s.,*
    Lyc., Phos., Puls., Sep., Sil.
  yellow-green: *Puls.*
Pain in chest: *Arn., Bell., Bry., Caust., Dros., Ign.,*
  Kali-b., Kali-c., Phos., Rumex, Spo.
  burning: *Phos., Rumex, Spo.*
  cutting: *Kali-c.*
  must hold chest to cough: *Arn., Bry., Dros.*
  racking: *Ign.*
  raw: *Caust.*
  sharp: *Bell.*
  short: *Ign.*
  sore, bruised: *Arn., Kali-b., Rumex, Spo.*
  stitching: *Bry., Ign., Kali-c., Rumex*
Pain in stomach: *Bry.*
With:
  bloodshot eyes: *Arn.*
  blue face: *Dros., Ip.*
  dry throat: *Cocc-c.*
  lump sensation in the throat: *Lach.*
  nausea: *Ip., Kali-c., Puls.*
  nosebleeds: *Arn., Dros., Ip.*
  retching: *Carb-v., Cina, Cocc-c., Dros., Hep-s., Ip.,*
    Puls.
  sleepiness: *Ant-t.*
  splitting headache: *Bry.*
  sweating: *Ars., Hep-s., Phos.*
  vomiting: *Ant-t., Bry., Dros., Hep-s., Ip., Kali-c.*
    when hawking up mucus: *Cocc-c., Nux-v.*
  vomiting of mucus: *Cocc-c., Dros.*
  voice hoarse: *Aco., All-c., Bell., Carb-v., Caust.,*
    Dros., Hep-s., Kali-b., Spo.
Better:
  drinking/eating: *Spo.*
  for being in warm room: *All-c.*
  fresh air: *Bry., Cocc-c., Puls.*
  heat: *Phos.*
  hot drinks: *Ars., Lyc., Nux-v., Rhus-t., Sil.*
  lying down: *Euphr.*
  lying on painful side: *Bry.*
  pressure: *Dros.*
  for sips of cold water: *Caust., Cupr.*
  sitting up: *Puls., Sep.*
    must sit up: *Ars., Con., Phos., Puls., Sep.*
    must sit up as soon as cough starts, to cough up
      mucus and then can rest: *Con.*
  walking slowly: *Ferr-m.*

Worse:
  around 11.30 p.m.: *Cocc-c.*
  around 3 a.m.: *Kali-c.*
  bending head forward: *Caust.*
  breathing in cold air: *Caust., Rumex*
  change of temperature: *Phos.*
    from warm to cold: *Phos., Rumex*
    from cold to warm: *Phos.*
  becoming cold: *Ars., Hep-s., Kali-c., Nux-v.,*
    Phos., Rhus-t., Rumex, Sil.
  cold air: *All-c., Caust., Cupr., Hep-s., Nux-v.,*
    Phos., Rumex
    single parts of the body becoming cold:
      Hep-s., Rhus-t.
  cold drinks: *Ars.*
  coughing: *Ign., Sul.*
  crying: *Arn.*
  damp, wet weather: *Dulc., Nat-s.*
  daytime: *Spo.*
  deep breathing: *Bell., Bry., Con., Kali-c.*
  drinking: *Bry., Dros.*
  dry, cold: *Aco., Hep-s.*
  eating: *Bry., Kali-b., Nux-v.*
  evening: *Ars., Calc-c., Carb-v., Hep-s., Ign.,*
    Kali-c., Merc-s., Nit-ac., Puls.
    evening in bed: *Calc-c., Coloc., Con., Hep-s., Ign.,*
      Lach., Lyc., Merc-s., Nat-m., Sep., Sul.
    evening before midnight: *Carb-v., Hep-s., Phos.*
  excitement: *Spo.*
  during fever: *Aco., Ars., Calc-c., Con., Ip., Kali-c.,*
    Nat-m., Nux-v., Phos.
  fresh air: *Ars., Phos., Rumex*
  getting hot: *Puls.*
  getting warm in bed: *Caust., Puls.*
  heat: *Kali-c., Kali-s., Puls.*
  left side: *Rumex*
  lying on left side: *Phos.*
  lying on right side: *Merc-s.*
  lying down: *Ap., Ars., Caust., Con., Dros., Kali-c.,*
    Lyc., Puls., Rumex, Sep., Sul.
    must sit up: *Ars., Con., Puls., Sep.*
  morning: *Calc-c., Euphr., Kali-c., Nux-v., Phos.,*
    Puls., Rumex, Sul.
    before getting up: *Nux-v.*
    after getting up: *Cina, Ferr-m., Phos.*
  movement: *Ferr-m.*
  movement of chest: *Bry., Chin., Nux-v.*
  moving arms: *Nat-m.*
  night: *Aco., Ars., Bar-c., Bell., Calc-c., Carb-v.,*
    Cham., Kali-c., Kali-s., Lach., Lyc., Merc-s., Puls.,
    Sep., Sul.
    on going to sleep: *Lyc.*
    before midnight: *Carb-v., Hep-s*
    after midnight: *Ars., Dros.*
  physical exertion: *Puls.*
  playing the piano: *Calc-c.*

reading aloud: *Phos.*
right lung: *Bry.*
during sleep: *Op.*
falling sleep: *Op.*
stuffy room: *Ant-c., Cocc-c., Kali-s., Puls.*
warm room: *Kali-s.*
talking: *Dros., Kali-c., Rumex*
teething: *Calc-p.*
touch: *Lach.*
uncovering: *Hep-s., Rhus-t., Rumex*
  hands: *Hep-s., Rhus-t.*
  feet or head: *Sil.*
walking: *Ferr-m., Rumex.*
on waking in the morning: *Kali-b., Nux-v., Op.,*
  Rumex, Sil.
warmth of bed: *Op.*
Causes:
  cold, dry wind: *Aco., Hep-s.*
  getting chilled: *Bell., Kali-c.*
  damp weather: *Dulc.*
  after measles: *Dros., Puls.*
  suppressed anger: *Stap.*
  swimming in cold water: *Rhus-t.*
Cracks at corners of mouth/around nostrils: *Ant-c.*
Cradle cap   *Calc-c., Lyc., Sul.*
Cramp   *Calc-c., Calc-p., Caust., Coloc., Cupr., Lyc.,*
Sep., Sul., Ver-a.
  Arm: *Mag-p.*
  Calf: *Calc-c., Calc-p., Coloc., Cupr., Lyc., Sep., Sul.,*
    Ver-a.
  Foot: *Caust., Cupr.*
  Fingers and hand when writing: *Mag-p.*
  Hand: *Calc-c., Mag-p.*
  Leg: *Coloc., Cupr., Sep., Sul., Ver-a.*
  Soles of feet: *Calc-c., Caust., Sul.*
  Thigh: *Coloc., Sul.*
  Toe: *Calc-c., Caust.*
  Wrist: *Mag-p*
  Better:
    heat: *Mag-p.*
  Worse:
    at night: *Calc-c., Caust., Lyc., Sul.*
    in bed: *Calc-c., Sul.*
    childbirth: *Cupr.*
    during labour (in hands or legs): *Bell., Cupr.,*
      Nux-v.
    in pregnancy: *Calc-c., Cupr., Sep., Ver-a.*
    preventing sleep: *Ver-a.*
    stretching leg in bed: *Calc-c.*
    when walking: *Calc-p., Sul.*
  Causes:
    childbirth: *Cupr.*
    prolonged use of hands: *Mag-p.*
Cravings   see **Likes**
Cries/Crying   see **Tearful**
Critical   *Ars., Sul.*

Croup   (see **Cough** for symptoms)   *Aco., Calc-s.,*
Hep-s., Kali-b., Lach., Phos., Spo.
  Only on waking: *Calc-s.*
  Recurrent: *Hep-s.*
  Worse:
    after sleep: *Lach.*
    on waking: *Lach.*
Cystitis   (see also **Incontinence**) *Aco., Ap., Ars.,*
Canth., Caust., Dulc., Lyc., Merc-c., Merc-s., Nux-v.,
Puls., Sars., Sep., Stap., Sul.
  Desire to urinate:
    constant: *Ap., Canth., Merc-c., Merc-s., Sul.*
    with dragging down pain in pelvis: *Sep.*
    frequent: *Ap., Canth., Caust., Lyc., Merc-c.,*
      Merc-s., Nux-v., Puls., Stap., Sul.
    ineffectual: *Ars., Canth., Caust., Lyc., Merc-s.,*
      Nux-v., Puls., Sars.
    painful: *Merc-c., Puls.*
    in pregnancy: *Puls.*
    urgent: *Canth., Nux-v., Puls., Sep., Sul.*
  Pains:
    aching: *Lyc.*
    burning: *Ap., Ars., Canth., Caust., Merc-c.,*
      Merc-s., Nux-v., Sul.
    cutting: *Canth., Lyc., Sars.*
    pressing: *Aco., Ap., Lyc., Nux-v., Sep.*
    severe: *Merc-c.*
    spasmodic: *Canth., Puls.*
    stinging: *Ap.*
    stitching: *Lyc.*
  Urination:
    burning: *Caust.*
    constant: *Ap.*
    difficult: *Caust., Merc-c.*
    dribbling: *Merc-c., Merc-s., Sars.*
    frequent: *Ap., Canth., Caust., Lyc., Merc-c.,*
      Merc-s., Nux-v., Puls., Sars., Sep., Stap.
    ineffectual: *Nux-v.*
    involuntary: *Caust., Dulc., Stap.*
    slow: *Sars.*
      can only pass urine while standing: *Sars.*
      waits long time for it to start: *Caust., Lyc., Sep.*
    with unfinished feeling: *Ars., Caust.*
  Urine:
    brown like beer: *Sul.*
    burning: *Nux-v., Sul.*
    cloudy: *Sep.*
    copious: *Puls., Sul.*
    dark: *Merc-c., Merc-s.*
    dark brown: *Sep.*
    green: *Merc-c., Sars.*
    hot: *Canth.*
    pale: *Sars.*
    red: *Canth., Merc-c., Sep.*
    scanty: *Canth., Merc-c., Merc-s., Nux-v., Sep.,*
      Stap., Sul.

smelly: *Sep.*, *Sul.*
with sediment: *Sars.*, *Sep.*
with mucus: *Sars.*
Better (pains):
  after urination: *Lyc.*
  heat: *Ars.*
  for sitting in a hot bath: *Ars.*
Worse (pains):
  for cold drinks: *Canth.*
  after getting up in the morning: *Sul.*
  after a few drops of urine have passed:
    Canth.
  after urinating: *Canth.*, *Puls.*
  at the beginning of urinating: *Canth.*, *Merc-s.*
  at the end of urination: *Sars.*
  before urinating: *Canth.*
  during a menstrual period: *Sars.*, *Sep.*
  when not urinating: *Merc-s.*
  while urinating: *Canth.*, *Caust.*, *Merc-c.*, *Nux-v.*,
    Sul.
  at night: *Sul.*
Causes:
  cold, wet weather: *Sars.*
  getting chilled: *Aco.*, *Sars.*
  getting cold and wet: *Dulc.*, *Puls.*

Dazed   (see also **Shock**; **Stupor**) *Cocc.*
Delirious   *Bell.*
Denial
  Of illness, of suffering: *Arn.*
  Of suffering in labour: *Arn.*
Depressed   (see also **Tearful**) *Alu.*, *Ars.*, *Calc-c.*,
  Calc-s., *Carb-a.*, *Caust.*, *Cham.*, *Chin.*, *Cimi.*, *Con.*,
  Eup-p., *Ferr-m.*, *Gels.*, *Ign.*, *Kali-p.*, *Lach.*, *Lil-t.*, *Lyc.*,
  Merc-s., *Nat-c.*, *Nat-m.*, *Nat-s.*, *Nit-ac.*, *Op.*, *Pho-ac.*,
  Puls., *Rhus-t.*, *Sep.*, *Sul.*, *Ver-a.*, *Zinc.*
  Cannot cry: *Gels.*, *Ign.*, *Nat-m.*
  Cries on own: *Ign.*, *Nat-m.*
  In pregnancy: *Chin.*, *Cimi.*, *Con.*, *Ign.*, *Lach.*,
    Nat-m., *Puls.*
  In labour: *Cimi.*, *Nat-m.*, *Puls.*
  Better:
    fresh air: *Puls.*
  Worse:
    before menstrual period: *Nat-m.*, *Puls.*
    stuffy room: *Puls.*
    on waking: *Alu.*, *Lach.*, *Lyc.*
    evening: *Puls.*
  Causes:
    suppressed grief: *Ign.*, *Nat-m.*, *Puls.*
Desires
  To be alone: *Alu.*, *Carb-a.*, *Cham.*, *Gels.*, *Ign.*, *Lach.*,
    Nat-m., *Sep.*
  To be carried (infants): *Bry.*, *Cham.*, *Cina*, *Kali-c.*,
    Kreos., *Lyc.*, *Puls.*
  Company: *Arg-n.*, *Ars.*, *Kali-c.*, *Lyc.*, *Phos.*
  In pregnancy and/or labour: *Lach.*, *Nat-m.*

In pregnancy: *Ars.*, *Bry.*, *Cina*, *Kreos.*, *Lyc.*, *Kali-c.*,
  Rhus-t., *Ver-a.*
Despair   *Ars.*, *Calc-c.*, *Coff.*, *Ign.*, *Lyc.*, *Sul.*,
  Ver-a.
  In pregnancy: *Nat-m.*
  In labour: *Coff.*, *Gels.*, *Sep.*
  Of getting well: *Ars.*, *Calc-c.*
Despondent   (see also **Depressed**) *Chin.*
Diaper rash   see **Nappy rash**
Diarrhoea   *Ant-c.*, *Ap.*, *Arg-n.*, *Ars.*, *Bor.*, *Bry.*,
  Calc-c., *Calc-p.*, *Cham.*, *Chin.*, *Colch.*, *Coloc.*, *Dulc.*,
  Ferr-m., *Gels.*, *Hep-s.*, *Ip.*, *Mag-c.*, *Mag-m.*, *Merc-c.*,
  Merc-s., *Nat-m.*, *Nat-s.*, *Nux-v.*, *Petr.*, *Pho-ac.*, *Phos.*,
  Podo., *Puls.*, *Rhe.*, *Rhus-t.*, *Sil.*, *Sul.*, *Sul-ac.*, *Ver-a.*
  Alternating with:
    constipation: *Podo.*
    headache: *Podo.*
  Abdomen/stomach:
    feels bloated: *Nat-m.*
    gurgling: *Nat-s.*, *Podo.*
    rumbling: *Nat-s.*, *Pho-ac.*, *Podo.*
  Breastfeeding babies: *Calc-p.*, *Cham.*
  Children (infants): *Ip.*, *Mag-m.*, *Merc-s.*, *Podo.*,
    Puls., *Sul.*
  Daytime only: *Nat-m.*, *Petr.*
  Drives person out of bed: *Sul.*
  In pregnancy: *Chin.*, *Phos.*, *Puls.*, *Sul.*
  Exhausting: *Ver-a.*
  Involuntary: *Ver-a.*
  Morning only: *Sul.*
  Painful: *Ars.*, *Cham.*, *Colch.*, *Dulc.*, *Mag-c.*, *Merc-c.*,
    Merc-s.
  Pains:
    burning: *Ars.*, *Merc-s.*, *Sul.*, *Ver-a.*
    colicky: *Mag-c.*
    cramping: *Mag-c.*, *Sul.*
    cutting: *Ver-a.*
    dull/aching: *Ver-a.*
    after passing a stool: *Ars.*, *Colch.*
    pressing: *Petr.*
    severe: *Merc-c.*
  Painless: *Ap.*, *Bor.*, *Chin.*, *Ferr-m.*, *Hep-s.*, *Nat-m.*,
    Phos., *Podo.*, *Sul.*
  Stools:
    blood-streaked: *Phos.*
    bloody: *Merc-c.*, *Merc-s.*
    changeable: *Puls.*
    copious: *Ver-a.*
    frequent: *Merc-c.*, *Phos.*, *Podo.*, *Ver-a.*
    frothy: *Mag-c.*
    grass green: *Ip.*
    green: *Arg-n.*, *Cham.*, *Coloc.*, *Mag-c.*, *Mag-m.*,
      Merc-c., *Merc-s.*, *Ver-a.*
    greenish-yellow: *Puls.*
    gushing: *Nat-m*: *Podo.*
    jelly-like: *Colch.*
    hot: *Cham.*

involuntary: *Podo.*
with mucus: *Bor., Colch.*
mushy: *Rhus-t.*
passed with wind: *Ferr-m.*
pasty: *Coloc., Rhe.*
profuse: *Pho-ac., Phos., Podo.*
slimy: *Mag-c., Merc-c., Merc-s., Puls., Sul.*
small, hard lumps: *Ant-c.*
smelling of rotten eggs: *Cham.*
smelly: *Arg-n., Ars., Merc-c., Merc-s., Nat-m.,*
  Nat-s., Podo., Sul.
soft: *Sul-ac.*
sour smelling: *Calc-c., Mag-c., Rhe., Sul.*
stringy: *Sul-ac.*
sudden: *Podo.*
thin: *Nat-s., Pho-ac.*
with undigested food: *Calc-c., Chin., Ferr-m.*
yellow: *Dulc., Merc-c., Merc-s., Sul-ac.*
watery: *Ant-c., Arg-n., Ars., Calc-c., Colch., Dulc.,*
  Nat-m., Nat-s., Pho-ac., Phos., Puls., Rhus-t.,
  Sul., Ver-a.
white: *Pho-ac.*
Straining frequent/painful: *Merc-c.*
Violent: *Ver-a.*
With:
  belching: *Ferr-m.*
  sour belching: *Sul-ac.*
  colic: *Coloc.*
  exhaustion: *Ars., Podo., Ver-a.*
  flatulence: *Arg-n., Ferr-m., Nat-s., Sil., Sul.*
  icy-cold hands and feet: *Ars., Phos., Ver-a.*
  indigestion: *Chin.*
  nausea: *Ars.*
  ravenous appetite: *Petr.*
  sweating: *Ars., Merc-s., Ver-a.*
    during/after passing stool: *Ver-a.*
    before/during/after stool: *Merc-s.*
  vomiting: *Arg-n., Ver-a.*
    sour: *Sul-ac.*
  wind:
    loud: *Nat-s.*
    smelly: *Nat-s., Sil., Sul.*
    spluttering: *Nat-s.*
Without weakness: *Pho-ac.*
Better:
  cold food: *Phos.*
  fresh air: *Puls.*
  heat: *Sil.*
  passing wind: *Nat-s., Sul.*
  warmth of bed: *Sil.*
  wrapping up warmly: *Sil.*
Worse:
  on alternate days: *Chin.*
  around 4 a.m.: *Podo.*
  5 a.m.: *Sul.*
  afternoon: *Chin.*
  before passing a stool (pains): *Mag-c., Merc-c.*

during passing a stool: *Merc-c.*
after passing a stool: *Merc-c., Merc-s.*
cold: *Ars., Merc-s.*
getting chilled: *Phos.*
after cold food/drinks: *Ars.*
after drinking: *Ars., Arg-n., Ver-a.*
after drinking milk: *Calc-c.*
after drinking water: *Ferr-m., Nux-v., Podo.*
immediately after drinking: *Arg-n., Podo.*
after eating: *Ars., Chin., Coloc., Podo., Puls.*
while eating: *Ferr-m.*
eating cold food: *Ars., Dulc.*
eating starchy food: *Nat-m., Nat-s., Puls.*
evening: *Merc-s.*
after eating fruit: *Ars., Coloc., Nat-s.*
after getting up in the morning: *Bry., Nat-s.*
hot weather: *Podo.*
during a menstrual period: *Ver-a.*
after midnight: *Ars.*
mid-morning: *Podo.*
morning: *Bry., Mag-c., Nat-s., Phos., Sul.*
movement: *Bry., Ferr-m., Ver-a.*
night: *Arg-n: Ars., Chin., Dulc., Ferr-m., Merc-s.,*
  Podo., Puls., Sul.
for being overheated: *Ant-c., Puls.*
rich food: *Puls.*
solid/dry food: *Pho-ac.*
starchy food: *Nat-s., Puls.*
standing: *Sul.*
stuffy room: *Puls.*
sugar/sweets: *Arg-n.*
Causes:
after an acute illness: *Chin.*
anger: *Coloc.*
anticipatory anxiety: *Arg-n., Gels.*
autumn: *Colch.*
bad or exciting news: *Gels.*
beer: *Sul.*
getting chilled: *Ver-a.*
damp, cold weather: *Dulc.*
getting cold or damp: *Colch., Dulc.*
excitement: *Arg-n.*
food poisoning: *Ars.*
fright/shock: *Gels.*
fruit: *Ars., Bry., Chin., Coloc., Nat-s., Puls., Ver-a.*
hot weather: *Bry., Chin., Pho-ac.*
ice-cream: *Ars.*
milk: *Calc-c., Mag-m.*
over-eating: *Ant-c.*
rich food: *Puls.*
sour wine: *Ant-c.*
sugar: *Arg-n.*
summer: *Pho-ac.*
teething: *Calc-c., Cham., Dulc., Ferr-m., Rhe., Sil.*
weaning: *Arg-n., Chin.*
getting wet: *Rhus-t.*
getting feet wet: *Rhus-t.*

Dictatorial (bossy)   *Ars., Kali-c., Lyc., Merc-s.*
   During labour: *Ars., Kali-c., Lyc.*
Disappointment   *Ign., Pho-ac., Puls., Staph.*
Discharges
   Bland (non-irritating): *Puls.*
   Blood-streaked: *Calc-s., Merc-s., Phos.*
   Burning: *Alu., Ars., Merc-s.*
   Like ammonia: *Nit-ac.*
   Like egg white: *Alu., Nat-m.*
   Smelly: *Ars., Carb-v., Merc-s., Pyr., Sul.*
   Sour: *Calc-c., Mag-c., Mag-m., Nat-p., Rhe., Sul.*
   Stringy/sticky: *Kali-b.*
   Thick: *Calc-c., Kali-b., Kali-s., Nat-m., Puls.*
   Watery: *Ars., Caust., Merc-s., Nat-m., Podo.,
      Sul.*
   White: *Alu., Kali-m., Nat-m.*
   Yellow: *Kali-s., Lyc., Merc-s., Puls., Sep.*
Discontented   *Calc-p., Merc-s., Nat-m., Sul.*
Dislikes   (see also **Desires; Aversions**)
   Bread in pregnancy: *Kali-c., Sep.*
   Bread: *Chin., Kali-c., Nat-m., Puls., Sul.*
   Butter: *Chin., Puls.*
   Cheese: *Nit-ac.*
   Coffee: *Calc-c., Nux-v.*
   Eggs: *Sul.*
   Fatty, rich food: *Chin., Petr., Puls.*
   Food in general: *Ars., Chin., Cocc., Colch., Coloc.,
      Nat-m., Nux-v., Puls., Sep.*
      with hunger: *Cocc., Nat-m., Nux-v.*
      sight of food: *Ars.*
      smell of food: *Cocc., Colch., Coloc., Ip., Sep.*
      thought of food in pregnancy: *Chin., Nat-m., Sep.*
   Fruit: *Chin., Ign., Phos., Puls.*
   Hot drinks/food: *Phos., Puls.*
   Meat: *Calc-c., Chin., Coloc., Nux-v., Petr., Puls.,
      Sep., Sil., Sul.*
   Milk: *Ign., Nat-c., Sep., Stap.*
   Pork: *Coloc.*
   Sweets: *Caust.*
   Tobacco: *Calc-c., Nux-v., Ign., Puls., Stap.*
   Water: *Nux-v., Stap., Stram.*
   Water in pregnancy: *Phos.*
Dislocation of a joint   *Rhus-t.*
Disobedient   *Chin.*
Dizziness   (see also **Faintness**) *Bell., Bor., Bry.,
   Calc-c., Cocc., Con., Ferr-m., Gels., Nat-c., Nat-m.,
   Nux-v., Petr., Phos., Puls., Sil., Sul., Ver-a.*
   In pregnancy: *Bell., Cocc., Gels., Nat-m., Nux-v.*
   Has to lie down: *Cocc., Phos., Puls., Sil.*
   With:
      headache: *Bell., Calc-c., Con., Nux-v., Sil.*
      nausea: *Cocc., Ferr-m., Petr.*
      turning sensation: *Con.*
      vomiting: *Ver-a.*
   Worse:
      getting up from bending down: *Bell., Ferr-m., Puls.*

getting up from lying down: *Cocc., Ferr-m.,
   Nat-m., Nux-v., Petr., Phos., Sul.*
getting up from sitting: *Ferr-m., Nux-v., Petr.,
   Phos., Puls., Sul.*
lying down: *Con.*
mental exertion: *Nat-c.*
moving/turning head quickly: *Calc-c., Con.*
slightest motion: *Bry.*
stooping: *Bell., Nux-v., Puls., Sul.*
stuffy room: *Nat-c.*
tobacco: *Nat-m., Nux-v.*
walking: *Nat-m., Nux-v., Puls., Sul.*
   Causes:
      downward motion (stairs, lifts, etc): *Bor.*
      high places: *Calc-c., Sul.*
      loss of sleep: *Cocc., Nux-v.*
      mental exertion: *Nat-c., Nat-m., Nux-v.*
      smoking: *Nat-m., Nux-v.*
Dreamy   (see also **Absent-minded**) *Nux-m., Op.*
Drowsy   (see also **Dazed**) *Gels., Op.*
Drowsy babies   *Nux-m.*
Dryness   (generally) *Ars., Bry., Nat-m.*
Dwells on the past   *Nux-v., Pho-ac.*

Earache   *Aco., Ap., Bell., Calc-c., Calc-s., Cham.,
   Hep-s., Kali-b., Kali-m., Kali-s., Lach., Lyc., Mag-p.,
   Merc-s., Nit-ac., Nux-v., Puls., Sil., Sul.*
   Discharge from ears:
      blood-streaked: *Calc-s., Merc-s.*
      smelly: *Calc-s., Hep-s., Kali-b., Merc-s., Puls.*
      thick: *Calc-s., Kali-b., Puls.*
      thin: *Kali-s.*
      yellow-green: *Puls.*
      yellow: *Kali-b., Kali-s., Puls.*
   Pains
      aching: *Cham., Puls., Sul.*
      behind the ear: *Sil.*
      boring: *Merc-s.*
      burning: *Merc-s.*
      lacerating: *Sul.*
      outward: *Puls.*
      pressing: *Cham., Merc-s., Puls.*
      pressing outwards: *Puls.*
      spreading down into neck: *Bell., Puls.*
      shooting: *Mag-p.*
      spasmodic: *Mag-p.*
      splinter-like: *Nit-ac.*
      stinging: *Ap.*
      stitching: *Bell., Cham., Hep-s., Kali-b., Nux-v.,
         Puls., Sul.*
      tearing: *Bell., Cham., Lyc., Merc-s., Puls., Sil., Sul.*
      throbbing: *Bell., Calc-c., Nit-ac., Puls.*
      unbearable: *Aco., Cham.*
   With:
      blocked feeling in ears: *Lyc., Merc-s., Puls., Sil.*

crackling in the ears: *Nit-ac.*
  when chewing: *Kali-s., Nit-ac.*
deafness: *Puls.*
deafness after a cold: *Kali-m.*
face-ache: *Bell.*
glands swollen: *Kali-m.*
itching in the ear: *Nux-v., Puls., Sil.*
  has to swallow: *Nux-v.*
noises in the ear: *Bell., Calc-c., Kali-m., Lyc.,*
  Puls., Sul.
  painful: *Sul.*
redness of the external ear: *Puls.*
sensitivity to wind: *Cham., Lach.*
sore throat: *Ap., Lach., Nit-ac.*
Better for:
heat: *Mag-p.*
firm pressure: *Mag-p.*
wrapping up warmly: *Hep-s.*
Worse:
bending down: *Cham.*
cold: *Hep-s., Mag-p.*
fresh air: *Merc-s.*
on left side: *Kali-b., Lach., Sul.*
noise: *Sul.*
night: *Merc-s., Puls.*
right side: *Bell., Nit-ac.*
swallowing: *Ap., Kali-m., Lach., Nit-ac., Nux-v.*
turning head: *Mag-p.*
wind: *Cham., Lach.*
warmth of bed: *Merc-s.*
Causes:
after a common cold: *Puls.*
after measles: *Puls.*
getting chilled: *Aco.*
cold dry wind: *Aco., Mag-p.*
Effects of drugs taken during or after labour   *Cham.,*
Nux-v., Op., Phos., Sec.
General 'de-tox': *Nux-v.*
Drowsy, sleepy and spaced out: *Op., Phos.*
Irritable and sleepless: *Cham., Nux-v.*
With vomiting (especially after a general
  anaesthetic): *Phos.*
Causes:
general anaesthetic: *Op., Phos.*
morphine or pethidine: *Cham., Op.*
syntometrine: *Sec.*
Euphoric   *Coff., Phos.*
Excitable   (see also **Complaints from** excitement)
Arg-n., Bell., Cham., Cimi., Coff., Lach., Nux-v.,
Phos., Puls.
During labour: *Coff.*
During pregnancy: *Gels.*
Exhaustion   *Alu., Ant-c., Ant-t., Arg-n., Ars., Bar-c.,*
Bry., Calc-c., Calc-p., Carb-a., Carb-v., Caust., Chin.,
Cocc., Colch., Con., Cupr., Ferr-m., Gels., Kali-c.,
Kali-p., Lach., Merc-c., Merc-s., Nat-c., Nat-m.,

Nat-p., Nit-ac., Nux-v., Pho-ac., Phos., Puls., Rhus-t.,
Sep., Sil., Spo., Stap., Sul., Sul-ac., Ver-a., Zinc.
During labour   see **Labour pains** with exhaustion
Extreme: *Ars., Bry.*
In pregnancy: *Alu., Calc-p., Sep., Sul., Ver-a.*
Nervous: *Chin., Cocc., Kali-p., Nat-c., Nat-p.,*
  Nit-ac., Nux-v., Pho-ac., Phos., Puls., Rhus-t., Sep.,
  Sil., Stap.
Paralytic: *Ars., Cocc., Gels., Pho-ac., Phos., Ver-a.*
Sudden: *Ars., Sep., Ver-a.*
With:
breath cold: *Carb-v.*
breathlessness: *Calc-c., Carb-v.*
cold extremities: *Carb-v., Nat-c., Ver-a.*
desire to lie down: *Alu., Ferr-m.*
dizziness: *Calc-c., Cocc.*
a faint feeling: *Alu., Ars.*
fever: *Ars., Phos.*
headache between the eyes: *Cupr.*
heaviness: *Merc-s., Nat-c., Nat-m., Rhus-t.*
  in the limbs: *Calc-p., Merc-s., Nat-c.*
nervousness: *Cocc.*
numbness: *Cocc., Con.*
profuse sweating: *Chin.*
restlessness: *Ars., Rhus-t.*
restless legs: *Zinc.*
sleepiness: *Ant-c.*
stiffness: *Cocc.*
trembling: *Arg-n., Cocc., Con., Gels., Stap., Sul-ac.*
vertigo: *Cocc.*
weak legs: *Calc-p., Nat-c., Zinc.*
Better:
being fanned: *Carb-v.*
fresh air: *Con., Ferr-m.*
during a menstrual period: *Sep.*
eating: *Nat-c., Phos., Sep.*
walking in fresh air: *Rhus-t.*
walking slowly: *Ferr-m.*
Worse:
afternoon: *Sul.*
after eating: *Ars., Bar-c., Pho-ac.*
for exercise: *Ferr-m.*
evening: *Caust., Nat-m.*
slightest exertion: *Ars., Bry., Calc-c., Con., Lach.,*
  Nat-c., Pho-ac., Phos., Rhus-t., Sep., Spo.
mental exertion: *Calc-c., Cupr., Lach., Nat-c., Puls.*
physical exertion: *Alu., Calc-c., Cocc., Nat-c.*
for fresh air: *Cocc.*
heat of sun: *Lach., Nat-c., Puls., Sul.*
hot weather: *Ant-c.*
after a menstrual period: *Ip.*
during a menstrual period: *Carb-a., Sep.*
morning: *Ars., Lach., Pho-ac., Sep.*
  in bed: *Puls.*
  after getting up: *Bry., Lach., Pho-ac., Sep.*
  on waking: *Nux-v.*

late morning: *Ant-c.*
mid-morning: *Bry.*
movement: *Ars., Spo.*
sitting down: *Rhus-t.*
standing: *Alu.*
after passing a stool: *Ars., Con., Merc-s., Nit-ac., Sul-ac., Ver-a.*
stuffy room: *Puls.*
exposure to sun: *Nat-c.*
after sweating: *Merc-s., Sep.*
talking: *Alu., Sul.*
after a walk: *Ruta.*
walking: *Alu., Ars., Bry., Calc-c., Carb-a., Cocc., Con., Ferr-m., Lach., Nit-ac., Pho-ac., Phos., Rhus-t., Sep., Sul.*
  in the fresh air: *Cocc., Rhus-t.*
  upstairs: *Calc-c.*
Causes:
  accident/injury: *Carb-v.*
  acute illness: *Carb-a., Carb-v.*
  anaemia: *Ferr-m.*
  breastfeeding: *Bry., Calc-c., Calc-p., Carb-a., Carb-v., Chin., Cocc., Pho-ac., Phos., Sep., Sil., Sul.*
  carbon monoxide poisoning: *Carb-v.*
  diarrhoea: *Ars., Carb-v., Chin., Nat-s., Nit-ac., Phos., Sil., Sul., Ver-a.*
  fever: *Phos.*
  flu: *Kali-p., Pho-ac., Sul.*
  food poisoning: *Ars., Carb-v.*
  hunger: *Sul.*
  after illness: *Carb-a., Carb-v., Chin.*
  irregular sleep: *Cocc., Nit-ac., Nux-v.*
  lifting: *Carb-a.*
  loss of body fluids (diarrhoea, vomiting): *Carb-v., Chin., Pho-ac.*
  loss of sleep (broken nights): *Cocc., Cupr., Nat-m., Nit-ac., Nux-v., Puls., Zinc.*
  mental exhaustion: *Cupr., Lach.*
  mental strain: *Nat-c.*
  nervous exhaustion: *Cocc.*
  nursing the sick: *Cocc., Nit-ac.*
  overexposure to sun: *Nat-c.*
  pain: *Ars.*
  surgery: *Carb-v.*
  sweating: *Bry., Carb-a., Chin., Ferr-m., Merc-s., Phos., Sep.*
  talking: *Alu., Sul.*
  vomiting: *Carb-v.*
  walking: *Alu., Sul.*

Exhilarated (see also **Excitable**) *Coff., Lach., Op.*
Expression
  Anxious: *Aco., Bor., Ver-a.*
  Confused: *Lyc.*
  Fierce: *Bell.*
  Frightened: *Aco.*

  Haggard: *Ars., Kali-c.*
  Sickly: *Ars., Cina, Lach., Lyc.*
  Sleepy: *Op.*
  Suffering: *Ars., Kali-c.*
Extremities cold *Cupr.*
Eye inflammation *Aco., All-c., Ap., Arg-n., Ars., Bell., Bry., Calc-c., Calc-s., Dulc., Euphr., Lyc., Merc-s., Nat-m., Nit-ac., Nux-v., Puls., Rhus-t., Sep., Sil., Sul., Zinc.*
  In babies: *Ap., Arg-n., Ars., Calc-c., Nit-ac., Puls., Sul.*
  Discharge:
    bland (non-irritating): *All-c.*
    burning: *Euphr.*
    profuse: *All-c.*
    purulent (mucus or pus): *Arg-n., Calc-c., Calc-s., Hep-s., Lyc., Merc-s., Puls.*
    smelly: *Arg-n., Puls.*
    thick: *Calc-s., Puls.*
    watery: *Euphr.*
    yellow: *Arg-n., Calc-s., Puls., Sil.*
  Eyelids:
    burning: *Ars., Euphr., Sul.*
    glued together: *Arg-n., Calc-c., Lyc., Puls., Rhus-t., Sep.*
    gritty: *Calc-c.*
    itching: *Puls., Rhus-t., Sul.*
     daytime: *Sul.*
    red: *Arg-n., Euphr., Sul.*
    swollen: *Ap., Euphr., Nit-ac., Rhus-t., Sep.*
  Eyes:
    aching: *Aco., Puls.*
    bloodshot: *Ars., Bell., Led.*
    burning: *Aco., Ap., Ars., Bell., Puls., Sep., Sul., Zinc.*
    dry: *Bell., Bry.*
    gritty (sandy sensation): *Ars., Calc-c., Nat-m., Sul., Zinc.*
    itching: *Puls., Sul.*
    red: *Aco., Ap., Arg-n.*
    sensitive to light: *Aco., Arg-n., Ars., Bar-c., Bell., Calc-c., Euphr., Lyc., Merc-s., Nat-m., Nat-s., Nux-v., Op., Rhus-t., Sul.*
    sore: *Ap., Bry., Rhus-t., Sil., Zinc.*
     worse for moving eyes: *Bry., Rhus-t.*
    stinging: *Ap.*
    stitching: *Ap., Kali-c., Lyc., Rhus-t., Sul.*
    watering: *All-c., Bell., Calc-c., Euphr., Lyc., Merc-s., Nat-m., Nit-ac., Puls., Rhus-t., Sul.*
  With a common cold: *Aco., All-c., Bell., Calc-c., Dulc., Euphr., Merc-s., Puls.*
  Better:
    cold: *Arg-n., Puls.*
    cold bathing: *Puls.*
    cold compresses: *Arg-n.*
    fresh air: *Puls.*

Worse:
  cold air: *Sil.*
  cold, dry wind: *Aco.*
  coughing: *Euphr.*
  evening: *Puls., Sep., Zinc.*
  heat of a fire: *Merc-s.*
  heat: *Ap., Bell.*
  light: *Bell, Euphr.*
  moving eyes: *Bry., Rhus-t.*
  night: *Zinc.*
  reading: *Sep.*
  warm room: *Puls.*
  warmth of bed: *Merc-s.*
  after a walk: *Sep.*
  washing eyes: *Sul.*
  wind: *Euphr.*
Causes:
  a foreign body in the eye: *Aco., Sil.*
  getting chilled: *Aco.*
  cold, wet weather: *Dulc., Rhus-t.*

Eye injuries   *Arn., Euphr., Led., Stap., Symph.*
Bruising:
  to eyeball: *Arn.*
  to surrounding areas: *Arn.*
  with swelling: *Arn.*
  with discolouration: *Led.*
Pains:
  in eyeballs: *Symph.*
  sore, bruised: *Arn., Symph.*
With eye inflammation: *Euphr.*
Wound punctured: *Stap.*
Better:
  cold compresses: *Led.*
Worse:
  touch: *Stap.*
Causes:
  a direct blow to the eyeball: *Symph.*

Eye strain   *Ruta.*

Eyelids heavy   *Caust., Gels.*

Eyes
Dull: *Ant-c.*
Glassy: *Op., Pho-ac.*
Shining: *Bell.*
Sunken: *Ant-c., Chin., Cina*

Face
Blue: *Carb-v., Cupr., Lach., Op., Ver-a.*
  during cough: *Dros., Ip.*
Dark red: *Bell., Bry., Op.*
Flushes easily: *Ferr-m.*
Pale: *Alu., Ant-t., Ars., Calc-c., Calc-p., Carb-v.,*
  Cina, Con., Cupr., Ferr-m., Lyc., Nat-c., Nat-p.,
  Op., Pho-ac., Tab., Ver-a., Zinc.
Pasty: *Chin., Ferr-m., Merc-s., Nat-m., Sep.*
Puffy: *Ap., Kali-c.*

Red: *Aco., Ap., Bell., Cham., Glon., Lach., Phos.,*
  Rhus-t., Sul.
  one-sided: *Cham., Ip.*
  from pain: *Ferr-m.*
  in spots: *Bell., Cham., Phos., Sul.*
  with toothache (teething): *Bell., Cham.*
Sallow: *Arg-n., Carb-v., Nat-m., Sul.*
Sickly: *Lyc.*
Yellow: *Sep.*

Faintness   (see also **Dizziness**)   *Alu., Carb-v.,*
  Kali-c., Op., Puls., Sep.
After excitement, fright: *Op.*
Coldness after the faint: *Sep.*
On waking/getting up: *Carb-v.*
Has to lie down: *Kali-c.*
Heat with the faintness: *Sep.*
In a warm room: *Puls.*
In pregnancy: *Kali-c., Puls., Sep.*
Worse:
  exercise: *Sep.*
  during a fever: *Sep.*
  during a menstrual period: *Sep.*
  standing: *Alu.*
  stuffy room: *Sep.*

Fatigue   see **Exhaustion**
Fault-finding   see **Critical**
Fearful   *Aco., Ap., Arg-n., Arn., Ars., Bor., Calc-c.,*
  Caust., Calc-p., Chin., Cimi., Coff., Ign., Lyc., Nat-c.,
  Nit-ac., Phos., Puls.
Animals: *Chin.*
Babies: *Bar-c., Calc-c., Caust., Lyc.*
  at night: *Ars., Bor., Calc-c., Caust., Cina, Kali-p.,*
    Stram.
  wakes terrified: *Stram.*
Being alone: *Ap., Arg-n., Ars., Kali-c., Phos.*
In a crowd: *Aco., Gels.*
Of the dark: *Phos., Stram.*
Of death: *Aco., Ap., Ars., Calc-c., Cimi., Gels.,*
  Nit-ac., Phos., Ruta.
  during labour: *Aco., Coff.*
  during pregnancy: *Aco.*
Of dogs: *Chin., Puls.*
In the evening: *Calc-c., Caust., Puls.*
Of downward movement: *Bor.*
Of falling: *Gels.*
In labour: *Aco., Ars., Coff., Kali-c., Op.*
Of painful death: *Coff.*
In pregnancy: *Aco., Caul., Cimi.*
Of public speaking: *Arg-n., Gels., Lyc.*
Paralysing: *Gels.*
Of strangers: *Bar-c., Lyc.*
Of sudden noises (sneezing, coughing, etc): *Bor.*
Of thunder: *Rhod.*
During a thunderstorm: *Phos., Rhod.*
At twilight: *Puls.*
Of being touched: *Arn.*

Fever *Aco., Ant-t., Ap., Ars., Bell., Bry., Cham., Cina, Eup-p., Ferr-m., Gels., Hep-s., Ign., Ip., Kali-c., Lyc., Merc-s., Nat-m., Nux-v., Op., Phos., Puls., Pyr., Rhus-t., Sep., Sil., Sul., Ver-a.*

  Heat:

    alternating with chills: *Aco., Ant-t., Ars., Bell., Bry., Hep-s., Merc-s., Nux-v., Pyr., Rhus-t., Sul.*

    burning: *Aco., Ap., Ars., Bell., Bry., Cham., Gels., Nat-m., Op., Phos., Puls., Rhus-t.*

    dry: *Aco., Ap., Ars., Bell., Bry., Nux-v., Phos., Rhus-t.*

    dry at night: *Aco., Ars., Bell., Phos.*

    dry in the evening: *Puls.*

    intense: *Ant-t., Op.*

    radiant: *Bell.*

  One-sided: *Bry., Cham., Lyc., Nux-v., Phos., Puls.*

    right side: *Phos.*

    left side: *Lyc.*

  Pulse:

    fast, strong: *Aco.*

  Without sweating: *Bell., Bry., Gels.*

  With:

    anxiety: *Aco., Ars., Ip., Sep.*

    appetite increased: *Phos.*

    backache: *Nux-v.*

    chest symptoms: *Ant-t.*

    chilliness: *Ap., Puls., Pyr., Ver-a.*

      better for fresh air: *Ip.*

      worse for heat: *Ip.*

      extreme: *Nux-v., Pyr.*

      internal: *Pyr.*

    deep sleep: *Op.*

    delirium: *Ars., Bell.*

    exhaustion: *Ars.*

    grinding of teeth: *Bell.*

    heat during sleep: *Ant-t.*

    hunger: *Cina*

    nausea: *Nat-m.*

    sensitive skin: *Ap.*

    shaking: *Pyr.*

    shivering: *Cham., Gels., Nux-v., Sul.*

    sweating see **Sweat**

    thirst see **Thirsty/Thirstless**

  Better:

    for complete rest: *Bry.*

    in bed: *Kali-c.*

    drinking cold water: *Caust.*

    fresh air: *Ip.*

    heat: *Hep-s., Kali-c.*

    hot drinks: *Rhus-t.*

    for sweating: *Gels.*

    for uncovering: *Aco., Ap., Ferr-m., Ign., Nat-m., Op., Puls.*

    for urinating: *Gels.*

  Worse:

    9 p.m.: *Bry.*

    afternoon: *Ap., Bell., Gels., Ign., Phos., Puls.*

    autumn: *Bry., Nat-m., Sep.*

    in bed: *Merc-s., Puls.*

    cold drinks: *Rhus-t.*

    draughts: *Nux-v.*

    after eating: *Kali-c.*

    evening: *Aco., Bell., Lyc., Phos., Puls., Rhus-t., Sil.*

      after lying down in bed: *Bry.*

    fresh air: *Merc-s., Nux-v.*

    front of the body: *Ign.*

    for heat: *Ap., Ip., Puls.*

    for light: *Bell.*

    mental exertion: *Sul.*

    after midnight: *Ars.*

    mid-morning: *Cham., Nat-m., Rhus-t.*

    morning: *Ap., Ars.*

      in bed: *Puls.*

    movement: *Nux-v., Rhus-t., Sil.*

    at night: *Aco., Ars., Bell., Cina, Merc-s., Phos., Puls., Rhus-t., Sil., Sul.*

    during sleep: *Op.*

    slightest movement of the bedclothes: *Nux-v.*

    in a stuffy room: *Ap., Puls.*

    for sweating: *Op., Sep., Ver-a.*

    for thinking: *Sul.*

    for being uncovered: *Bell., Hep-s., Nux-v., Puls., Pyr., Rhus-t., Sep., Sil.*

    warm covers: *Ap., Ign., Puls.*

    washing: *Ap., Puls.*

  Causes:

    anger: *Cham., Sep.*

    getting chilled: *Aco.*

    teething in babies: *Aco.*

Fingernails

  Split: *Ant-c., Sil.*

  Weak nails, split easily: *Sil.*

  White spots on nails: *Sil., Zinc.*

  Caused by:

    injury: *Ant-c.*

Flatulence *Arg-n., Ars., Calc-c., Carb-a., Carb-v., Cham., Chin., Colch., Lyc., Mag-c., Nat-s., Nit-ac., Nux-v., Podo., Puls., Sil., Sul.*

  Abdomen/stomach feels:

    bloated: *Arg-n., Ars., Calc-c., Carb-a., Carb-v., Cham., Chin,., Colch., Lyc., Mag-c., Nux-v., Sul.*

      above the navel: *Chin.*

      below the navel: *Carb-v., Lyc.*

    gurgling: *Podo., Puls., Sul.*

      before stool: *Podo.*

    intolerant of tight clothing (belts etc.): *Arg-n., Calc-c., Lyc., Mag-c., Nux-v.*

    rumbling: *Carb-v., Chin., Lyc., Nat-s., Nux-v., Puls., Sil., Sul.*

      before stool: *Mag-c.*

  Wind:

    loud: *Arg-n., Nat-s.*

during stool: *Nat-s., Podo.*
smelly: *Ars., Carb-v., Nat-s., Nit-ac., Puls., Sil., Sul.*
  of rotten eggs: *Sul.*
obstructed (difficult to expel): *Arg-n., Chin.,*
  Colch., Nit-ac., Puls., Sil.
With:
  diarrhoea: *Carb-v., Nat-s.*
  urging for stool but only spluttering wind is
    passed: *Nat-s.*
Better:
  passing wind: *Carb-v., Lyc., Nat-s., Nux-v., Puls.,*
    Sul.
Worse:
  after eating: *Arg-n., Lyc., Nux-v.*
  after breakfast: *Nat-s.*
  before/after stool: *Lyc.*
Causes:
  abdominal surgery: *Carb-a., Carb-v., Chin.*
  eating fruit: *Chin.*
Flu   *Ars., Bry., Dulc., Eup-p., Gels., Ip., Nux-v., Pyr.,*
Rhus-t.
Chills: *Ip.*
Eyeballs aching: *Bry., Eup-p., Gels.*
Eyelids red: *Eup-p.*
Pains:
  aching: *Ip., Pyr., Rhus-t.*
  back: *Ip.*
  bones: *Eup-p., Ip., Nux-v., Pyr., Rhus-t.*
  bones feel broken: *Eup-p.*
  joints: *Nux-v., Rhus-t.*
  legs: *Ip., Pyr., Rhus-t.*
  muscles: *Gels.*
  shooting: *Rhus-t.*
  sore, bruised: *Ip., Nux-v., Rhus-t.*
Skin sore: *Eup-p.*
With:
  chilliness, extreme, can't get warm: *Gels., Nux-v.,*
    Pyr.
  common cold: *Ars., Nux-v.*
  exhaustion: *Gels., Rhus-t.*
  fever: *Ars., Nux-v., Pyr., Rhus-t.*
  headache: *Eup-p.*
  heaviness: *Gels.*
  nasal catarrh: *Eup-p.*
  numbness: *Gels.*
  restlessness: *Ars., Pyr.*
  shivering/chills in back: *Eup-p., Gels., Pyr.*
  sneezing: *Eup-p., Rhus-t.*
  extreme thirst: *Pyr.*
Better:
  warm compresses: *Nux-v.*
  for movement: *Pyr.*
  for sweating: *Eup-p., Gels.*
  for urinating: *Gels.*
  for walking: *Pyr.*
  warmth of bed: *Nux-v., Pyr.*

Worse:
  in bed: *Nux-v.*
  cold: *Nux-v.*
  during the chilly stage: *Pyr.*
  exertion: *Gels.*
  morning: *Nux-v.*
  walking: *Gels.*
  sitting: *Pyr.*
Causes:
  change of temperature: *Ars.*
  cold, damp weather: *Dulc.*
Flushed   see **Face flushes easily**
Food poisoning   *Ars., Carb-v., Puls.*
With:
  diarrhoea: *Ars., Puls.*
  flatulence: *Carb-v.*
  nausea: *Ars.*
  vomiting: *Ars.*
Causes:
  fish: *Carb-v., Puls.*
  meat: *Ars., Carb-v., Puls.*
Forgetful   (see also **Absent-minded; Confused**) *Arg-n.,*
Arn., Ars., Caust., Cocc., Colch., Con., Glon., Kali-p.,
Lyc., Merc-s., Nat-c., Petr., Pho-ac., Sep., Stap., Ver-a.
  Following injury: *Arn.*
Fractures   see **Broken bones**
Frightened   see **Fearful**
Full feeling   *Aesc.*
Fussy   see **Critical; Capricious**

Gas   see **Flatulance**
Gastric flu   *Ars., Bry., Eup-p., Ip., Nux-v.*
Pains:
  aching in stomach: *Bry.*
With:
  biliousness: *Bry.*
  fever: *Bry., Eup-p.*
  flu symptoms (see also **Flu**): *Ars., Bry., Eup-p., Ip.,*
    Nux-v.
  nausea/retching/vomiting of bile or food: *Eup-p.*
Better:
  after chills during fever: *Eup-p.*
  for belching: *Bry.*
Worse:
  evening: *Bry.*
  coughing: *Bry.*
  lying down in bed: *Bry.*
  movement: *Bry.*
  walking: *Bry.*
Gentle   *Puls.*
German measles   see **Measles**
Glands   (see also **Sore throat**, Tonsils swollen)
Sensitive: *Bar-c., Bell.*
Swollen: *Bar-c., Bell., Calc-c., Merc-s., Puls., Rhus-t.,*
  Sil., Sul.
    painless: *Calc-c.*

Gloomy   (see also **Depressed**; **Despondent**; **Morose**)
Nat-c.

Groin pains
In pregnancy: *Bell-p.*
Legs feel weak: *Bell-p.*

Guilt   *Ars., Ign.*

Gum boils   (see also **Abscesses**) *Sil.*

Gums
Bleeding: *Arn., Lach., Merc-c., Nat-m., Pho-ac.,
Phos., Stap., Zinc.*
after tooth extraction: *Arn., Lach., Phos.*
Pale: *Ferr-m., Merc-c., Stap., Zinc.*

Haemorrhages   see **Bleeding**
Haemorrhoids   see **Piles**
Hair loss   *Calc-c., Carb-v., Lach., Lyc., Nat-m., Nit-ac.,
Pho-ac., Phos., Sep., Sul.*
In handfuls: *Phos.*
Causes:
acute illness: *Carb-v., Phos.*
childbirth: *Calc-c., Carb-v., Lyc., Nat-m., Nit-ac.,
Sep., Sul.*
grief: *Pho-ac.*
pregnancy: *Lach.*

Headache   *Aco., All-c., Ant-c., Ap., Arg-n., Ars.,
Bell., Bry., Calc-c., Calc-p., Carb-v., Chin., Cimi.,
Cocc., Coff., Coloc., Eup-p., Ferr-m., Gels., Glon., Ign.,
Ip., Kali-b., Kali-c., Kali-p., Kali-s., Lach., Lyc.,
Mag-c., Mag-m., Mag-p., Merc-s., Nat-c., Nat-m.,
Nat-p., Nat-s., Nit-ac., Nux-v., Petr., Pho-ac., Phos.,
Puls., Rhod., Rhus-t., Ruta., Sep., Sil., Stap., Sul.,
Zinc.*
Extremities icy cold: *Sep.*
Eyes/eyelids:
red: *Glon.*
sensitive to light: *Nat-s.*
smarting: *Pho-ac.*
sore, watering: *Nat-m.*
Face:
pale: *Nat-p.*
red: *Glon.*
Head feels:
constricted: *Nit-ac., Sul.*
full: *Ap., Sul.*
heavy: *Carb-v., Gels., Lach., Nat-c., Nux-v., Petr.,
Pho-ac.*
hot: *Ap., Lach., Sul.*
Nervous: *Chin., Coff., Kali-p., Puls., Zinc.*
Pains:
aching: *Gels.*
back of head: *Bell., Carb-v., Cimi., Cocc., Eup-p.,
Gels., Nux-v., Petr., Pho-ac., Rhus-t., Sil., Stap.*
above eyes: *Kali-c.*
behind eyeballs: *Bry.*
in bones: *Eup-p., Nit-ac., Sep.*

burning: *Aco., Ars., Calc-c., Merc-s., Phos., Sil.,
Sul.*
bursting: *Aco., Bell., Bry., Calc-c., Glon., Lach.,
Phos., Sep., Sul., Zinc.*
eyes: *Bell., Rhod.*
forehead: *Ars., Bell., Bry., Cocc., Ferr-m., Ign.,
Kali-c., Kali-s., Lach., Lyc., Merc-s., Nat-m.,
Nat-p., Nux-v., Phos., Puls., Sil., Stap., Sul.,
Zinc.*
hammering: *Bell., Ferr-m., Glon., Nat-m., Sil.,
Sul.*
left side of face: *Coloc.*
maddening: *Calc-c.*
nape of neck: *Cocc., Pho-ac.*
one-sided: *Coff., Kali-p., Pho-ac., Puls.*
pressing: *Carb-v., Chin., Lach., Lyc., Merc-s.,
Nat-c., Nat-m., Nit-ac., Nux-v., Petr., Pho-ac.,
Phos., Puls., Sep., Sil., Stap., Sul.*
pressing out: *Cimi.*
pressing up: *Cimi.*
pulling: *Stap.*
pulsating: *Bell.*
recurring at regular intervals: *Ars., Kali-b.,
Mag-c., Nit-ac.*
rheumatic: *Rhus-t.*
right side of head: *Mag-p.*
shooting: *Kali-c., Mag-c., Mag-p., Sep.*
sides of head: *Kali-s., Phos., Ruta., Zinc.*
sinuses: *Kali-b., Sil.*
sore, bruised: *Chin., Cocc., Eup-p., Gels.,
Ip., Merc-s., Nux-v., Puls., Ruta., Sil.,
Stap.*
spasmodic: *Mag-c., Mag-p.*
splitting: *Nat-m.*
spreading to:
back of head: *Gels., Lach.*
forehead: *Gels.*
top of head: *Sil.*
to ear: *Coloc.*
eyes: *Mag-m., Nit-ac., Sil.*
stabbing: *Ap., Ign.*
start and stop suddenly: *Bell.*
stitching: *Kali-s.*
stupefying: *Nux-v.*
sudden: *Ap.*
tearing: *Coloc., Kali-c., Mag-c., Nux-v., Rhod.,
Sep., Zinc.*
temples: *Bell., Lach., Lyc., Mag-m., Nat-m., Zinc.*
throbbing: *Aco., Ars., Bell., Chin., Eup-p., Ferr-m.,
Glon., Lach., Lyc., Nat-m., Phos., Puls., Sep., Sil.,
Sul.*
top of head: *Cimi., Lach., Pho-ac., Sul.*
violent: *Bell., Bry., Glon., Ign., Lach., Rhus-t.,
Sil.*
in waves: *Sep.*
Pupils dilated: *Gels.*

Scalp feels:
  sensitive: *Chin.*
  sore: *Ap.*
  tight: *Ap.*
Urination frequent: *Gels.*
Vision blurred: *Gels.*
With:
  belching: *Mag-m.*
  biliousness: *Nux-v.*
  cold feet: *Gels.*
  dizziness: *Nux-v.*
  eye strain: *Ruta.*
  faintness: *Glon.*
  fever: *Eup-p.*
  heaviness: *Petr.*
  hot flushes: *Glon.*
  hunger before/during headache: *Phos.*
  nausea: *Ant-c., Cocc., Petr., Sul.*
  sweating on forehead: *Nat-c.*
  thirst: *Mag-m.*
  thirstlessness: *Ferr-m.*
  vomiting: *Ip.*
Better:
  for binding up the head: *Arg-n.*
  closing eyes: *Sil.*
  for cold: *Phos., Sul.*
  for cold compresses: *Bry., Glon., Phos., Sul.*
  after eating: *Lach., Sep.*
  evening in bed: *Nux-v.*
  excitement: *Nux-v., Pho-ac.*
  for fresh air: *Ars., Cimi., Kali-s., Lyc., Phos., Puls., Sep., Zinc.*
  gentle walking: *Rhus-t.*
  getting up: *Nux-v., Phos., Rhod.*
    in the morning: *Nux-v.*
  heat: *Mag-p., Sil.*
  for lying down: *Calc-c., Ferr-m., Puls., Sil.*
  in a quiet, dark room: *Sil.*
  with head high: *Puls.*
  for lying in a darkened room: *Bell.*
  massage: *Phos.*
  movement: *Rhus-t.*
  for firm pressure: *Chin., Ferr-m., Mag-p., Nat-m., Puls.*
  for pressure: *Bell., Bry., Glon., Mag-c., Nux-v.*
  for resting head: *Bell.*
  after sleep: *Phos.*
  sunset: *Glon.*
  urinating: *Gels.*
  walking: *Mag-c., Phos., Puls., Rhod.*
    in the fresh air: *Puls., Rhod.*
  wrapping up head: *Nux-v., Rhod., Rhus-t., Sil.*
Worse:
  10 a.m.–3 p.m.: *Nat-m.*
  for bending down: *Bell., Merc-s., Puls., Sep., Sul.*
  blowing nose: *Puls., Sul.*

  getting chilled: *Sil.*
  getting cold: *Bell., Calc-p., Kali-c., Mag-p., Nux-v., Phos.*
  getting head cold: *Sep., Sil.*
  getting feet cold: *Sil.*
  for coughing: *Bry., Lyc., Nat-m., Phos., Sul.*
  damp weather: *Rhod.*
  daylight: *Phos., Sil.*
  after drinking wine: *Zinc.*
  after eating: *Nat-c., Nat-m., Nux-v., Puls., Sul.*
  emotions: *Nat-m.*
  evening: *Kali-s.*
  excitement: *Nat-m.*
  moving eyes: *Nux-v.*
  during a fever: *Nat-m.*
  after getting up: *Bry., Sul.*
  getting up from lying down: *Pho-ac., Sil.*
  for heat: *Ars., Bell., Glon., Puls.*
  hot drinks: *Phos., Puls.*
  jarring movement: *Glon., Nit-ac., Sil.*
  left side: *Kali-c., Lach.*
  for light: *Bell., Calc-c.*
  lying down: *Lach., Mag-c.*
  during menstrual period: *Bell., Glon., Lyc., Nat-m., Sep.*
  mental exertion: *Glon., Nat-c., Nat-m.*
  in the morning: *Sul.*
  moving head: *Ferr-m., Gels.*
  movement: *Gels., Nit-ac.*
  at night: *Merc-s., Nit-ac.*
  for noise: *Calc-c., Coff., Nit-ac.*
  getting overheated: *Lyc.*
  in pregnancy: *Bell., Puls., Sep.*
  pressure: *Lach., Mag-m., Nit-ac.*
  reading/writing: *Nat-m.*
  on the right side of the head: *Calc-c.*
  running: *Puls.*
  shaking head: *Nux-v.*
  smoky room: *Ign.*
  sneezing: *Sul.*
  standing: *Puls.*
  stuffy room: *Kali-s., Phos., Puls.*
  summer: *Glon.*
  exposure to sun: *Bell.*
  sunrise: *Glon.*
  sweating: *Eup-p.*
  talking: *Nat-m.*
  thinking: *Nat-c., Nat-m.*
  travelling: *Sep.*
  before/during a thunderstorm: *Rhod.*
  touch: *Coloc., Stap.*
  turning head quickly: *Nat-c.*
  for tying up hair: *Bell.*
  on waking: *Lach., Nat-m., Nit-ac.*
  for walking: *Bell., Glon., Lach., Nit-ac., Sul.*
  walking upstairs: *Sil.*

walking heavily: *Sil.*
warm room: *Kali-s.*
warmth of bed: *Lyc., Sul.*
wine: *Zinc.*
wrapping up head: *Lyc., Mag-m., Phos.*
Causes:
  anaemia: *Calc-p.*
  artificial light (working in): *Sep., Sil.*
  breastfeeding: *Bry., Calc-c., Puls., Sep.*
  change of weather: *Bry., Rhus-t.*
  getting chilled: *Aco., Mag-p.*
  cold air: *Bell., Rhod., Rhus-t., Sil.*
  cold, damp weather: *Bry., Calc-c., Sul.*
  cold wind: *Calc-p., Nux-v., Rhus-t.*
  common cold: *Merc-s., Nux-v.*
  damp weather: *Nux-v., Rhus-t., Sil., Sul.*
  draughts: *Sil.*
  emotions: *Stap.*
  excitement: *Coloc., Puls., Stap.*
  excited conversation: *Sul.*
  eye strain: *Kali-c., Lyc., Pho-ac., Ruta., Sil.*
  fright: *Aco.*
  getting head wet (haircut): *Bell.*
  getting wet: *Calc-c., Rhus-t.*
  grief: *Pho-ac., Stap.*
  head injury: *Nat-s.*
  ice-cream: *Puls.*
  ironing: *Bry.*
  irregular sleep: *Cocc.*
  lifting: *Rhus-t.*
  loss of sleep: *Cocc., Nux-v.*
  mental exertion: *Calc-c., Calc-p., Kali-p., Nat-c., Nat-p., Nux-v., Pho-ac.*
  mental strain: *Chin., Lyc., Nat-c., Nux-v., Pho-ac.*
  nerves: *Chin., Cocc.*
  overeating: *Nux-v.*
  overexposure to sun: *Bell., Bry., Glon., Lach.*
  overwork: *Calc-p., Cocc., Kali-p., Sil., Zinc.*
  physical exertion: *Calc-p.*
  rheumatism: *Merc-s.*
  running: *Puls.*
  shock: *Aco.*
  summer: *Nat-c.*
  sunstroke: *Nat-c.*
  before a thunderstorm: *Phos.*
  travelling (car/coach/train etc.): *Cocc., Sil.*
  vexation: *Coloc., Stap.*
  winter: *Sul.*
Head injuries   see **Injuries** to head
Healing after childbirth   see **Bruises; Injuries** (cuts/wounds); **Back pain; Sprains** and **Strains**
Heartburn (see also **Indigestion**)
  In pregnancy: *Bry., Calc-c., Merc-s., Nat-m., Nux-v., Tab., Zinc.*
  With:
    indigestion: *Calc-c., Merc-s., Nat-m., Nux-v.*

sour belches: *Nux-v.*
sweetish belches: *Nat-m., Zinc.*
watery belches: *Nat-m., Tab.*
Worse:
  at night: *Merc-s.*
Heavy feeling (see also **Sluggish**)
  Generally: *Aesc., Gels., Phos., Sep.*
Hernia in babies
  Inguinal: *Lyc., Nux-v.*
    right side: *Lyc.*
    left side: *Nux-v.*
  Umbilical: *Bry., Calc-c.*
  Cause:
    constipation: *Nux-v.*
Herpes   See **Cold sores**
Hiccups in babies   *Bor., Mag-p., Nux-v.*
  Violent: *Mag-p., Nux-v.*
  Worse after eating or drinking: *Mag-p., Nux-v.*
Hitting (in angry babies)   *Bell., Cham., Cina., Lyc., Nux-v., Stram., Ver-a.*
Hives   *Ap., Dulc., Rhus-t., Urt-u.*
  Rash:
    biting: *Urt-u.*
    burning: *Rhus-t., Urt-u.*
    itching: *Rhus-t., Urt-u.*
    lumpy: *Dulc.*
    stinging: *Rhus-t., Urt-u.*
  With:
    fever: *Ap.*
    joint pain: *Rhus-t., Urt-u.*
    sweating: *Ap.*
  Better:
    rubbing: *Urt-u.*
  Worse:
    cold: *Rhus-t.*
    exercise: *Urt-u.*
    heat: *Dulc., Urt-u.*
    night: *Ap., Urt-u.*
    after scratching: *Dulc., Rhus-t.*
  Causes:
    getting chilled/wet: *Rhus-t.*
    getting cold: *Dulc.*
    cold air: *Rhus-t.*
    during a fever: *Rhus-t.*
    insects: *Urt-u.*
    stinging nettles: *Urt-u.*
Hoarseness (painless)   *Calc-c.*
Homesick   *Ign., Pho-ac.*
Hot flushes   *Cocc., Kali-c., Lach., Nat-s., Phos., Sep., Sul., Sul-ac., Ver-a.*
  Flush moves up the body: *Sep.*
  in pregnancy: *Sul., Ver-a.*
  With:
    headache: *Lach.*
    palpitations: *Lach.*

hot sweats: *Lach.*
Worse:
    during the afternoon: *Sep.*
    during the evening: *Sep.*
    after sweating: *Sep.*
Humiliation   *Coloc., Lyc., Staph.*
Hurried   *Arg-n., Hep-s., Lil-t., Sul-ac.*
    While eating: *Hep-s., Sul-ac.*
    At work: *Sul-ac.*
    While speaking: *Arg-n., Hep-s.*
    While waiting: *Arg-n.*
    While walking: *Arg-n., Sul-ac.*
    While writing: *Sul-ac.*
Hyperactive   *Stram.*

Idealistic   *Ign.*
Impatient (see also **Irritable**)   *Cham., Hep-s., Nux-v., Sul.*
Impulsive   *Arg-n., Hep-s., Nux-v.*
Incontinence (involuntary urination)   *Ars., Caust., Nat-m., Puls., Sep.*
    In pregnancy: *Ars., Caust., Nat-m., Puls., Sep.*
    After childbirth: *Ars.*
    Worse for:
        coughing, laughing, sneezing or walking: *Caust., Nat-m., Puls., Sep.*
        getting chilled: *Caust.*
        day and night: *Ars.*
Indecisive   *Bar-c., Ign., Lyc., Op.*
Indifferent (see also **Apathetic**)   *Carb-v., Nat-m., Nat-p., Pho-ac., Rhe., Sep., Stram.*
    During a fever: *Op., Pho-ac.*
    Babies: *Rhe.*
      to playing: *Rhe.*
    To everything: *Carb-v.*
    To own children: *Sep.*
    To family: *Sep.*
    To loved ones: *Sep.*
    To personal appearance (i.e. scruffy): *Sul.*
    To work: *Sep.*
Indigestion (see also **Heartburn; Flatulence; Taste**)   *Ant-c., Arg-n., Ars., Bry., Calc-c., Carb-v., Caust., Chin., Ign., Kali-b., Kali-c., Kali-m., Kali-p., Lyc., Mag-c., Nat-c., Nat-m., Nat-p., Nat-s., Nux-v., Phos., Puls., Sul.*
    Abdomen/stomach feels:
        bloated: *Ant-c., Arg-n., Calc-c., Carb-v., Chin., Kali-c., Mag-c., Nat-p., Nat-s., Nux-v., Sul.*
        empty: *Ant-c., Ign., Kali-p., Lyc., Nux-v., Puls., Sul.*
        at 11 a.m.: *Sul.*
        full: *Ant-c., Caust., Kali-c., Lyc.*
          very quickly (when eating): *Lyc.*
        hard: *Calc-c.*
        painful: *Arg-n.*

    rumbling: *Mag-c.*
Belches:
    acrid: *Lyc.*
    bitter: *Chin., Nat-s., Nux-v., Puls.*
    difficult: *Arg-n.*
    empty: *Ant-c., Arg-n., Carb-v., Caust., Kali-b., Lyc., Puls, Sul.*
    greasy: *Mag-c.*
    incomplete, ineffectual: *Chin., Nat-m.*
    loud: *Arg-n.*
    sour: *Calc-c., Carb-v., Chin., Ign., Kali-b., Lyc., Mag-c., Nat-c., Nat-m., Nat-p., Nat-s., Nux-v., Sul.*
    tasting of food just eaten: *Ant-c., Caust., Chin., Nat-m., Puls.*
Nervous: *Kali-p.*
Pains in the stomach:
    burning: *Ars., Carb-v., Phos., Sul.*
    cramping: *Carb-v., Caust., Lyc., Nat-m., Nux-v.*
    pressing: *Calc-c., Caust., Chin., Lyc., Nat-m., Nux-v., Puls.*
    sore, bruised: *Kali-c., Nat-c., Nux-v., Phos.*
With:
    diarrhoea: *Kali-m.*
    flatulence: *Arg-n., Calc-c., Carbo-v., Sul.*
      after breakfast: *Nat-s.*
        obstructed: *Chin.*
    headache: *Ars.*
    heartburn: *Ars., Bry., Calc-c., Lyc., Mag-c., Merc-s., Nat-p., Nux-v., Puls.*
    nausea: *Arg-n., Carb-v., Mag-c., Nat-c.*
    stools pale: *Kali-m.*
    violent hiccups: *Nat-m.*
Better:
    belching: *Arg-n., Carb-v., Ign., Kali-b., Kali-c., Lyc.*
    hot drinks: *Ars., Nux-v.*
    after passing a stool: *Nat-s.*
    passing wind: *Carb-v.*
    warmth of bed: *Nux-v.*
Worse:
    after belching: *Chin.*
    after cabbage: *Mag-c.*
    after drinking: *Chin., Sul.*
    after eating: *Arg-n., Carb-v., Chin., Kali-b., Kali-c., Lyc., Nux-v., Phos., Puls., Sul.*
    fruit: *Chin.*
    milk: *Mag-c., Sul.*
    at night: *Puls.*
    onions: *Lyc.*
    pregnancy: *Puls.*
    rich/fatty food: *Carb-v., Puls.*
    starchy food: *Kali-m., Nat-m., Nat-s.*
    sweet foods/sugar: *Arg-n.*
    tight clothing: *Carb-v., Lyc., Nux-v.*
Causes:
    abdominal surgery: *Chin.*

coffee: *Nux-v.*
grief: *Ign.*
mental strain: *Nux-v.*
nervous exhaustion: *Kali-p.*
overeating: *Nux-v.*
overwork: *Kali-p.*
rich/fatty food: *Nux-v., Puls.*

Inflammation of navel in newborn babies   *Hep-s., Sil.*

Inflammation of penis in babies   *Arn.*

Injuries   (see also **Bites/stings; Broken bones; Bruises; Burns; Sprains; Strains**)   *Aco., Arn., Bell., Calc-s., Calen., Con., Hep-s., Hyp., Lach., Led., Phos., Ruta., Sil., Stap.*

Cuts/wounds:
  bleed freely: *Aco., Bell., Lach., Phos.*
  blood:
    bright red: *Phos.*
    slow to clot: *Phos.*
  crushed: *Hyp.*
  inflamed: *Hep-s., Sil.*
    with redness around: *Hep-s.*
    with dirt/splinter still inside: *Sil.*
    with pus inside: *Sil.*
    with pus oozing: *Calc-s.*
  painful: *Calen., Hep-s., Hyp., Sil., Stap.*
    shooting: *Hyp.*
    sore/bruised: *Arn., Hep-s., Ruta.*
    splinter-like: *Hep-s.*
    stitching/tearing: *Stap.*
  painful out of proportion to the injury: *Calen.*
  suppurate: *Calc-s., Calen., Sil.*
  with bruising: *Arn.*
To fingers/toes (crushed): *Hyp.*
Lacerated wounds (torn): *Calen., Hyp., Led., Stap.*
Punctured wounds (with a knife, or nail, etc.): *Hyp., Led.*
Slow to heal: *Calc-s., Hep-s., Hyp., Lach., Sil.*
To glands (breasts, etc.): *Con.*
  cold, inflamed, sensitive, stony hard lumps; swollen: *Con.*
To head: *Arn., Nat-s.*
To muscles: *Arn.*
To nerves/nerve-rich parts of the body: *Hyp., Stap.*
To palm of hand or sole of foot: *Led.*
To shins: *Ruta.*
With:
  shock (anxiety and fear): *Aco.*
  foreign body: *Sil.*
Scars:
  become lumpy: *Sil.*
  become red: *Lach.*
  are painful, break open and/or suppurate: *Sil.*
Better:
  cold compresses: *Led.*

Worse:
  heat: *Led.*
  touch: *Hep-s., Stap.*
Causes:
  accident: *Hyp., Stap.*
  after dental treatment: *Arn., Hyp., Stap.*
  childbirth: *Stap.*
  circumcision: *Stap.*
  episiotomy: *Hep-s., Hyp., Sil., Stap.*
  nails: *Led.*
  splinter: *Hyp., Led., Sil.*
  surgery: *Arn., Hyp., Sil., Stap.*

Insect bites   see **Bites/stings**

Insomnia   *Aco., Ars., Bell., Bell-p., Calc-c., Calc-p., Cham., Cocc., Coff., Con., Cypr., Kali-c., Kali-p., Ign., Lyc., Mag-c., Mag-m., Nat-c., Nat-m., Nit-ac., Nux-v., Op., Pho-ac., Phos., Puls., Rhus-t., Sep., Sil., Sul.*

Dreams:
  anxious: *Aco., Ars., Calc-c., Cocc., Kali-c., Nat-c., Nat-m., Nit-ac., Phos., Puls.*
  nightmares: *Ars., Cocc., Con., Kali-c., Sil., Sul.*
    vivid: *Sil., Sul.*
  unpleasant: *Sul.*
    vivid: *Aco., Cham., Coff., Nat-m., Nux-v., Puls.*
In pregnancy: *Aco., Cham., Coff., Con., Ign., Nux-v., Puls.*
In restless babies: *Cypr.*
Sleep:
  disturbed: *Sul.*
  restless: *Aco., Ars., Bell., Cocc., Puls., Rhus-t., Sil., Sul.*
  unrefreshing: *Mag-c., Mag-m., Nit-ac., Pho-ac., Sul.*
Sleepless: *Pho-ac.*
  after midnight: *Pho-ac., Rhus-t., Sil.*
  after 2 a.m.: *Nit-ac.*
  after 3 a.m.: *Bell-p., Mag-c., Nux-v.*
  after waking: *Sil.*
  before midnight: *Con., Kali-c.*
  daytime (babies): *Lyc.*
Waking:
  around 3 a.m.: *Nux-v., Sep.*
  difficult: *Calc-p.*
  early: *Nat-c., Nux-v.*
  frequent: *Pho-ac., Puls., Sul.*
  from cold: *Puls.*
  late: *Calc-p., Nux-v., Sul.*
  to play in the night (babies): *Cypr.*
With:
  empty feeling in pit of stomach: *Kali-p.*
  grinding of teeth: *Bell.*
  sleepiness: *Bell., Cham., Op., Phos., Puls., Sep.*
Better:
  short naps: *Sul.*
Worse:
  around 1–2 a.m.: *Kali-c.*

after 2 a.m.: *Nit-ac.*
after 3 a.m.; *Bell-p.*, *Sep.*
after 3, 4 or 5 a.m.: *Sul.*
after midnight: *Ars.*, *Sil.*
before midnight: *Calc-c.*, *Calc-p.*, *Kali-c.*, *Puls.*
Causes:
anxiety: *Ars.*, *Cocc.*, *Kali-p.*
coffee: *Cham.*, *Nux-v.*
cramps in pregnancy: *Cham.*, *Coff.*, *Nux-v.*
excitement: *Kali-p.*, *Nux-v.*
grief: *Nat-m.*
mental strain: *Kali-p.*, *Nux-v.*
movements of the baby (in pregnancy): *Con.*
nervous exhaustion: *Cypr.*, *Kali-p.*
overactive mind: *Ars.*, *Calc-c.*, *Coff.*, *Nux-v.*, *Puls.*
overexcitement: *Coff.*
overwork: *Nux-v.*
repeating thoughts: *Puls.*
shock: *Ars.*, *Ign.*
worry: *Calc-c.*
Introspective/Introverted (see also **Broody; Morose; Uncommunicative**) *Cocc.*, *Ign.*, *Nat-c.*, *Nat-m.*, *Puls.*
Irritable (see also **Angry**) *Ant-c.*, *Ant-t.*, *Ap.*, *Ars.*, *Bor.*, *Bry.*, *Calc-p.*, *Calc-s.*, *Carb-v.*, *Caust.*, *Cham.*, *Cina*, *Ferr-m.*, *Hep-s.*, *Kali-c.*, *Kali-s.*, *Lil-t.*, *Lyc.*, *Mag-c.*, *Nat-c.*, *Nat-m.*, *Nit-ac.*, *Nux-v.*, *Petr.*, *Pho-ac.*, *Phos.*, *Puls.*, *Rhe.*, *Rhus-t.*, *Sep.*, *Sil.*, *Stap.*, *Sul.*, *Sul-ac.*, *Ver-a.*, *Zinc.*
And anxious: *Nux-v.*
And dislikes consolation: *Nat-m.*, *Sep.*, *Sil.*
Babies: *Calc-p.*, *Cham.*, *Chin.*, *Cina*, *Lyc.*, *Mag-c.*, *Sil.*, *Stap.*
Worse:
after a sleep: *Lyc.*
before stools: *Bor.*
daytime: *Lyc.*
mornings: *Chin.*, *Lyc.*
when sick: *Lyc.*
when touched: *Ant-t.*
with teething: *Cham.*, *Rhe.*
During pregnancy: *Cham.*
During labour: *Ars.*, *Cham.*, *Kali-c.*, *Nux-v.*, *Sep.*

Jaundice in babies *Chel.*, *Chin.*, *Nat-s.*
Jealous *Ap.*, *Lach.*, *Puls.*
Joint pain *Ap.*, *Arn.*, *Bell-p.*, *Bry.*, *Calc-c.*, *Calc-p.*, *Caul.*, *Caust.*, *Cham.*, *Cimi.*, *Colch.*, *Dulc.*, *Ferr-m.*, *Hep-s.*, *Kali-b.*, *Kali-c.*, *Kali-s.*, *Led.*, *Lyc.*, *Merc-s.*, *Nit-ac.*, *Puls.*, *Rhod.*, *Rhus-t.*, *Ruta.*, *Sul.*
Feet cold: *Calc-p.*, *Kali-s.*
Joints:
icy cold: *Led.*
hot: *Led.*
stiff: *Led.*

In pregnancy: *Cimi.*
Pains:
aching: *Rhus-t.*
acute: *Colch.*
alternating with:
indigestion: *Kali-b.*
cough: *Kali-b.*
arms: *Ferr-m.*, *Kali-c.*, *Rhod.*
upper: *Ferr-m.*
in back: *Caust.*
bones: *Nit-ac.*, *Puls.*, *Ruta.*
burning: *Ap.*, *Caust.*, *Merc-s.*, *Sul.*
cramping: *Calc-c.*
drawing: *Rhod.*
feet: *Calc-p.*, *Colch.*, *Led.*, *Ruta.*
fingers: *Hep-s.*
flying around: *Caul.*
gnawing: *Caust.*
hands: *Colch.*, *Led.*, *Ruta.*
hips: *Hep-s.*, *Kali-c.*, *Kali-s.*
in pregnancy: *Calc-p.*
right: *Led.*
irregular: *Caul.*
in joints: *Caust.*, *Puls.*
legs: *Kali-c.*, *Kali-s.*, *Nit-ac.*, *Rhod.*
lower back: *Ruta.*
in neck: *Caust.*
parts lain on: *Ruta.*
pressing: *Caust.*
pulling: *Hep-s.*, *Puls.*
shoulders: *Ferr-m.*, *Hep-s.*, *Kali-c.*, *Rhod.*
left: *Led.*
in small joints: *Caul.*
in one spot: *Kali-b.*
sore/bruised: *Arn.*, *Hep-s.*, *Kali-b.*, *Kali-c.*, *Puls.*, *Rhus-t.*, *Ruta.*
shooting: *Rhus-t.*
splinter-like: *Nit-ac.*
stinging: *Ap.*
stitching: *Bry.*, *Caust.*, *Ferr-m.*, *Kali-c.*, *Nit-ac.*
tearing: *Caust.*, *Colch.*, *Ferr-m.*, *Hep-s.*, *Kali-c.*, *Lyc.*, *Merc-s.*, *Nit-ac.*, *Rhod.*, *Rhus-t.*, *Sul.*
violent: *Cham.*
wandering: *Kali-b.*, *Kali-s.*, *Puls.*
With:
heaviness: *Rhus-t.*
lameness: *Rhus-t.*, *Ruta.*
numbness: *Cham.*, *Kali-c.*
restless legs: *Kali-c.*
stiffness: *Caust.*, *Rhus-t.*
swelling: *Ap.*, *Bry.*, *Colch.*
weakness of arms: *Kali-c.*
Better:
after a common cold: *Led.*
cold compresses: *Led.*, *Puls.*
cold bathing: *Led.*

continued movement: *Rhus-t.*
fresh air: *Kali-s., Puls.*
gentle movement: *Ferr-m., Puls.*
heat: *Caust., Hep-s., Rhus-t.*
movement: *Dulc., Kali-c., Kali-s., Lyc., Rhod.*
pressure: *Bry.*
complete rest: *Bry.*
stretching out limb: *Rhod.*
uncovering: *Led.*
walking: *Cham., Kali-c., Kali-s., Lyc., Puls., Rhus-t.*
warm compresses: *Rhus-t.*
warmth: *Caust., Colch.*
warmth of bed: *Caust., Lyc., Rhus-t.*
Worse:
around 2–3 a.m.: *Kali-c.*
in bed: *Merc-s.*
beginning to move: *Ferr-m., Lyc., Puls., Rhus-t.*
bending arm backwards: *Ferr-m.*
change of weather: *Rhod.*
getting chilled: *Rhus-t.*
cold: *Bry., Calc-c., Calc-p., Cimi., Colch., Hep-s.*
damp weather: *Rhus-t.*
dry cold: *Caust.*
cold, wet weather: *Calc-p., Colch.*
after a common cold: *Puls.*
during a fever: *Lyc., Rhus-t.*
getting up from sitting: *Caust.*
heat: *Kali-s., Led., Puls.*
lifting arm up: *Ferr-m.*
lying on the painful part: *Kali-c.*
night: *Dulc., Led., Merc-s., Nit-ac., Rhus-t.*
slightest movement: *Bry.*
movement: *Colch., Led.*
sitting down: *Dulc., Lyc., Rhus-t., Rhod.*
stormy weather: *Rhod.*
summer: *Kali-s.*
touch: *Arn.*
walking: *Ruta., Sul.*
warm weather: *Colch.*
warmth of bed: *Led., Puls., Sul.*
wet weather: *Calc-c., Merc-s., Puls., Rhod.*
Causes:
getting chilled after being very hot: *Bell-p.*
getting cold: *Dulc., Hep-s.*
damp: *Dulc.*
wet weather: *Calc-c.*

Joking
During labour: *Coff.*
Jumpy (see also **Anxious; Restless**)   *Bar-c., Bor., Kali-c., Kali-p., Nat-c., Nat-s., Phos., Sil.*

Labour   *Aco., Arn., Bell., Calc-c., Caul., Cham., Cimi., Coff., Cupr., Gels., Ip., Kali-c., Kali-p., Lyc., Mag-p.,*

Nat-m., Nux-v., Op., Puls., Sec., Sep., Ver-a.
Fast (too fast): *Aco., Lyc.*
Late: *Aco., Caul., Cimi., Gels., Lyc.*
with anticipatory anxiety: *Gels., Lyc.*
with fear of labour: *Aco., Cimi.*
Long (too long): *Arn.*
Premature: *Nat-m., Nux-v., Op.*
Premature caused by shock: *Op.*
Slow: *Bell., Caul., Nat-m., Sec.*
Labour pains (contractions)   *Aco., Bell., Cimi., Caul., Cham., Coff., Cupr., Gels., Ip., Kali-c., Kali-p., Mag-p., Nat-m., Nux-v., Op., Puls., Sec., Sep., Ver-a.*
In back: *Cham., Cimi., Coff., Gels., Nux-v., Puls., Sep.*
In back/buttocks and/or thighs: *Gels., Kali-c.*
In hips: *Cimi.*
Pains:
distressing: *Bell., Caul., Cham., Coff., Gels., Kali-c., Sep.*
false: *Bell., Caul., Gels., Puls.*
flying around abdomen: *Cimi.*
ineffectual:
cervic doesn't dilate: *Coff., Kali-c., Puls.*
cervix doesn't soften: *Bell., Caul., Cham., Cimi., Gels., Nux-v., Sec.*
irregular: *Caul., Coff., Puls.*
long (each contraction lasts a long time): *Sec.*
severe (violent): *Aco., Bell., Cham., Coff., Nux-v., Sep.*
short (each contraction lasts a short time): *Caul., Puls.*
stopping or slowing down: *Bell., Caul., Cham., Cimi., Coff., Kali-c., Nat-m., Nux-v., Op., Puls., Sec., Sep.*
from exhaustion: *Caul.*
with cramps in hip and/or shivering: *Cimi.*
with talkativeness: *Coff.*
unbearable: *Cham.*
weak: *Bell., Caul., Cimi., Gels., Kali-c., Nat-m., Op., Puls., Sec.*
With:
chilliness after a contraction: *Kali-c.*
cramps:
in hands or legs: *Bell., Cupr., Mag-p., Nux-v.*
in fingers or toes: *Cupr.*
exhaustion: *Bell., Caul., Cham., Kali-c., Kali-p., Nat-m., Nux-v., Op., Puls., Sec., Sep., Ver-a.*
faint feeling: *Cimi., Nux-v., Puls., Sec., Ver-a.*
irritability: *Caul.*
nausea: *Ip., Puls., Ver-a.*
constant: *Ip.*
red face: *Bell., Op.*
thirst: *Caul.*
trembling: *Caul., Cimi., Gels.*
if the contractions stop: *Sec.*

urging to pass a stool: *Nux-v.*
vomiting: *Cupr., Puls., Ver-a.*
Lack of self-confidence (see also **Shy**)   *Bar-c., Lyc., Sil.*
Laryngitis   see **Sore throat**
Lazy   *Sul.*
Lethargic   see **Apathetic; Exhaustion; Sluggish**
Likes
boiled eggs: *Calc-c.*
bread and butter: *Merc-s.*
chocolate: *Lyc., Phos.*
cold drinks: *Aco., Bry., Cham., Chin., Cina, Eup-p., Merc-c., Merc-s., Nat-s., Phos., Ver-a.*
cold food: *Phos., Puls.*
cold food in pregnancy: *Ver-a.*
fat/fatty foods: *Nit-ac.*
fruit: *Pho-ac., Ver-a.*
ham, salami, smoked foods: *Caust.*
hot drinks: *Ars., Bry.*
hot food: *Ars., Bry.*
ice-cream: *Phos., Ver-a.*
ice-cold drinks: *Phos., Ver-a.*
milk: *Phos., Rhus-t.*
refreshing things: *Pho-ac., Ver-a.*
salt, salty foods: *Nat-m., Phos.*
salty foods in pregnancy: *Nat-m., Ver-a.*
sour food: *Hep-s., Ver-a.*
sour foods in pregnancy: *Sep., Ver-a.*
spicy food: *Chin., Nux-v., Phos., Sul.*
strange things in pregnancy (like raw spaghetti/rice, chalk, coal): *Alu., Calc-c.*
sugar: *Arg-n.*
sweets: *Arg-n., Chin., Lyc., Sul.*
vinegar: *Sep.*
Lips
Cracked: *Ars., Nat-m., Sul.*
Blue: *Cupr., Lach.*
Dry: *Ant-c., Ars., Bry., Puls., Rhus-t., Sul.*
Licks: *Ars.*
Red: *Sul.*
Swollen: *Ap.*
Lively (see also **Excitable**)   *Coff., Lach., Nat-c., Op.*
Lochia   *Calc-c., Kreos., Puls., Sec., Sil.*
Burns: *Kreos.*
Dark: *Kreos., Sec.*
Flows while baby breastfeeds: *Sil.*
Intermittent: *Calc-c.*
Lasts too long: *Calc-c., Sec.*
Lumpy: *Kreos.*
Returns: *Calc-c., Kreos., Puls.*
Scanty: *Puls., Sec.*
Smelly: *Kreos., Sec.*
Lonely   *Puls., Stram.*
Loquacious   see **Talkative**
Loss of libido   *Caust., Nat-m., Sep.*

Lumbago   see **Backache**
Mastitis   see **Breastfeeding problems; Breasts inflamed**
Measles   *Aco., Ap., Ars., Bell., Bry., Euphr., Gels., Puls., Sul.*
Onset:
slow: *Bry., Gels.*
sudden: *Aco., Bell.*
Skin rash:
burns: *Aco., Bell., Sul.*
hot: *Bell.*
itches: *Aco., Bell., Sul.*
maddeningly: *Sul.*
red: *Bell., Sul.*
slow to appear: *Ap., Bry., Sul.*
With:
common cold: *Euphr., Puls.*
cough: *Aco., Bell., Bry., Euphr., Puls., Sul.*
eye inflammation: *Ap., Bell., Euphr., Puls.*
fever: *Aco., Ap., Bell., Bry., Gels., Sul.*
heachache: *Bry., Gels.*
Worse for heat: *Sul.*
Melancholic   *Calc-c., Con.*
Memory weak   *Arg-n., Caust., Cocc., Colch., Con.*
Migraine   see **Headache**, one-sided
Mild, gentle   *Cocc., Puls., Sil.*
Mischievous   *Chin., Merc-s., Nux-v., Stram.*
Moaning, complaining   *Aco., Coff.*
During labour: *Coff.*
In babies: *Bor., Cham., Cina*
who can't have what they want: *Cham.*
Moody (changeable)   *Ferr-m., Ign., Lyc., Puls., Sul-ac., Zinc.*
Morose   (see also **Depressed; Despondent**)   *Bry.*
Mouth
Burning: *Ars.*
Dry: *Ars., Bry., Merc-s., Nat-m., Puls.*
with thirst: *Bry., Nat-m.*
without thirst: *Puls.*
Mouth ulcers   *Lyc., Merc-s., Nit-ac.*
Ulcers:
edges of tongue: *Nit-ac.*
gums: *Merc-s.*
painful: *Nit-ac.*
on the tongue: *Merc-s.*
under the tongue: *Lyc.*
Pains:
stinging/throbbing: *Merc-s.*
Mumps   *Aco., Ap., Ars., Bar-c., Bell., Bry., Carb-v., Jab., Lach., Lyc., Merc-s., Phyt., Puls., Rhus-t., Sil.*
Glands (parotid):
hard: *Merc-s., Phyt.*
swelling moves from the right side to the left: *Lyc.*
swollen/painful: *Bell., Carb-v., Jab., Lach., Lyc., Merc-s., Phyt., Puls., Rhus-t., Sil.*

Onset sudden: *Aco., Bell.*
Pains spread to breasts, ovaries: *Carb-v., Jab.,
Phyt., Puls.*
With:
  face red: *Jab.*
  fever: *Aco., Bell., Lyc., Merc-s., Puls., Rhus-t.*
  headache: *Bell.*
  copious saliva: *Jab., Merc-s., Phyt.*
  profuse sweating: *Jab., Merc-s., Phyt.*
  sore throat: *Bell., Lach., Lyc., Phyt.*
  vomiting: *Puls.*
Better:
  for heat: *Rhus-t., Sil.*
Worse:
  blowing nose: *Merc-s.*
  at night: *Merc-s.*
  on the left: *Lach., Rhus-t.*
  on the right: *Bell., Merc-s.*
  for cold: *Rhus-t., Sil.*

Nappy rash (Diaper rash)   *Ap., Petr., Rhus-t., Sul.*
  Burns: *Rhus-t., Sul.*
  Bleeding: *Petr., Sul.*
  Cracked/dry: *Petr.*
  Flaky: *Rhus-t.*
  Hot: *Ap., Sul.*
  Itches: *Petr., Rhus-t., Sul.*
  Red: *Ap., Petr., Sul.*
  Raw: *Sul.*
  Shiny/sore: *Ap.*
  Weepy: *Petr.*
  Better:
    covering: *Rhus-t.*
    uncovering: *Ap., Sul.*
  Worse:
    bathing/washing, heat: *Ap., Sul.*
    cold: *Rhus-t.*
    in the folds of the skin: *Petr.*
    touch: *Ap.*
Naughty see **Mischievous**
Nausea see also **Taste** *Ant-c., Ant-t., Ars., Asar.,
Cocc., Colch., Con., Ip., Kreos., Lyc., Nux-v., Petr.,
Phos., Puls., Sep., Sul., Tab., Ver-a.*
  Constant: *Ant-c., Asar., Ip., Kreos., Nux-v.*
  Deathly: *Ars., Ip., Tab.*
  Intermittent: *Ant-t., Sep., Tab.*
  Persistent: *Ip.*
  Violent: *Ip., Tab.*
    during pregnancy: *Ant-c., Asar.*
  Abdomen/stomach feels:
    bloated: *Colch.*
    empty: *Cocc., Phos., Sep.*
  Appetite lost: *Cocc., Colch.*
  Belches: *Ant-c., Cocc.*
    empty: *Ant-c., Ip.*

  sour: *Phos.*
  tasting of food eaten: *Ant-c.*
Pains gnawing: *Sep.*
With:
  copious saliva: *Ip., Kreos., Nux-v., Petr.*
  dizziness: *Petr.*
  faintness: *Cocc., Colch.*
  face pallid: *Ip.*
  headache: *Petr.*
  inability to vomit: *Nux-v.*
  retching: *Asar., Colch., Con., Ip., Nux-v.*
  vomiting: *Ars., Asar., Colch., Con., Ip., Kreos.,
  Lyc., Nux-v., Petr., Puls., Sep., Sul., Tab.,
  Ver-a.*
Better:
  for belching: *Ant-t.*
  for cold drinks: *Phos., Puls.*
  after eating (temporarily): *Sep.*
  fresh air: *Lyc., Puls., Tab.*
  for vomiting: *Ant-t.*
Worse:
  after drinking: *Ars., Cocc., Puls.*
  after eating: *Ant-c., Cocc., Colch., Con., Ip.,
  Kali-c., Lyc., Nux-v., Puls., Sep., Sul.*
  afternoon: *Ars., Cocc.*
  bending down: *Ip.*
  before breakfast: *Sep., Tab.*
  cold drinks: *Ars., Kali-c., Lyc.*
  coughing: *Ip., Kali-c., Puls.*
  eating acidic foods: *Ant-c.*
  eating bread or starchy food: *Ant-c.*
  fasting: *Lyc., Tab.*
  fresh air: *Petr.*
  hot drinks: *Phos., Puls.*
  ice-cream: *Ars., Ip., Puls.*
  milk: *Calc-c., Nit-ac., Sep.*
  morning: *Puls., Sep.*
  morning in bed: *Nux-v.*
  movement: *Cocc., Ip., Kali-c., Tab., Ver-a.*
  noise: *Asar., Cocc.*
  pork: *Sep.*
  putting hands in warm water: *Phos.*
  rich food: *Puls.*
  sight of food: *Cocc., Colch., Ip.*
  sitting up in bed; *Cocc.*
  smell of eggs or fish: *Colch.*
  smell of food: *Ars., Cocc., Colch., Ip., Sep.*
  stuffy room: *Lyc., Puls., Tab.*
  sweating: *Nux-v.*
  tobacco: *Ip., Lyc., Nux-v.*
  water: *Phos.*
Causes:
  pregnancy: *Ant-c., Ars., Asar., Colch., Con., Ip.,
  Kreos., Lyc., Nux-v., Petr., Puls., Sep., Sul., Tab.,
  Ver-a.*
  travelling: *Cocc., Nux-v., Tab.*

Nervous   see **Anxious**
Nettle rash   see **Hives**
Nose
  Child picks constantly: *Cina*
Nosebleeds   *Arn., Carb-v., Cocc., Ferr-m., Ham.,*
  Lach., Phos., Sep., Sul.
  Babies: *Ferr-m.*
  Blood:
    bright red: *Phos.*
    dark: *Carb-v., Ham.*
    persistent: *Phos.*
    thin: *Ham.*
  In pregnancy: *Cocc., Sep.*
  With:
    sweating: *Phos.*
  Worse:
    before a menstrual period: *Lach.*
    blowing nose: *Phos., Sul.*
    morning: *Ham., Lach.*
    at night: *Carb-v.*
  Causes:
    blowing nose: *Lach.*
    injury: *Arn.*

Obstinate   see **Stubborn**
Oedema (swelling)
  Of ankles and feet: *Ap., Calc-c., Ferr-m., Lyc.,*
    Merc-c., Nat-m., Puls., Rhus-t., Zinc.
  Of hands and fingers: *Ap., Calc-c., Ferr-m., Lyc.,*
    Merc-c., Nat-m., Puls., Rhus-t.
Onset of complaint
  Slow: *Bry., Gels.*
  Sudden: *Aco., Bell.*
Oversensitivity   see **Sensitive**

Pains   (see also **Abdominal pain in pregnancy;**
  Groin pains; Backache, etc.)
  Absent: *Op.*
  Appear suddenly: *Bell.*
  Appear suddenly and disappear suddenly: *Bell.,*
    Kali-b., Nit-ac.
  Bones: *Eup-p., Merc-s., Nit-ac., Pho-ac., Ruta.*
  Burning: *Ap., Ars., Canth., Caust., Phos., Rhus-t.,*
    Sul.
  Cramping: *Calc-c., Cupr., Mag-p., Nux-v.*
  Flying around: *Cimi., Nit-ac.*
  Glands: *Arn., Bell., Lyc., Merc-s., Phos.*
  Legs: *Bry.*
  Needle-like: *Arg-n., Hep-s., Nit-ac.*
  Parts lain on: *Puls., Pyr., Ruta.*
  Pressing: *Canth., Merc-s., Rhus-t., Sep.*
  Shooting: *Bell., Cimi., Hyp., Rhus-t.*
  Shoot upwards: *Phyt.*

  Sore/bruised: *Arn., Bry., Chin., Cimi., Eup-p.,*
    Ham., Pyr., Rhus-t., Ruta.
  Splinter-like   see **Needle-like**
  In a spot: *Kali-b.*
  Stinging: *Ap., Bry., Kali-c., Sil.*
  Stitching: *Bry., Kali-c.*
  Throbbing: *Bell.*
  Unbearable: *Aco., Cham.*
  Wandering: *Kali-b., Kali-s., Led., Puls.*
Pale   see **Face,** pale
Palpitations   *Aco., Arg-n., Ars., Calc-c., Lach.*
  In pregnancy: *Con., Lil-t., Nat-m., Sep.*
Panic (see also **Anxious; Fearful**)   *Arg-n.*
Perspiration   see **Sweat**
Phlebitis   *Arn., Bry., Ham., Puls., Rhus-t.*
Piles   *Aesc., Ars., Ham., Ign., Kali-c., Lach., Lil-t.,*
  Lyc., Nat-m., Nit-ac., Nux-v., Puls., Sul.
  Bleeding: *Aesc., Ars., Lach., Lyc., Nat-m., Nux-v.,*
    Sul.
  Bluish: *Lach.*
  Burning: *Ars., Sul.*
  External: *Aesc., Lach., Lyc., Sul.*
  Internal: *Ars., Ign., Nux-v., Puls., Sul.*
  Itching: *Aesc., Lyc., Nux-v., Sul.*
  Large: *Aesc., Kali-c., Lach., Nux-v., Sul.*
  With:
    backache: *Aesc.*
    constipation: *Aesc., Lyc., Nat-m., Nux-v., Sul.*
    dragging down sensation: *Lil-t.*
  Better:
    bathing in warm water: *Aesc., Ars.*
    bathing in cold water: *Nux-v.*
  Worse:
    coughing or passing a stool: *Ign., Kali-c., Nit-ac.*
    touch: *Kali-c., Stap., Sul.*
    standing/walking: *Aesc., Ign., Lil-t., Sul.*
Pink eye   see **Eye inflammation**
Play
  Baby wants to play at night: *Cypr.*
  Baby doesn't want to play: *Bar-c., Cina, Hep-s.,*
    Lyc., Nux-m., Rhe., Sil.
Prickly heat   *Nat-m., Sul., Urt-u.*
Prolapse   *Calc-c., Lil-t., Puls., Rhus-t., Sec., Sep.*
  With:
    bearing down sensation: *Lil-t., Sep.*
    constipation: *Sep.*
    pressure in abdomen and small of back: *Puls.*
  Better:
    lying down or sitting with legs crossed: *Sep.*
  Causes:
    forceps delivery: *Sec.*
    straining in labour: *Rhus-t., Sec.*
Pulse rapid   *Pyr.*
Pupils
  Contracted: *Op.*
  Dilated: *Bell.*

Quarrelsome   (see also **Dislikes** contradiction;
Irritable)   *Ign., Nux-v., Petr., Sul.*
   During labour: *Bell., Cham.*

Rage   *Bell., Lyc., Stram., Ver-a.*
Rage during labour   *Bell.*
   With a desire to bite or hit: *Bell., Stram.*
   Babies on being picked up: *Stram.*
Resentful (see also **Unforgiving; Complaints from**
suppressed anger)   *Ign., Lyc., Nat-m., Stap.*
Restless   *Aco., Ap., Arg-n., Ars., Bell., Calc-p.,
Canth., Caust., Cham., Cimi., Cina, Coff., Coloc.,
Cupr., Eup-p., Ferr-m., Lil-t., Lyc., Mag-m., Merc-s.,
Rhus-t., Sil., Sul., Zinc.*
   Babies: *Ars., Cham., Cina, Cupr., Merc-s., Rhus-t.,
      Stram., Sul.*
      better for being carried: *Ars., Cham., Cina*
      in teething babies: *Rhe.*
      wanders aimlessly: *Stram., Ver-a.*
   During labour: *Aco., Coff., Lyc.*
   Evening: *Caust., Zinc.*
   In bed: *Ars., Cupr., Ferr-m., Mag-m., Rhus-t.*
   Legs in pregnancy: *Caust., Rhus-t., Sul., Zinc.*
   Sleep: *Cina*
      body twitching/limbs jerking/grinding of teeth:
         Cina
   With anxiety: *Ars.*
   Worse:
      for heat: *Sul.*
Retained placenta   *Arn., Cimi., Puls., Sec.*
   After a long labour: *Arn.*
   With:
      a bearing down sensation: *Sec.*
      the shakes: *Cimi.*
      ineffective contractions: *Puls.*
Retention of urine   *Aco., Ap., Arn., Ars., Caust.,
Nat-m., Op., Stap.*
   In newborn babies: *Aco., Op.*
   In babies: *Aco., Ap.*
      who catch cold: *Aco.*
   Causes:
      childbirth: *Arn., Ars., Caust., Op., Stap.*
      presence of strangers: *Nat-m.*
      shock: *Op.*
Retention of urine (after childbirth)   *Arn., Ars.,
Caust., Op., Stap.*
   After a difficult birth or forceps delivery: *Arn.,
      Stap.*
   With:
      frequent, painful urging to pass urine – only
         passes a little each time: *Caust.*
      involuntary urination: *Arn., Ars., Caust.*
      no desire to pass urine: *Ars.*
      painful urging: *Arn., Nux-v.*
      painless urging: *Op.*

Rheumatism   see **Joint pain**
Rhinitis   see **Common cold**
Roseola (see also **Measles**)   *Aco., Bell., Puls.*
Rushed feeling   see **Hurried**

Sad   see **Depressed; Tearful**
Saliva
   Increased: *Merc-s., Ver-a.*
      during sleep: *Merc-s.*
Scared   see **Fearful**
Scarlet fever   *Ap., Bell., Lach., Merc-s., Rhus-t.*
   Rash:
      bluish: *Lach.*
      itches and burns: *Rhus-t.*
Scars   *Thios*
Sciatica   *Coloc., Ferr-m., Mag-p., Puls., Rhus-t.*
   Pains:
      tearing: *Coloc.*
   Better:
      fresh air: *Puls.*
      gentle movement: *Ferr-m.*
      heat: *Mag-p., Rhus-t.*
      movement: *Rhus-t.*
      walking: *Ferr-m., Rhus-t.*
      walking slowly: *Ferr-m.*
   Worse:
      beginning to move: *Rhus-t.*
      cold: *Mag-p., Rhus-t.*
      cold compresses: *Rhus-t.*
      lying on painful part: *Rhus-t.*
      right side: *Coloc.*
      warm room: *Puls.*
      washing in cold water: *Rhus-t.*
      wet weather: *Rhus-t.*
Screaming   *Aco., Ant-t., Bell., Bor., Calc-p., Cham.,
Chin., Cina, Coff., Kali-p., Kreos., Lyc., Nux-v., Rhe.*
   If touched: *Ant-t.*
   In babies: *Bor., Cina, Lyc., Kreos.*
   With pain: *Aco., Bell., Cham., Coff.*
   On waking: *Cham., Chin., Cina, Kali-p., Lyc.,
      Mag-c., Zinc.*
   In sleep: *Calc-p.*
   During sleep: *Bor., Lyc.*
   On waking: *Lyc.*
Sense of smell
   Acute: *Colch., Nux-v., Op.*
   Lost: *Calc-c.*
Senses
   Acute: *Asar., Coff., Op.*
   Dull: *Op.*
   Hyperacute: *Asar.*
Sensitive   *Aco., Asar., Bell., Cham., Chin., Cimi.,
Coff., Con., Hep-s., Ign., Kali-c., Lach., Lyc., Nat-c.,
Nat-m., Nat-p., Nit-ac., Nux-v., Phos., Puls., Sep.,
Sil., Stap.*

Babies: *Aco., Bell., Cham., Kali-p., Phos., Puls., Stap.*
To light: *Bell., Con., Nux-v., Phos.*
To music: *Nat-c., Nux-v., Sep.*
To noise: *Aco., Asar., Bell., Chin., Coff., Con., Kali-c.,
Nit-ac., Nux-v., Op., Sep., Sil., Zinc.*
To noise during labour: *Bell., Cimi., Coff., Nux-v.*
To pain: *Cham., Coff., Ign., Lach., Nit-ac., Phos.,
Sep., Sil., Stap.*
during pregnancy: *Asar., Cimi.*
To rudeness: *Hep-s., Nux-v., Stap.*
To touch: *Lach.*

Sentimental   *Ant-c., Ign.*

Shock   *Aco., Arn., Hyp., Ign., Lach., Op., Pho-ac.,
Phos., Stap., Stram.*
With:
anger: *Stap.*
anxiety: *Aco.*
fear: *Aco., Stram.*
indignation: *Stap.*
stupor: *Op.*
vomiting: *Phos.*
Causes:
emotional trauma: *Ign., Pho-ac.*
injuries: *Aco., Arn., Hyp., Lach., Op., Stap.*
surgery: *Aco., Arn., Op., Phos., Stap., Stram.*
childbirth: *Aco., Arn., Stram.*

Shrieking during labour   *Bell., Cimi.*

Shy   *Bar-c., Lyc., Nat-c., Puls., Sil.*

Side   see **Symptoms**

Sighing   *Calc-p., Cimi., Ign.*

Sinusitis   see **Common cold**

Skin complaints of pregnancy
Broken veins: *Arn.*
Brown pigmentation patches on face: *Sep.*
Dryness: *Calc-f.*
Itching: *Sul.*
Spots: *Sep.*
Stretch marks: *Calc-f.*

Sleepless   see **Insomnia**

Sleepy   see **Drowsy**

Slowness   *Asar., Bar-c., Calc-c., Calc-p., Con., Phos.*
In babies: *Bar-c., Calc-c., Calc-p.*
learning to walk: *Calc-c.*
to develop: *Bar-c.*
to teethe: *Calc-c., Calc-p.*
to learn: *Calc-p.*

Sluggish, dull (see also **Apathetic; Confused;
Exhaustion**)   *Ant-c., Asar., Bar-c., Bry., Calc-c.,
Calc-p., Calc-s., Carb-v., Gels., Kali-c., Lach., Lyc.,
Merc-c., Nat-c., Nat-p., Nit-ac., Nux-m., Pho-ac., Phos.,
Puls., Sep., Sil., Stap., Sul., Ver-a., Zinc.*
Babies: *Bar-c., Calc-p., Sul.*
On waking: *Lach.*
Better for:
fresh air: *Lyc.*

Snuffles in newborn babies   *Dulc., Lyc., Nux-v., Puls.*

Sore throat   *Aco., All-c., Ap., Arg-n., Ars., Bar-c., Bell.,
Bry., Calc-c., Caust., Dros., Dulc., Hep-s., Ign., Kali-m.,
Lach., Lyc., Merc-c., Merc-s., Nat-m., Nit-ac., Nux-v.,
Phos., Phyt., Puls., Rhus-t., Rumex, Sil., Spo., Sul.*
Air passages irritated: *Rumex*
In babies: *Dros.*
Constant: *Caust.*
Glands:
swollen: *Bell., Sil.*
Gums:
bleeding, swollen: *Merc-c.*
Larynx:
inflamed: *Dros.*
irritated: *Dros., Puls.*
tickling: *Dros., Puls., Rhus-t.*
Mouth dry: *Ap.*
Noises in ears:
roaring: *Bar-c.*
on swallowing: *Bar-c.*
Pains:
burning: *Aco., Ap., Ars., Bar-c., Caust., Merc-c.,
Nat-m., Nit-ac., Spo., Sul.*
dry: *Caust.*
pressing: *Nit-ac.*
raw: *Caust., Hep-s., Lyc., Merc-c., Nit-ac., Nux-v.,
Phos., Puls., Sul.*
scraping: *Puls.*
severe: *Bell.*
sore: *Lyc., Merc-s., Phos., Rumex, Spo., Sul.*
splinter-like: *Arg-n., Hep-s., Lach., Nit-ac.*
spreading up to ears: *Hep-s., Lach., Merc-s.,
Nit-ac., Nux-v.*
spreading up to neck: *Merc-s.*
stitching: *Aco., Bell., Bry., Ign., Merc-s., Nit-ac.,
Nux-v., Puls., Sil., Sul.*
Throat:
burning: *Caust.*
constricted: *Bell.*
dark red: *Phyt.*
dry: *Calc-c., Caust., Lyc., Nat-m., Puls., Rhus-t.,
Sil., Spo., Sul.*
inflamed: *Bar-c.*
irritated: *Arg-n., Bell., Rumex*
raw: *Arg-n., Bar-c., Bell., Caust., Rumex, Sul.*
sore: *Rumex*
Tonsils:
swollen/inflamed: *Bar-c., Hep-s., Kali-m., Lyc.,
Merc-s., Nit-ac., Phos., Phyt., Sil., Sul.*
ulcerated: *Ars., Merc-s., Nit-ac.*
white: *Kali-m.*
Voice:
hoarse: *Arg-n., Bry., Dros., Nat-m., Phos., Rhus-t.,
Spo., Sul.*
lost: *Arg-n., Rumex*
With:
choking sensation: *Caust., Ign., Lach., Sul.*

desire to swallow: *Caust.*
fever: *Bry.*
hair sensation at the back of tongue: *Sil.*
lump sensation in throat: *Ign.*, *Lach.*, *Lyc.*,
  Nat-m., *Nux-v.*
saliva increased: *Bar-c.*, *Merc-c.*
ulcers in the throat: *Ars.*, *Merc-c.*
wind: *Dros.*
Better:
  cold drinks: *Phyt.*
  eating: *Merc-c.*
  hot drinks: *Ars.*, *Hep-s.*
  swallowing: *Ign.*
  swallowing liquids: *Bar-c.*
  swallowing solids: *Lach.*
  warm compresses: *Hep-s.*
  warm drinks: *Lyc.*
Worse:
  breathing in cold air: *Hep-s.*, *Rumex*
  breathing in: *Phos.*
  cold air: *Nux-v.*
  cold drinks: *Ars.*, *Hep-s.*, *Rhus-t.*
  getting cold: *Sil.*
  coughing: *Hep-s.*, *Phos.*, *Spo.*, *Sul.*
  evening: *Ign.*
  heat: *Lach.*, *Puls.*
  hot drinks: *Phyt.*
  left side: *Lach.*
  morning and evening: *Phos.*
  night: *Bar-c.*, *Lyc.*, *Merc-s.*
  not swallowing: *Ign.*
  pressure: *Lach.*, *Merc-c.*, *Phos.*
  right side: *Bell.*, *Lyc.*, *Merc-s.*
  singing: *Spo.*
  swallowing: *Ars.*, *Bry.*, *Dros.*, *Hep-s.*, *Merc-s.*,
    Nit-ac., *Nux-v.*, *Rhus-t.*, *Sil.*, *Spo.*, *Sul.*
  swallowing saliva (empty swallowing): *Bar-c.*,
    Lach.
  swallowing food: *Bar-c.*
  swallowing liquids: *Bell.*, *Lach.*, *Merc-c.*
  sweet drinks/food: *Spo.*
  talking: *Caust.*, *Phos.*, *Spo.*
  touch: *Lach.*, *Spo.*
  turning the head: *Hep-s.*
  uncovering: *Nux-v.*, *Rhus-t.*, *Sil.*
  winter: *Hep-s.*
Causes:
  change of weather: *Calc-c.*
  exposure to wind: *Hep-s.*
  getting cold: *Bell.*, *Hep-s.*
  singing: *Arg-n.*
  straining voice: *Rhus-t.*
  talking: *Arg-n.*
  getting chilled: *Aco.*, *Bell.*
Speedy   see **Hurried**
Spiteful   *Nux-v.*

Splinters (see also **Injuries**)   *Sil.*
  Wound inflamed: *Sil.*
Spots in babies   *Carb-v.*, *Sil.*, *Sul.*
Sprains   *Arn.*, *Calc-c.*, *Rhus-t.*, *Ruta.*
  Ankle: *Arn.*, *Calc-c.*, *Rhus-t.*, *Ruta.*
  Foot: *Arn.*, *Rhus-t.*
  Hand: *Calc-c.*
  Wrist: *Arn.*, *Calc-c.*, *Rhus-t.*, *Ruta.*
  First stage: *Arn.*
  Pains:
    bruised, constant: *Ruta.*
  With:
    bruising: *Arn.*
    exhaustion, lameness: *Ruta.*
    stiffness: *Rhus-t.*
    swelling: *Arn.*
    trembling: *Rhus-t.*
  Worse:
    exercise: *Ruta.*
    lifting: *Calc-c.*
    pressure/standing/walking: *Ruta.*
  Causes:
    falling: *Rhus-t.*
    lifting: *Calc-c.*, *Rhus-t.*
      heavy weights: *Calc-c.*
    twisting: *Rhus-t.*
Sticky eyes   see **Eye inflammation**
Stiff neck   *Rhus-t.*
Stomach-ache   see **Colic**
Strains   *Arn.*, *Carb-a.*, *Rhus-t.*, *Ruta.*
  Ankle: *Ruta.*
  Back: *Carb-a.*
  Muscles: *Carb-a.*
  Periosteum: *Ruta.*
  Tendons: *Carb-a.*, *Ruta.*
  Wrist: *Carb-a.*, *Ruta.*
  Pains:
    bruised, constant: *Ruta.*
    joints: *Rhus-t.*
    sore, bruised: *Arn.*, *Rhus-t.*
  With:
    exhaustion, lameness: *Ruta.*
    stiffness, trembling: *Rhus-t.*
  Better:
    continued movement: *Rhus-t.*
  Worse:
    beginning to move: *Rhus-t.*
    exercise, standing, walking: *Ruta.*
  Causes:
    childbirth: *Arn.*
    lifting: *Carb-a.*
    over-exertion: *Arn.*
Stubborn   *Calc-c.*, *Cham.*, *Nux-v.*
  Babies: *Ant-c.*, *Calc-c.*, *Cham.*, *Chin.*, *Cina*
Stupor (see also **Dazed**)   *Nux-m.*, *Op.*,
  Sec.

Styes   *Puls., Stap.*
  Worse:
    upper eyelids: *Puls.*
Sudden onset   see **Onset**
Sulky (see also **Moody; Morose**)   *Ant-c.*
Sunburn   see **Burns**
Sunstroke   *Bell., Glon.*
  With:
    fever: *Bell.*
    headache: *Bell.*
Sweat
  Absent during fever: *Ars., Bell., Bry., Gels.*
  Clammy: *Ars., Cham., Ferr-m., Lyc., Merc-s.,*
    Pho-ac., Phos., Ver-a.
  Cold: *Ant-t., Ars., Carb-v., Chin., Cocc., Ferr-m.,*
    Hep-s., Ip., Lyc., Merc-c., Merc-s., Sep., Ver-a.
  Exhausting: *Carb-a., Ver-a.*
  From fright: *Nux-v., Op.*
  Head: *Calc-c., Sil.*
  Hot: *Aco., Cham., Con., Ign., Ip., Nux-v., Op., Sep.*
  Oily: *Mag-c.*
  On covered parts of the body: *Aco., Bell., Chin.*
  One-sided: *Bar-c., Lyc., Nat-c., Nux-v., Petr., Puls.*
  From pain: *Lach., Merc-s., Nat-c., Nat-s., Sep.*
  Profuse: *Ant-t., Ars., Calc-c., Carb-a., Carb-v.,*
    Chin., Ferr-m., Hep-s., Kali-c., Kali-p., Lyc.,
    Merc-s., Op., Pho-ac., Sep., Sil., Sul., Ver-a.
  Scanty: *Eup-p.*
  Single parts of the body: *Chin., Cocc., Ign., Kali-c.,*
    Nit-ac., Phos., Puls., Op., Sep.
  Smelly: *Carb-a., Hep-s., Lyc., Merc-s., Nit-ac.,*
    Nux-v., Petr., Puls., Sep., Sil., Sul.
  Sour: *Ars., Calc-c., Colch., Hep-s., Lyc., Mag-c.,*
    Merc-s., Nit-ac., Sep., Sil., Sul., Ver-a.
  With:
    diarrhoea: *Ver-a.*
    fever: *Pyr.*
    shivering: *Nux-v.*
  Better:
    uncovering: *Cham., Lyc.*
  Worse:
    after eating: *Kali-c.*
    at night: *Con., Puls., Sil.*
    closing eyes: *Con.*
    during sleep: *Con., Sil.*
    lying down: *Con., Ferr-m., Rhus-t.*
    mental exertion: *Calc-c., Hep-s., Lach., Sep., Stap.*
    pain: *Lach., Merc-s., Nat-c., Sep.*
    slightest physical exertion: *Calc-c., Chin., Ferr-m.,*
      Kali-c., Kali-p., Lyc., Nat-c., Nat-s., Nit-ac.,
      Phos., Rhus-t., Sep., Sul.
    when tired: *Kali-p.*
    uncovering: *Rhus-t.*
  Causes:
    fright: *Op.*
Swelling   see **Oedema**

Sympathetic   *Caust., Phos.*
Symptoms
  Changeable: *Puls.*
  Contradictory: *Ign.*
  One-sided: *Pho-ac.*
  Left-sided: *Lach., Sep., Sul.*
  Right-sided: *Ap., Bell., Calc-c., Lyc., Nux-v., Puls.*
  Moving from:
    left side to right side: *Lach.*
    right side to left side: *Ap., Lyc.*

Talkative   *Cimi., Lach.*
Tantrums   *Bell., Lyc., Nit-ac., Stram., Ver-a.*
Taste   Mouth tastes:
  Bad: *Calc-c., Merc-s., Nat-s., Nux-v., Puls., Sul.*
    in the morning: *Nat-s., Nux-v., Puls.*
  Bitter: *Aco., Ars., Bry., Carb-v., Chin., Merc-s.,*
    Nat-m., Nat-s., Nux-v., Sul.
  Metallic: *Cocc., Cupr., Merc-s., Nat-c., Rhus-t., Zinc.*
  Salty: *Nat-m.*
  Sour: *Arg-n., Calc-c., Lyc., Mag-c., Nux-v., Phos.*
  Sweet: *Cupr.*
Tearful (see also **Depressed; Dislikes**
  consolation)   *Ap., Bell., Bor., Calc-c., Calc-s., Caust.,*
  Cham., Ign., Lyc., Nat-m., Puls., Rhe., Rhus-t., Sep.,
  Spo., Stram., Ver-a.
  Babies: *Bell., Bor., Calc-c., Cham., Lyc., Puls., Rhe.,*
    Stram.
    at night: *Bor., Rhe.*
    when teething: *Phyt.*
    who can't have what they want: *Cina*
  During a fever: *Aco., Bell., Puls., Spo.*
  During pregnancy: *Ign., Lach., Nat-m., Puls.*
  During labour: *Coff., Puls.*
  Better for fresh air: *Puls.*
  Difficulty crying: *Nat-m.*
  Involuntary: *Ign.*
  Cries on own: *Ign., Nat-m.*
  Whilst breastfeeding: *Puls.*
Teeth
  Crumbling/decaying: *Calc-f., Calc-p.*
Teething   painful in babies: *Aco., Bell., Bor., Calc-c.,*
  Calc-p., Cham., Kreos., Mag-m., Mag-p., Phyt., Puls.,
  Rhe., Sil.
  Cheeks:
    hot and red: *Aco., Bell., Cham.*
    pale and cold: *Cham.*
    red spot on one cheek: *Cham.*
    swollen: *Bell.*
  Slow (babies late to teethe): *Calc-c., Calc-p., Sil.*
  Teeth decay as soon as they come through: *Kreos.*
  Pains:
    cries out in sleep: *Cham.*
    severe: *Kreos.*

unbearable: *Cham.*
With:
  colic: *Mag-m.*
  cough: *Cham.*
  crying: *Phyt.*
  diarrhoea: *Calc-c., Cham., Rhe., Sil.*
  difficulty teething: *Calc-c., Calc-p., Cham., Sil.*
  fever: *Aco.*
  green stools: *Calc-p., Cham., Mag-m.*
  restless sleep: *Aco., Bell., Cham., Kreos.*
  toothache: *Sil.*
Better:
  biting gums together hard: *Phyt.*
  cold drinks/water: *Puls.*
  external heat: *Mag-p.*
  walking in the fresh air: *Puls.*
Worse:
  heat of bed, warm food/drinks: *Cham., Puls.*
  pressure: *Cham.*

Tennis elbow *Ruta.*

Thin *Calc-p.*

Thirstless *Ant-c., Ant-t., Ap., Bell., Cina, Colch., Gels., Nux-m., Pho-ac., Puls.*

Thirsty *Aco., Ars., Bell., Bry., Cham., Eup-p., Merc-c., Merc-s., Nat-m., Phos., Pyr., Sil., Sul., Ver-a.*
  Thirst with chills: *Ign.*
  Thirst:
    for cold drinks/hot drinks see **Likes**
    extreme: *Merc-c., Nat-m., Sul.*
    for large quantities: *Ars., Bry., Nat-m., Phos., Sul., Ver-a.*
      at infrequent intervals: *Bry.*
    for sips: *Ars.*
    for small quantities often: *Ars.*
    unquenchable: *Eup-p., Phos.*
    for water: *Phos., Sul.*

Throat see **Sore throat**

Thrush (genital)/Yeast infection *Bor., Merc-s., Nat-m., Nit-ac., Sep.*
  Discharge:
    burning: *Bor., Merc-s., Nat-m., Nit-ac., Sep.*
    copious: *Sep.*
    like cottage cheese: *Sep.*
    greenish: *Merc-s.*
    like egg white: *Bor., Nat-m., Sep.*
    smelly: *Merc-s., Nit-ac., Sep.*
    thin: *Nit-ac.*
    yellow: *Sep.*
    white: *Bor., Nat-m.*
  With:
    dryness: *Sep.*
    itching: *Merc-s., Nat-m., Nit-ac., Sep.*
  Worse:
    before menstrual period: *Sep.*
    between menstrual periods: *Bor., Sep.*
    at night: *Merc-s.*

Thrush (genital in pregnancy) *Alu., Cocc., Kreos., Petr., Puls., Sep.*
  Discharge:
    burning: *Alu., Kreos., Petr., Puls., Sep.*
    cream-like: *Puls.*
    like egg white: *Alu., Petr., Sep.*
    lumpy: *Sep.*
    milky: *Kreos., Puls., Sep.*
    profuse: *Alu., Cocc., Kreos., Petr., Sep.*
    smelly: *Kreos., Sep.*
    thick: *Puls.*
    thin, watery: *Cocc., Kreos.*
    white: *Alu.*
  With:
    itching (vulva/vagina): *Kreos., Sep.*

Thrush (oral) in babies, of gums and/or tongue: *Bor., Kali-m., Merc-s., Nat-m., Sul-ac.*
  In breastfeeding babies: *Bor., Kali-m.*
  Tongue/gums: *Sul-ac.*
    coated white: *Kali-m., Nat-m.*
    hot/dry/bleeds easily: *Bor.*
  With:
    excess saliva: *Bor., Merc-s.*
  Worse:
    for feeding: *Bor.*
    for touch: *Bor.*

Tidy *Ars., Nux-v.*

Time passes
  quickly: *Cocc.*
  slowly: *Glon.*

Timid see **Shy**

Tired see **Apathetic; Exhaustion; Sluggish**

Tongue
  Brown-coated: *Bry.*
  Cold: *Ver-a.*
  Cracked: *Merc-s., Nit-ac.*
  Dirty white: *Bry.*
  Fiery red: *Ap.*
  Green: *Nat-s.*
  Red: *Bell., Phos.*
  Red-edged: *Ars., Sul.*
  Red stripe down centre (white edges): *Caust.*
  Red-tipped: *Arg-n., Ars., Phyt., Rhus-t., Sul.*
  Strawberry: *Bell.*
  Swollen: *Ap.*
  White-coated: *Ant-c., Ant-t., Bell., Calc-c., Kali-b., Kali-m., Puls., Rhus-t., Sul.*
  Yellow-coated: *Kali-s., Merc-c., Merc-s., Nat-p., Puls.*
    at the back: *Nat-p.*

Toothache *Coff., Nux-v., Sep.*

Touchy see **Irritable; Sensitive**

Travel sickness *Bor., Cocc., Nux-v., Petr., Sep., Stap., Tab.*
  With:
    biliousness: *Sep.*

diarrhoea: *Cocc.*
dizziness: *Cocc.*
faint-like feeling: *Cocc., Nux-v.*
headache: *Cocc., Nux-v., Petr., Sep.*
nausea: *Bor., Cocc., Nux-v., Petr., Sep., Tab.*
  deathly, intermittent, violent nausea: *Tab.*
  vomiting: *Bor., Cocc., Petr., Sep., Tab.*
Better:
  lying down: *Cocc., Nux-v.*
  fresh air: *Tab.*
Worse:
  for downward movement: *Bor.*
  after drinking: *Cocc.*
  after eating: *Cocc., Nux-v., Sep.*
  fresh air: *Cocc., Nux-v., Petr.*
  morning: *Sep.*
  movement: *Cocc., Tab.*
  sitting up: *Cocc.*
  stuffy room: *Tab.*
  tobacco: *Nux-v., Tab.*
Causes:
  pregnancy: *Sep.*
  travelling: *Petr.*
Trembling   *Agar., Arg-n., Cimi., Cocc., Gels., Zinc.*
  From emotion: *Cocc.*
Twitchy   *Agar., Zinc.*

Uncommunicative (see also **Broody;**
  Introspective)   *Carb-a., Cocc., Glon., Pho-ac., Phos.,*
  Ver-a., Zinc.
Unforgiving   *Nit-ac.*
Urethritis   see **Cystitis**
Urinary tract infections   see **Cystitis**
Urine   see **Retention of urine**
Urticaria   see **Hives**

Varicose veins   *Bry., Calc-c., Calc-f., Carb-v., Ferr-m.,*
  Ham., Lyc., Puls., Zinc.
  Of leg and thigh: *Carb-v., Ferr-m., Ham., Lyc.,*
    Puls., Zinc.
  Of foot: *Ferr-m., Puls.*
  Of vulva: *Bry., Calc-c., Carb-v., Ham., Lyc., Zinc.*
  Painful: *Ferr-m., Ham., Lyc., Puls., Zinc.*
  Pains – stinging: *Ham., Puls.*
  Swollen: *Ferr-m., Ham.*
  Worse during pregnancy: *Calc-c., Calc-f., Carb-v.,*
    Ferr-m., Ham., Lyc., Puls., Zinc.
Vomiting (see also **Food poisoning; Travel**
  sickness)   *Ant-c., Ant-t., Ars., Asar., Bry., Calc-c.,*
  Cham., Chin., Colch., Ferr-m., Ip., Nux-v., Phos., Sep.,
  Sil., Sul-ac., Symph-r., Tab., Ver-a.
  Abdomen/stomach feels cold: *Colch., Ver-a.*
  In breastfed babies: *Ant-c., Sil., Sul.*

Constant: *Symph.*
Difficult: *Ant-t.*
Easy: *Ars., Cham.*
Exhausting: *Tab.*
Frequent: *Ars., Chin.*
In pregnancy: *Ant-c., Nux-v., Sep., Symph-r., Tab.*
Pains in the stomach:
  burning: *Colch., Phos.*
  cramping/griping: *Ver-a.*
  sore, bruised: *Colch.*
Sudden (while eating): *Ferr-m.*
Violent: *Ars., Asar., Phos., Symph-r., Tab., Ver-a.*
Vomit   *Ant-c., Ant-t., Ars., Bry., Calc-c., Cham.,*
  Chin., Colch., Ferr-m., Ip., Nat-c., Nux-v., Phos.,
  Sep., Sil., Sul-ac., Tab., Ver-a.
  bile: *Ant-c., Ars., Cham., Ip., Nux-v., Phos., Sep.,*
    Ver-a.
  bitter: *Bry., Nux-v., Phos.*
  curdled milk: *Ant-c., Calc-c., Sil.*
  food: *Ars., Chin., Ferr-m., Ip.*
  green: *Ip.*
  mucus: *Nux-v., Phos., Ver-a.*
  smelly: *Ars., Nux-v., Sep.*
  sour: *Ant-t., Calc-c., Chin., Nux-v., Sul-ac., Tab.,*
    Ver-a.
  violent: *Phos., Tab.*
  watery: *Ars., Bry., Ver-a.*
  yellow: *Phos., Ver-a.*
With:
  diarrhoea: *Ars., Ver-a.*
  dizziness: *Ver-a.*
  faintness after vomiting: *Ars.*
  fever: *Ant-t.*
  headache: *Ip.*
  hiccuping after vomiting: *Ver-a.*
  nausea, retching: *Symph-r.*
  retching after vomiting: *Colch., Symph-r.*
  sweating while vomiting: *Ars.*
Better:
  lying on back: *Symph-r.*
Worse:
  after midnight: *Ferr-m.*
  before breakfast: *Tab.*
  bending down: *Ip.*
  coughing: *Ant-t., Bry., Ip.*
  coughing up phlegm: *Nux-v.*
  after drinking: *Ant-c., Ant-t., Ars., Phos., Ver-a.*
  after eating: *Ant-t., Ars., Chin., Ip., Phos., Sep.,*
    Sil., Ver-a.
  a short while after eating/drinking: *Phos.*
  eggs: *Ferr-m.*
  expectorating: *Nux-v.*
  milk: *Ant-c., Nat-c., Sil.*
  morning: *Sep.*
  movement: *Ars., Bry., Symph-r., Tab.*
  night: *Ferr-m.*

smell of eggs: *Colch.*
Causes:
  anger: *Cham., Nux-v.*
  ice-cream: *Ars.*
  measles: *Ant-c.*
  meat: *Ars.*
  pregnancy: *Nux-v., Sep., Tab.*
  travelling: *Tab.*

Warts *Thu.*
  Bleeding: *Thu.*
  Large: *Thu.*
  Stinging: *Thu.*
Weakness see **Exhaustion**
Weaning to dry up milk: *Lac-c., Puls.*
Weary *Gels., Ruta.*
  of life: *Nat-s.*
Weepy see **Tearful**
Weight gain
  Poor in babies: *Bar-c., Calc-p., Mag-c., Sil.*
  Early in babies: *Calc-c.*
  Easy: *Calc-c.*
Whiny *Ap., Puls.*
Whooping cough see **Cough**
Wind see **Flatulence**
Worms *Cina*
Worse generally (see also **Complaints from**)
  After midnight: *Ars., Podo.*
  Around:
    1 a.m.: *Ars.*
    2–4 a.m.: *Kali-c.*
    10 a.m.: *Nat-m.*
    10–11 a.m.: *Sul.*
    3 p.m.: *Bell.*
    3–5 p.m.: *Ap.*
    4–8 p.m.: *Lyc.*
    9 p.m.: *Bry.*
  Afternoon: *Lyc.*
  Autumn: *Colch., Rhus-t.*
  Bathing: *Sul.*
  Before breakfast: *Tab.*
  Beginning to move: *Ferr-m., Rhus-t.*
  Change of temperature: *Ars., Kali-s.*
  Change of weather see **Complaints from** Change
    of weather
  Cloudy weather: *Rhus-t.*
  Coffee: *Caust., Cham., Ign., Nux-v.*
  Cold: *Agar., Ars., Bar-c., Bor., Calc-c., Calc-p.,*
    Caust., Chin., Cimi., Colch., Dulc., Hep-s., Hyp.,
    Kali-b., Kali-c., Kali-p., Mag-p., Merc-s., Nit-ac.,
    Nux-m., Nux-v., Pho-ac., Phos., Puls., Pyr., Rhod.,
    Rhus-t., Sep., Sil.
  Cold and heat: *Merc-s.*
  Cold, dry weather: *Asar., Caust., Hep-s., Kali-c.,*
    Nux-v.

Cold food: *Nux-v.*
Cold drinks/food: *Canth., Rhus-t.*
Cold wind: *Bell., Hep-s., Nux-v., Spo.*
Cold, wet weather: *Pyr., Rhod., Rhus-t.* (see also
  Damp)
Consolation see **Averse** to consolation
Damp (see also Cold, wet): *Ars., Calc-c., Calc-p.,*
  Colch., Dulc., Nat-s., Rhus-t., Sil.
Draughts: *Calc-c., Calc-p., Caust., Kali-c., Rhus-t.,*
  Sil., Sul.
After eating: *Kali-b., Nat-m., Zinc.*
Before eating: *Nat-c., Phos.*
Evening: *Caust., Cham., Euphr., Lyc., Mag-c.,*
  Merc-s., Nat-p., Pho-ac., Phos., Sul-ac., Zinc.
Excitement: *Kali-p.*
Exertion (physical): *Ars., Calc-c., Carb-v., Cocc.,*
  Kali-p., Stap., Sul.
Exposure to sun: *Ant-c., Glon., Nat-c., Nat-m.,*
  Puls.
Fasting: *Sep., Stap., Sul., Tab.*
First lying down: *Con.*
Flatulent foods (beans, etc.): *Bry., Lyc.*
Foggy weather: *Rhus-t.*
Fresh air: *Calc-c., Calc-p., Caust., Cham., Chin.,*
  Cocc., Coff., Hep-s., Nat-c., Nit-ac., Nux-m.,
  Nux-v., Petr., Sil.
Frosty weather: *Sep.*
Fruit: *Ver-a.*
Getting feet wet: *Bar-c., Puls., Sil.*
Getting head wet: *Bell.*
Getting overheated: *Ant-c., Kali-c.*
Getting up: *Op.*
Getting wet: *Caust., Sep.*
Heat: *Ap., Arg-n., Asar., Calc-s., Glon., Kali-s.,*
  Lach., Led., Lil-t., Nat-m., Puls., Sec., Sul.,
  Sul-ac.
Heat and cold: *Merc-s.*
Hot food/drinks: *Asar.*
Humidity: *Carb-v., Lach., Nat-s.*
Jarring movement: *Arn., Bell., Glon., Nit-ac.*
Light touch: *Chin., Merc-s.*
Loss of sleep: *Cocc., Nit-ac., Nux-v.*
Lying down: *Con., Dros., Dulc., Ferr-m., Merc-s.,*
  Nat-s., Rhus-t.
Lying on the injured part: *Arn.*
Lying on the painful part/side: *Hep-s., Ruta.*
Lying on the side: *Kali-c.*
Before a menstrual period: *Con., Lach., Nat-m.*
Before/during/after a menstrual period: *Sep.*
Mental exertion: *Calc-p., Kali-p., Sep.*
Mid-morning: *Nat-c., Nat-m., Podo., Sul-ac.*
Midnight: *Dros.*
Milk: *Calc-c., Calc-s., Mag-m., Nat-c., Sul.*
Morning: *Lach., Nat-s., Nux-v., Petr., Pho-ac.,*
  Phos.
Morning on waking: *Kali-b., Lach.*

Movement: *Aesc., Asar., Chin., Cocc., Colch., Led., Spo.*
Night: *Aco., Chin., Cina, Coff., Colch., Dulc., Ferr-m., Hep-s., Ip., Kali-b., Kali-c., Lil-t., Mag-c., Mag-m., Merc-s., Nit-ac., Sep., Zinc.*
Onions: *Lyc.*
On one side of body: *Pho-ac.*
Physical exertion: *Calc-s., Gels., Nat-c., Nat-m., Sep.*
Pressure: *Bar-c., Cina, Hep-s., Hyp., Lach., Lyc., Mag-p., Merc-c.*
Rest: *Puls., Sep.*
Rich, fatty food: *Carb-v., Puls.*
Riding in a car: *Bor.*
Sight of food: *Colch.*
Sitting still: *Dulc.*
After sleep: *Lach., Spo.*
During sleep: *Op.*
Slightest movement: *Bry.*
Standing: *Sul.*
Starchy food: *Nat-m., Nat-s.*
Stormy weather: *Nat-c., Rhod.*
  before a storm: *Rhod.*
  during a storm: *Nat-c.*
Stuffy rooms: *Asar., Calc-s., Lyc., Puls., Sul.*
Sugar/sweets: *Arg-n.*
Sun   see **Complaints from** sunstroke
Summer: *Kali-b.*

Sweating: *Pho-ac., Sep.*
Swimming in cold water: *Ant-c., Mag-m., Mag-p., Rhus-t.*
Thinking: *Calc-c.*
Tight clothes: *Calc-c., Lach., Lyc., Nux-v., Spo.*
Tobacco: *Ign., Nux-v., Spo., Stap.*
Touch: *Aco., Ap., Arn., Bell., Cocc., Coff., Colch., Cupr., Ham., Hep-s., Kali-c., Led., Mag-p., Nit-ac., Nux-v., Sep., Sil., Stap.*
Travelling: *Petr.*
Twilight: *Puls.*
Uncovering: *Hep-s., Kali-c., Mag-p., Nux-v., Rhus-t., Sil.*
Vomiting: *Cupr.*
On waking: *Ars., Lach., Nit-ac.*
Walking: *Aesc., Caust., Glon., Lach., Nit-ac., Nux-v.*
  in the fresh air: *Caust., Cocc., Led., Mag-p.*
  in the wind: *Sep.*
Warmth of bed: *Dros., Op., Sul.*
Wet weather: *Ars., Asar., Calc-p., Nat-s., Puls., Sil.*
Wind: *Cham., Lyc., Nux-v., Phos., Puls., Rhod.*
Wine: *Coff., Led., Zinc.*
Winter: *Nux-v.*
Worry: *Kali-p.*
Writing: *Sep.*
Wounds   see **Injuries**

Yeast infection   see **Thrush (genital)**

LIST OF REMEDIES AND ABBREVIATIONS

Aconitum napellus	Aco.	Kali bichromicum	Kali-b.
Aesculus hippocastanum	Aesc.	Kali carbonicum	Kali-c.
Agaricus muscarius	Agar.	Kali muriaticum	Kali-m.
Allium cepa	All-c.	Kali phosphoricum	Kali-p.
Alumina	Alu.	Kali sulphuricum	Kali-s.
Antimonium crudum	Ant-c.	Kreosotum	Kreos.
Antimonium tartaricum	Ant-t.	Lac caninum	Lac-c.
Apis mellifica	Ap.	Lac defloratum	Lac-d.
Argentum nitricum	Arg-n.	Lachesis	Lach.
Arnica montana	Arn.	Ledum palustre	Led.
Arsenicum album	Ars.	Lillium tigrinum	Lil-t.
Asarum europum	Asar.	Lycopodium	Lyc.
Baryta carbonica	Bar-c.	Magnesia carbonica	Mag-c.
Belladonna	Bell.	Magnesia muriaticum	Mag-m.
Bellis perennis	Bell-p.	Magnesia phosphorica	Mag-p.
Borax veneta	Bor.	Mercurius corrosivus	Merc-c.
Bryonia alba	Bry.	Mercurius solubilis	Merc-s.
Calcarea carbonica	Calc-c.	Natrum carbonicum	Nat-c.
Calcarea fluorica	Calc-f.	Natrum muriaticum	Nat-m.
Calcarea phosphorica	Calc-p.	Natrum phosphoricum	Nat-p.
Calcarea sulphurica	Calc-s.	Natrum sulphuricum	Nat-s.
Calendula officinalis	Calen.	Nitricum acidum	Nit-ac.
Cantharis vesicatoria	Canth.	Nux moschata	Nux-m.
Carbo animalis	Carb-a.	Nux vomica	Nux-v.
Carbo vegetabilis	Carb-v.	Opium	Op.
Castor equi	Cast.	Petroleum	Petr.
Caulophyllum	Caul.	Phosphoric acid	Pho-ac.
Causticum	Caust.	Phosphorus	Phos.
Chamomilla	Cham.	Phytolacca decandra	Phyt.
Chelidonium majus	Chel.	Podophyllum	Podo.
China officinalis	Chin.	Pulsatilla nigricans	Puls.
Cimicifuga	Cimi.	Pyrogen	Pyr.
Cina		Rheum	Rhe.
Cocculus indicus	Cocc.	Rhododendron	Rhod.
Coccus cacti	Cocc-c.	Rhus toxicodendron	Rhus-t.
Coffea cruda	Coff.	Rumex crispus	Rumex
Colchicum autumnale	Colch.	Ruta graveolens	Ruta
Colocythis	Coloc.	Sabina	Sab.
Conium maculatum	Con.	Sarsaparilla	Sars.
Cuprum metallicum	Cupr.	Secale	Sec.
Cypripedium	Cypr.	Sepia	Sep.
Dioscorea	Dios.	Silica	Sil.
Drosera rotundifolia	Dros.	Spongia tosta	Spo.
Dulcamara	Dulc.	Staphysagria	Stap.
Eupatorium perfoliatum	Eup-p.	Stramonium	Stram.
Euphrasia	Euphr.	Sulphur	Sul.
Ferrum metallicum	Ferr-m.	Sulphuric acid	Sul-ac.
Gelsemium sempervirens	Gels.	Symphoricarpus racemosa	Symph-r.
Glonoine	Glon.	Symphytum	Symph.
Hamamelis virginica	Ham.	Tabacum	Tab.
Hepar sulphuris calcareum	Hep-s.	Thiosinaminum	Thios.
Hypericum perfoliatum	Hyp.	Thuja occidentalis	Thu.
Ignatia amara	Ign.	Urtica urens	Urt-u.
Ipecacuanha	Ip.	Veratrum album	Ver-a.
Jaborandi	Jab.	Zincum metallicum	Zinc.

APPENDICES

FIRST-AID KITS

You may wish to make up some basic kits, building on them as you need them and as you gain in knowledge and experience. I have included a few below which you can use as models. Some pharmacies can prepare 10 remedies of your choice in a box: small boxes take 10 small bottles, containing 40 soft tablets, and larger boxes take the same number of bottles each containing 60 soft tablets. Many pharmacies also produce many different types of first-aid kit. Their smallest, a plastic wallet holding 24 vials of sugar granules, will fit in a pocket and is ideal for travellers. You can order it in remedies of your choice.

What potency?

If you are just starting out with homeopathy I recommend that you stock your kit in the 6th or the 12th potency. If you are more experienced you may choose to stock some remedies in the 30th potency (a higher potency) such as *Cantharis* for burns. You will need fewer doses of the higher potencies (see dosage chart on p. 20) as they are stronger, homeopathically, and you need, therefore, to be more careful in how often you repeat them (so as not to prove them accidentally, see p. 10).

Reminders for successful first-aid prescribing

- Choose a remedy that fits the whole picture including one or more emotional, general and physical symptoms if possible. You may be prescribing on a single symptom, e.g. *Arnica* for a

bruised forehead, in which case the following points still apply.
- Choose a potency that fits the severity of the complaint (if you have a choice). See p. 19.
- Tip a pill or a few granules from the bottle into the lid, then tip into the hand of the person taking the remedy. If there is no lid carefully tip a few granules straight on to the hand. Do not put back into the bottle any that have been touched or fallen on the floor. See p. 19 for giving remedies to babies.
- Repeat the doses according to the urgency of the situation, e.g. every 5 minutes if in great distress and less often if the need is less (see dosage chart p. 20).
- Give the remedy less often once there is some improvement.
- Stop the remedy once there is a marked improvement.
- Repeat the same remedy if there is a relapse (if the same symptoms recur).
- If you have given 6 doses and there has been no effect it may be the wrong remedy: reassess the whole picture and change the remedy, try a different potency, or ring your homeopath for advice.
- Keep notes of what you prescribed, why you prescribed it and what happened (including the name of the 'patient' and the date).

ACCIDENTS AND INJURIES

These are remedies that you may need urgently and

would like to have to hand. I have included a few keynotes for each one to remind you of its uses.

Aconite shock with fear. Any complaint that starts suddenly, especially after a shock, or exposure to the cold or cold wind.

Apis bites or stings with swelling, hives, general inflammations (coughs, colds, flus, fevers, ear-aches, sore throats, etc.).

Arnica delayed shock, injury with bruising, head injury, first stage sprains with swelling, jet-lag.

Calendula cuts and wounds, bites.

Cantharis burns with or without blisters, cystitis.

Hepar sulphuricum inflamed cuts and wounds, general inflammations.

Hypericum painful injuries to nerves, in areas such as the coccyx, fingers, toes.

Ledum puncture wounds, bites; prevents infection.

Rhus tox sprains and strains, joint pain and inflammation.

Ruta sprains and strains, eyestrain.

EVERYDAY COMPLAINTS

Arsenicum food poisoning; anxious, restless, thirsty for sips, burning pains, better for heat.

Belladonna complaints start suddenly; delirious, dry heat, great pain.

Bryonia sprains, joint pain; complaints start slowly, worse for slightest movement.

Chamomilla teething; unbearable pain; very angry.

Gelsemium complaints start slowly; apathetic, thirstless, better for urinating.

Magnesia phosphorica homeopathic 'aspirin', better for heat and pressure.

Mercurius solubilis sweaty and smelly, an increase of saliva, glands swollen.

Nux vomica food poisoning, gastric disorders (bili-ous), insomnia; irritable.

Pulsatilla teething, food poisoning; weepy, thirstless, better for fresh air.

Sulphur teething, sunburn; restless, thirsty, worse for heat.

LABOUR

If this isn't your first baby, think back to your pre-vious labour or labours and plan to have remedies for the situations that were difficult then. If you are in a relationship engage the help of your partner in put-ting together your labour kit: ideally, they will pres-cribe on you in labour and will need to be familiar with the remedies and their uses.

Ask yourself if there is anything you are scared of

happening in this coming birth. Be honest in answering this question. Don't worry about whether your fear is appropriate or not. Just jot it down and notice if it recurs. If it does and you can find a remedy for it in this book, make sure you have it in your labour kit. You may want to include your partner's fears as well.

What do you know about yourself under stress? In pain? What difficulties are you likely to encounter? If you know that pain makes you vomit, for example, include a remedy for vomiting in labour: read up the pictures and choose one that may fit *you*.

Include your 'constitutional remedy' if you know it (see pp. 6–7), that remedy which helps you what-ever you have wrong with you.

Labour takes an enormous amount of energy. Because of this I advise you to stock your labour kit throughout in the 30th potency. If a remedy works, keep taking it, between contractions if necessary, for as long as it helps. A remedy may help *and* it may need to be repeated, for longer than I suggest for an acute illness, because labour is a stress to the body that may continue for many hours. Remedies may be 'used up' quickly and need to be repeated. You can also alternate remedies (see p. 20) in labour where you want to give, say, *Arnica* for bruising and *Gel-semium* for backache labour.

During labour if your instincts tell you to do some-thing that isn't in the rule book, such as giving a remedy, deciding it isn't right and giving another one straight away, don't worry. No harm can come to mother or baby. The worst that can happen is that it will have no effect. If your instincts are right, how-ever, there will be an improvement.

Make a list of each remedy you order and its keynotes (see below as well as in each remedy picture in the Materia Medica). List the prescribing guide-lines above (p. 301) as a reminder. Keep this list with the kit.

Use the list below to help you decide which reme-dies to order: these are the ones most often called for in my experience. Order *soft* tablets, as it can be irritating to have to chew hard tablets in labour especially if you don't like sugar.

Aconite labour is fast and violent, with great fear/anxiety of death.

Arnica take throughout to prevent bruising, every four hours or more frequently if there is relief from pain.

Caulophyllum Induction is threatened because you are late for dates: take one every four hours for up to two days – if it doesn't work, either your baby isn't ready to be born or you aren't ready for the birth (see p. 112). Labour is slow, contractions are ineffective or stop, but before they become very painful; with exhaustion and shaking, neuralgic (twinging) pains.

Arsenicum vomiting in labour; with typical anxiety and fussiness.

Chamomilla labour exceedingly painful; backache labour; generally obnoxious, angry, impossible to please, asks for things that aren't then wanted.

Coffea contractions are ineffective or stop and/or are extremely painful; fear alternating with excitement, restless, makes jokes, laughs, is generally talkative and hilarious, sensitive to noise.

Gelsemium backache labour; lethargic, lifeless, dazed, thirstless.

Kali carbonicum backache labour; irritable *and* anxious and bossy.

Kali phosphoricum 6X is the best potency for this remedy, as you may need to take a lot. Simple tiredness in labour with no other symptoms.

Pulsatilla gives up during labour; weepy, clingy, pathetic, loses courage, thirstless, hot and craves fresh air or is better for it.

Sepia gives up in labour; very exhausted – sags on every level.

Don't forget *Rescue Remedy*. Have a glass of water with 5 drops of Rescue Remedy added beside you all the time. Take at any time if panicky or fearful.

POST-NATAL KIT FOR THE BABY

The following remedies may be needed in the early weeks after your baby's birth.

Aconite shock
Argentum nitricum sticky eyes
Borax jumpy babies; thrush
Calcarea carbonica snuffles in slow, sweaty babies
Colocynthis colic, when baby pulls knees up
Dioscorea colic, when baby arches whole body back
Kali muriaticum thrush in the mouth
Nux moschata sleepy babies
Pulsatilla sticky eyes, snuffles in clingy babies
Stramonium shock with screaming

POST-NATAL KIT FOR THE MOTHER

Aconite shock
Arnica to heal bruised muscles anywhere; after pains
Belladonna engorged breasts; throbbing pains, red streaks, breasts hot

Bellis perennis bruised soreness not helped by *Arnica*
Bryonia engorgement; pains stitching, breasts pale and hard, worse for movement
Calendula speeds the healing of a tear or episiotomy
Castor equi sore, cracked nipples
China exhaustion from breastfeeding; anaemia
Hypericum pain in coccyx after the birth especially after forceps; painful piles
Magnesia phosphorica afterpains
Nitric acid exhaustion from broken nights; irritable
Phosphoric acid exhaustion from breastfeeding; apathetic
Phytolacca cracked nipples; blocked duct; breast lumpy; abscess/mastitis
Pulsatilla afterpains; weepy and pathetic
Secale if Syntometrine injection administered take one dose after the birth
Silica cracked nipples
Staphysagria pains after the birth, with resentment and a feeling of assault

Remember to look in the External Materia Medica for help with what to put on a tear, painful piles or cracked nipples to help them to heal.

NB The above lists are to help you plan your own kits. Many other remedies may be needed for your pregnancy, birth or the post-natal period: if you don't find what you are looking for above use the Repertory and the Materia Medica to hunt out the remedies you need. If you are not able to find them or are struggling to self-prescribe effectively do seek the advice of a professional homeopath, who has access to hundreds more remedies and the skill to choose between them.

You can order remedies by phone from most homeopathic pharmacies – they will be sent out the same day, by first-class post with an invoice. Or you can pay by credit card.

NB Homeopathic remedies have an indefinite shelf life, providing they are properly stored. If you are a traveller, don't put your homeopathic remedies through an airport X-ray machine as this has been known to antidote them; carry them in your pocket as the metal detector you walk through will not affect them.

FURTHER READING

BIRTH

Burck, Frances, *Babysense*, revised edition, New York: St. Martin's Press: New York, 1991.

Harrison, Helen, *The Premature Baby Book*, New York: St. Martin's Press, 1983.

Mueser, Anne, and George Verrilli, M.D., *While Waiting*, New York: St. Martin's Press, 1981. Also available in Spanish under the title *Mientras Espera*.

Mueser, Anne, and George Verrilli, M.D., *Welcome Baby*, New York: St. Martin's Press, 1981.

BREASTFEEDING

La Leche League International, *The Womanly Art of Breastfeeding*, 1974.

Mason, Diane and Diane Ingersoll, *Breastfeeding and the Working Mother*, New York: St Martin's Press, 1986.

HOMEOPATHY

Castro, Miranda, *The Complete Homeopathy Handbook*, New York: St. Martin's Press, 1991.

Cummings. Stephen, and Dana Ullman, *Homeopathic Medicines*, Los Angeles: Jeremy P. Tarcher, Inc., 1984.

Panos, Maesimund, and Jane Heimlich, *Homeopathic Medicine at Home*, Los Angeles: Jeremy P. Tarcher, Inc., 1980.

ORGANISATIONS

Alcoholics Anonymous
General Service Office
475 Riverside Drive
New York, NY 10115
(212) 870–3400

The Family Resource Coalition
Department P
230 North Michigan Avenue
Room 1625
Chicago, IL 60601
(312) 726–4750

How to Grow a Parent Group
SDG Enterprises
P.O. Box 97
Western Springs, IL 60558

International Foundation for Homeopathy
1141 NW Market Street
Seattle, WA 98107

International Lactation Consultant Association
P.O. Box 4013
University of Virginia Station
Charlottesville, VA 22903

La Leche League International, Inc.
P.O. Box 1209
Franklin Park, IL 60131
708–455–7730 or 1–800 LA LECHE

Mothers' Center for Development Project
129 Jackson Street
Hempstead, NY 11550

National Center for Homeopathy
1500 Massachusetts Avenue, N.W.
Washington, DC 20005

ORGANISATIONS

HOMEOPATHIC ORGANISATIONS

Each of the following organisations publish a directory of homeopathic practitioners to help you to find a registered homeopath in your area. In addition, some offer memberships to lay persons interested in homeopathy.

American Foundation for Homeopathy
1508 S. Garfield
Alhambra, CA 91801

American Institute of Homeopathy
(703) 246-9501
Medical doctors who practice homeopathy
Directory available

American Association of Homeopathic Pharmacists
P.O. Box 61067
Los Angeles, CA 90061

Council for Homeopathic Certification
1709 Seabright Avenue
Santa Cruz, CA 95062
(408) 421-0565
Wide range of practitioners who practice classical
   homeopathy to a uniformly high standard
Includes medical doctors, naturopathic doctors,
   professional homeopaths, physical therapists, etc.
Directory available

Foundation for Homeopathic Education and
   Research
(510) 649-8930
Collects and disseminates new and on-going
   scientific research in the field of homeopathic
   medicine

Homeopathic Academy of Naturopathic Physicians
(503) 761-3298
Naturopaths who practice classical homeopathy
Directory available

Homeopathic Information Resources
Oneida River Park Drive
Clay, NY 13041

Homeopathic Nurses Association
3403 17th Ave. So.
Minneapolis, MN 55407

Homeopathic Pharmacopoeia of the United States
P.O. Box 40360
4974 Quebec St. N.W.
Washington, D.C. 20016

International Foundation for Homeopathy
(206) 776-3172
Practitioners who have trained with the IFH
Memberships available to lay persons

National Board of Homeopathy in Dentistry, Inc.
P.O. Box 423
Marengo, IL 60152

The National Center for Homeopathy
801 N. Fairfax, #306
Alexandria, VA 22314
(703) 548-7790
Memberships available to professionals *and* lay
   persons
Directory available of licensed health care
   practitioners who practice homeopathy
The NCH publishes a monthly newsletter,
   organizes an annual conference, and conducts
   nationwide study groups and a summer school
   program for professionals and lay persons
   interested in homeopathy

New England Journal of Homeopathy
356 Middle Street
Amherst, MA 01002

HOMEOPATHIC PHARMACIES

The following supply homeopathic remedies singly and/or in the form of home care kits—this is particularly useful if you are not able to purchase homeopathic remedies locally. Many also sell books.

Boericke and Tafel, Inc.
2381 Circadian Way
Santa Rosa, CA 95407
(800) 876-9505 (West Coast)
(800) 272-2820 (East Coast)

Boiron-Borneman, Inc. (Pennsylvania)
(800) BOIRON-1

Dolisos America, Inc. (Nevada)
(702) 871-7153

Ehrhart and Karl
33 N. Wabash Ave.,
Chicago, IL 60602
312-332-1046

Hahnemann Medical Pharmacy (California)
(510) 527-3003

Homeopathy Overnight (Maine)
(800) ARNICA-30

Luyties Pharmacal Co.
4200 Laclede St.
St. Louis, MO 63108
(800) 325-8080

Propulsora Homeopathia De Mexico
Calle Mirto 116 y 118
Mexico, D.F. Mexico 06400

Standard Homeopathic Co.
210 W. 131st St., Box 61067
Los Angeles, CA 90061
(213) 321-4284

Washington Homeopathic Products, Inc. (Maryland)
(800) 336-1695

HOMEOPATHIC BOOKS

These companies sell homeopathic books (for the beginner to the advanced homeopath), tapes, and even computer software.

Homeopathic Educational Services
(510) 649-0294

Minimum Price Books
(800) 663-8272

HOMEOPATHIC TRAINING PROGRAMS

The following organisation accredits homeopathic training programs, as well as providing a list (updated regularly) of courses, seminars, and post-graduate training programs that are available in the United States.

Academy for Classical Homeopathy
7549 Louise Ave.,
Van Nuys, CA 91406
(818) 776-0078
Clinical Practice of Classical Homeopathy Course

Atlantic Academy of Classical Homeopathy
21 West 58th St., Suite 6E
New York, NY 10019
(718) 518-4593

Bastyr College of Natural Health Sciences
144 NE 54th
Seattle, WA 98105
(206) 523-9585

British Institute of Homeopathy
702 Washington St., Suite 204
Marina Del Rey, CA 90292
(213) 306-5408
Home Study Course

Council for Homeopathic Education
Clocktower Building
3 Main Street
Chatham, NY 12037
(518) 392-6456

Four Winds Seminars
187 Hillside Drive
Fairfax, CA 94930
(415) 457-8452

Hahnemann Academy of North America
2801 Rodeo Rd., Suite B-135
Santa Fe, NM 87505
(505) 959-7018

Hahnemann College of Homeopathy
1918 Bonita Ave.,
Berkeley, CA 94704
(415) 849-1925
Professional Training Course

Homeopathic Association of Greater Chicago
P.O. Box 3791
Oak Brook, IL 60522
(708) 325-2804 or (708) 529-7552

International Foundation for Homeopathy
2366 Eastlake Dr., E.
Seattle, WA 98102
(206) 324-8230
Professional Course
Advanced Acute Course

National Center for Homeopathy
801 N. Fairfax, #306
Alexandria, VA 22314
(703) 548-7790
Summer courses for licensed practitioners and the public

National College of Naturopathic Medicine
11231 SE Market St.
Portland, OR 97216
(503) 255-4860

New England School of Homeopathy
356 Middle Street
Amherst, MA 01002
(203) 763-1255
Courses for professionals and lay practitioners

Pacific Academy of Homeopathic Medicine
1678 Shattuck Ave. #42
Berkeley, CA 94709
(510) 549-3475

Pan-American Homeopathic Medical Congress
Edificio 166, Entrada D
Unidad Kennedy
Mexico G, D.F.

INDEX